NOT ALL IN

NOT ALL IN

Race, Immigration, and Health Care Exclusion in the Age of Obamacare

TIFFANY D. JOSEPH

JOHNS HOPKINS UNIVERSITY PRESS
Baltimore

Johns Hopkins University Press
2715 North Charles Street
Baltimore, Maryland 21218
www.press.jhu.edu

Library of Congress Cataloging-in-Publication Data

Names: Joseph, Tiffany D., author.
Title: Not all in : race, immigration, and health care exclusion in the age
of Obamacare / Tiffany D. Joseph.
Description: [Baltimore] : [Johns Hopkins University Press], [2025] |
Includes bibliographical references and index.
Identifiers: LCCN 2024025708 | ISBN 9781421451114 (hardcover) |
ISBN 9781421451121 (ebook)
Subjects: LCSH: Medical policy—Social aspects—Massachusetts—Boston. |
Medical care—Social aspects—Massachusetts—Boston. | Health insurance—
Social aspects—Massachusetts—Boston. | Latin Americans—Medical care—
United States. | Immigrants—Medical care—United States. | Latin Americans—
Health and hygiene—Massachusetts—Boston. | Immigrants—Health and
hygiene—Massachusetts—Boston. | Racism in medicine—
Massachusetts—Boston.
Classification: LCC RA395.A4 M44 2024 |
DDC 362.109744/61—dc23/eng/20240826
LC record available at https://lccn.loc.gov/2024025708

A catalog record for this book is available from the British Library.

Special discounts are available for bulk purchases of this book.
For more information, please contact Special Sales at specialsales@jh.edu.

For my boys and Mama,
and
in memory of my dad N. L. Joseph, whose smile, helpful spirit,
and wisdom I miss every day.

America's healthcare system is neither healthy, caring, nor a system.
—*Walter Cronkite*

We may have all come on different ships, but we're in the same boat now.
—*Dr. Martin Luther King Jr.*

CONTENTS

TABLES AND FIGURES

Tables

Figures

ACKNOWLEDGMENTS

A project of this scope would not have been possible without the immense support of various funding agencies, institutions, and individuals. I am incredibly grateful to the grant reviewers and administrators who saw merit in and recommended funding for this project from the following organizations (in alphabetical order): the Ford Foundation Senior Fellowship, the Fund for the Advancement of the Discipline supported by the American Sociological Association and the National Science Foundation, the Mellon Emerging Faculty Leaders Award (formally the Nancy Weiss Malkiel Junior Faculty Fellowship) from the Institute for Citizens and Scholars, and the Robert Wood Johnson Foundation Scholars in Health Policy Program. Research reported in this publication was also supported by the National Library of Medicine of the National Institutes of Health Grant for Scholarly Works in Biomedicine and Health under award number G13LM013543. The content is solely the responsibility of the author and does not necessarily represent the official views of the National Institutes of Health or the other funding sources for this book project.

I am also very thankful for the institutional support from my current employer, Northeastern University, and my former employer, Stony Brook University. At Northeastern, I was a recipient of multiple Health Equity Pilot Awards from the Institute of Health Equity and Social Justice Research, the Multigenerational Research Team Grant from the College of Social Sciences and Humanities, multiple Project-Based Exploration for the Advancement of Knowledge Awards, and additional research funds from the College of Social Sciences and Humanities and Provost's Office. At Stony Brook University, I was a recipient of the Fine Arts, Humanities, and Social Sciences Research Funds Award and Faculty Research Award Fellowship.

Just as important as financial support are the people who played important roles throughout this project. I begin by recognizing the 207 respondents of the interviews I conducted among Greater Boston's Brazilian, Dominican, and Salvadoran communities, with Boston Health Coalition (BHC) healthcare providers, and with employees from dozens of immigrant and health advocacy organizations and city and state government agencies. Your openness and generosity with your time, knowledge, and experiences formed the basis for this book. To the immigrant respondents, I appreciate your courage in sharing your stories of resilience and struggle. I hope this book can shed light on and improve the myriad challenges that immigrants face. I would like to give special mention to Zilda Sacramento-Bourne, who assisted with immigrant recruitment efforts. To the many BHC health professionals working tirelessly to provide quality health care, thank you for sharing your insights working on the front lines of a complicated and imperfect system. To the advocates providing and connecting communities with essential services such as health care and fighting for more inclusive laws, thanks for your activism and for providing a close look at how policies shape people's lives. I am especially appreciative of the providers and advocates who were willing to be interviewed multiple times throughout the project. Special acknowledgment goes to Andrew Cohen, Iván Espinoza-Madrigal, Heloisa Galvão, María González-Albuixech, Amy Grunder, Alex Pirie, and Anderson Pinto, who graciously and patiently answered my emails about shifting policies, coverage eligibility rules, and their impact on immigrant communities.

This book also would not have been possible without the numerous graduate and undergraduate research assistants from Harvard, Stony Brook, and Northeastern University, who assisted with data organization, coding, and analysis; conducted literature searches; and proofread earlier chapter drafts. I am really grateful for your diligent efforts (alphabetical order): Maria Baez, Colleen Binder, Ellen Bostwick, Emily Breen, Mateus Cello, Tibrine Da Fonseca, Fatoumata Diallo, Valeria Do Vale, Rylie Ellam, Samantha Gomes, Kevin Ha, Ashley Houston, Roy Jeong, Kenadi Kaewmanaprasert, Jaeyoon Lee, Rachel Louie, Michaiah Parker, Olivia Scioletti, Aileen Shin, Alissah Sillah, Shadia Tannir, Vibhustuti Thapa, Jessica Torres, João Vogel, and Madeline Wong.

Many colleagues provided mentorship, guidance, and encouragement over the course of this project. I would like to start by thanking my supportive colleagues in Northeastern University's Sociology and Anthropology Department, College of Social Sciences and Humanities, Institute for Health Equity and Social Justice, and Partnership for Immigrants' Rights, especially (in alphabetical order) Nicole Aljoe, Jennifer Akula, Shalanda Baker, Amilcar Barreto, Linda Blum, Phil Brown, Elizabeth Bucar, Margaret Burnham, Anjanette Chan Tack, Danielle Crookes, Silvia Dominguez, Elizabeth Ennen, Suzanne Gaverich, Matthew Hunt, Régine Jean-Charles, Carla Kaplan, Doreen Lee, Alisa Lincoln, Isabel Martinez, Cassie McMillan, Uta Poiger, Carmel Salhi, Laura Senier, Jennie Stephens, Nina Sylvanus, Berna Turam, Wajma Yusufzai, and Liza Weinstein. I would also like to thank Diedra Wrighting and the ADVANCE Office for providing valuable resources, such as the Women of Color in the Academy Writing Group and a National Center for Faculty Diversity and Development (shout-out to founder Kerry Ann Rockquemore) institutional membership, which provided protected time for writing and productivity strategies, without which this project would not have been completed. I am particularly grateful to Laura Senier, who connected me with Daniel Dawes, the editor of this Health Equity in America Book Series, and Robin Coleman, acquisitions editor at Johns Hopkins University Press (JHUP), the home for this book. Their patience and invaluable support, along with that of other JHUP staff, have been crucial at every stage of the writing process. I also had a book conference, where Debby Carr, Wendy Parmet, and Anahí Viladrich reviewed and provided extensive feedback on earlier drafts of the book proposal and empirical chapters. Their insightful and constructive feedback pushed me to make the book stronger for the external reviewers (thank you, too!) who gave my proposal and manuscript a thumbs-up for JHUP. I also worked with an amazing editor, Grey Osterud, throughout the book-writing process, who helped me get this manuscript into tip-top shape.

I am also thankful to other trusted colleagues around the country whose conversations and constructive feedback were incredibly helpful as I developed the research design, contemplated relevant scholarship, conducted interviews, and drafted papers and presentations based on this research (in alphabetical order): Margarita Alegría, Denise Anthony, Asad Asad, Moya Bailey, Vilna Bashi Treitler, Jason Beckfield, Larry Bobo, Eduardo Bonilla-Silva, Sarah Burgard, Rebekah Burroway, Heide Castañeda, Orly Clergé, Alan Cohen, Benjamin Cook, David Cook-Martín, Susan Eckstein, Erika Edwards, Gregory Elliott, Joseph Ewoodzie, Katy Fallon, Patricia Fernández-Kelly, David FitzGerald, Cybelle Fox, Angela García, Marco Garrido, Daniel Gillion, Tanya Golash-Boza, Roberto Gonzales, Heba Goyawed, Colleen Grogan, Tod Hamilton, Anna Haskins, Laura Hirshfield, Jennifer Hochschild, Elizabeth Hordge-Freeman, Jedediah Horwitt, James House, Mosi Ifatunji, Tony Jack, the late James Jackson, Kimberly Kay Hoang, Nazli Kibria, Sage Kochavi, Nicole Kreisberg, Michèle Lamont, Peggy Levitt, Daniel Levy, Donald Light, Laura López-Sanders, William López, Helen Marrow, Cecilia Menjívar, James Morone, Aldon Morris, Anthony Ocampo, Francisco Pedraza, David Pellow, Catherine Player, Rashawn Ray, Victor Ray, Naomi Rosenthal, Rubén Rumbaut, Gabriel Sanchez, Michael Sauder, Saher Selod, Susan Sered, Carrie Shandra, John Shandra, Hilary Silver, Kristen Shorette, John Solomos, Lisa Sun-Hee Park, Michael Schwartz, Anna Skarpelis, Kathy Swartz, Veronica Terriquez, Kevin J. A. Thomas, Meredith Van Natta, Robert Vargas, Jocelyn Viterna, Derron Wallace, Natasha Warikoo, Mary Waters, Nicholas Wilson, France Winddance Twine, Alford Young Jr., Ruth Zambrana, Kathrin Zippel, and Gilda Zwerman.

Over the past decade, I have also presented papers around the country that eventually became publications and chapters in this book. The feedback received at the following institutions were valuable as I drafted this book manuscript: Boston University; Brown University; Dartmouth College; Duke University; Emory University; Harvard University (Comparative Inequality Workshop; Migration and Immigrant Incorporation Workshop; Petrie-Flom Center for Health Law Policy, Biotechnology, and Bioethics); Northeastern University; Princeton University (Center for Migration and Development, Princeton Institute for International and Regional Studies Migration Lab); Rutgers University (School of Public Health); Stony Brook University; University of California, Los Angeles; University of Chicago (Center for Health and Administrative Studies); University of Kansas; University of New Mexico; University of North Carolina at Chapel Hill; University of Southern California; University of Wisconsin; Vanderbilt University; and Wellesley College. Presenting previous versions of this work at the following conferences and seminars also made this manuscript stronger: American Anthropological Association, American Sociological Association, Eastern Sociological Association, Intersectional Qualitative Research Methods Institute, National Institute of Minority Health and Health Disparities Research Institute, and The OpEd Project.

Last, but certainly not least, I want to thank God, the author and finisher of my faith, for providing everything I needed when I needed it to bring this project from start to finish. To my husband, Enderson Nogueira, thanks for being the best and most supportive life partner and providing me with the love and encouragement amid the ups and downs of this project. To my sons, Alessandro and Sebastian, you are my inspiration for making the world a better place. To my mom, Sarah Joseph, and late dad, N. L. Joseph, thanks for nurturing me and supporting my dreams and ambitions even though they took me far away from home. To my extended family in the United States and abroad—the Josephs, Nogueiras, Cashes—and my cherished friends who are family, especially (in alphabetical order) Makini Chism-Straker, Moira Flavin, Michelle Glasgow Woods, A. Kilolo Harris Evans, Anna Hidalgo, Tammy Hotniansky, Julie Huang, Jennifer Jackson, Marcelle Rainone, Gita Sjahrir, Tulani Thaw, Ligaya Rebolos Lee, and Mary Ziegler, thanks for your love and encouragement over the years amid our conversations about this project and the state of health care and life in general in the United States. To the readers of this book, thanks for taking the time to read it; I hope it will inspire you to create the positive change you want to see in the world.

LEXICON

American (adjective): Pertaining to American people, society, and culture, but not the nation-state.

ethnicity (noun): A social construction based on common culture and shared interests among groups of people, such as language, ancestry, and religion; sometimes also known as "nationality" or "national origin" when referring to immigrants in a host country.

ethno-racial (adjective): Term that refers to the intersection between ethnicity and race, whereby certain characteristics associated with ethnic groups become racialized or tied to physical features associated with race; also used when discussing both racial and ethnic categories and groups— for example, "the ethno-racial demographics of the United States are changing."

health coverage (noun): Programs that provide access to specified health services.

health insurance (noun): Programs that cover the full or partial cost of health services.

immigrants (noun): Foreign-born individuals who migrate to the United States temporarily or permanently, regardless of documentation status before they arrive. This is not to be confused with the US government definition of "immigrants," who are individuals seeking to become legal permanent residents or green card holders. The US government refers to foreign-born individuals admitted to the United States on a temporary basis for specific purposes (i.e., with a visa) as nonimmigrant aliens.

lawful permanent residents (LPRs) (noun): Term that refers to immigrants with a legal status that allows them to remain in the United States. LPRs are also known as green card holders. Since the 1996 welfare reform, there has been a ban on public benefits based on length of time in the country. For simplicity in the text, I sometimes use "short-term LPRs" to refer to LPRs residing in the country less than five years and "long-term LPRs" to refer to LPRs residing in the country for five or more years.

race (noun): A social construction that has historically grouped people with similar physical characteristics—such as skin color, hair texture, nose shape—into categories and that has contributed to unequal power and social relations between people of different racial groups. Such relations are shaped by laws and policies and how resources are distributed in a society.

racialization (noun) or racialized (verb): The process through which groups of people are ascribed, are placed into, or become associated with particular racial groups or categories; also refers to how the racial categories ascribed to different types of human bodies are given social meaning.

structural racism (noun): The generation and reproduction of racial inequality among different racial groups, even in socioeconomic and institutional structures that appear to be race-neutral.

systemic racism (noun): A system that creates racial inequality in multiple domains among different racial groups.

United States (noun), US (adjective): Pertaining to the United States as a polity or its policies.

US-born (adjective): Term that refers to individuals born in the United States, who are US citizens based on birth.

Terms for immigrants' premigration self-identification and classification (adjectives):

Brazilian: Amarelo, Pardo—these are skin color or racial categories in the Brazilian census that respectively can be used to refer to those who self-classify as "Yellow," or have Asian ancestry, or who self-classify as "racially mixed," with Black, White, or Indigenous ancestry or a combination of these. Other Brazilian census categories include White (**Branco**), Black (**Negro**), and Indigenous (**Indígena**).

Dominican: Moreno, Mulato, Indio—these are skin color or racial categories in the Dominican census that can be used to refer to someone who self-classifies as "racially mixed" with Black and White ancestry, Indigenous ancestry, or a combination of these. This racially mixed ancestry is typically more Black and White, as most of the Indigenous population died before the importation of African enslaved individuals in the Dominican Republic. Other Dominican census categories include White **(Blanco)**, Black **(Negro)**, Asian **(Asiático)**.

Salvadorans: Mestizo—this is a skin color or racial category in the Salvadoran census that can be used to refer to someone who self-classifies as "racially mixed" with White and Indigenous ancestry. Other categories include White **(Blanco)**, Amerindian **(Indígena)**, and Black **(Negro)**, although there is a very small African-descended population in El Salvador.

Terms for immigrants' post-migration self-identification by ethnicity in the United States:

Hispanic: A term used for self-identified ethnicity in the US census, which includes US-born individuals with Latin American ancestry. In this book, the term refers to Spanish-speaking individuals with Latin American ancestry and does not include Brazilians.

Latin American: The umbrella term for immigrants from Mexico, the Caribbean, and Central and South America used by the US census, as in "people of Latin American origin/ethnicity."

Latinx, rather than Latino/a, for *both* ethnicity and national origin: Gender-neutral umbrella term indicating ethnicity and national origin for individuals of Latin American origin and descent in the United States regardless of nativity, documentation status, or language spoken; includes Brazilians.

NOT ALL IN

Introduction

Massachusetts is one of the best states for health. Many people come here for innovative surgeries, to see doctors, and there is nowhere else like here. Massachusetts is a state that invests a lot in health and medical services. There are lots of good hospitals in Boston.
—*Victoria, Dominican immigrant interviewed in 2012*

But for immigrant patients in general, having to bear the issue of discriminations, language issues, frequently work[ing] one or two or three jobs, whether it's by their own decision or just having to do it—they bring all of that to their medical care. It's really not separate. So you have to have a good understanding of the social context in which folks are living.
—*Greg, healthcare provider interviewed in 2013*

Despite describing the Massachusetts healthcare system as one of the best, Victoria, a 50-year-old Dominican immigrant with a green card who has been in the country for more than 30 years, has had some problematic experiences with healthcare providers.[1] When I spoke with Victoria in Cambridge in fall 2012, she was insured through MassHealth, the state's Medicaid program. Though it covered most of her healthcare needs, she found the co-pays for her numerous prescription medications difficult to afford. She was not in good health: she had high blood pressure, anemia, an eye ailment, and depression. These conditions meant that she had to go on medical leave from her job in human services in 1999 and had been unable to work since then. Victoria acknowledged that the stresses of life as a Dominican immigrant had contributed to her deteriorating health over her decades in the United States: dealing with family issues, being culturally different, eventually learning English, and coping with the harsh climate had taken their toll. With medium-brown skin tone and short, slightly curly dark-brown and streaked-blonde hair, she regards herself as Latina and feels that most other people see her that way.[2] She believes that this perception negatively influences her interactions with healthcare providers. During our conversation, Victoria recounted her troubling experience with a culturally insensitive White American psychiatrist.[3] "I was suffering from depression," but she "thought I was using drugs because I was very hyper. I thought it was the medicine they prescribed me." When the psychiatrist discontinued the antidepressant, Victoria continued, "I went into a really deep depression. If she had been Hispanic, she could have better explained to me what was happening." Victoria had also seen her relatives receive substandard treatment from White medical providers. She prefers having Hispanic doctors and has gone out of her way to make that happen. She feels she receives better treatment from them and that they are more patient and explain things in a culturally competent way that she can understand.

Negative experiences with the healthcare system are all too common among Latinx immigrants in greater Boston. As a Latina with darker skin whose first language is not English, she is racialized as non-White, and research shows that experiences of racism increase the likelihood of having negative health outcomes.[4] These factors also make her disproportionately likely to encounter interpersonal and structural discrimination in the healthcare system. Despite being college educated, she has limited income. Social Security and Disability Insurance (SSDI) along with Medicaid provide some subsistence, but not enough to live comfortably in an expensive metropolitan area. Victoria's story exemplifies how the intersection of race, ethnicity, and documentation status—which I refer to as "racialized legal status"—shapes the lives of millions of people living in the United States.[5] "Racialization" refers to the social process by which people are classified by others as belonging to a distinct racial group, which is important in shaping their identity and position in society.[6] For example, people who do not know Victoria perceive her as non-White. Others assume correctly that she is an immigrant but may then assume erroneously that she is undocumented and treat her as undeserving of the benefits she is entitled to receive. Victoria's story reflects that of many other immigrants—especially those of color—whose health declines the longer they remain in this country and who experience exclusion based on their noncitizen status or their race and ethnicity. Understanding racialized legal status is crucial not only because it shapes immigrants' encounters with health care, but also because it affects the wider sociopolitical climate. Deeply embedded structural racism and White supremacy continue to damage the lives of people of color, while being a noncitizen routinely results in systematic exclusion from decent housing, jobs that pay a living wage, and even driver's licenses. The concept of racialized legal status enables us to make sense of the ways that discrimination associated with race, ethnicity, and documentation status compounds and intensifies the difficulties that Latinx immigrants and other immigrants of color face every day. This book shows how and why racialized legal status matters as immigrants try to take care of their health and navigate the complex US healthcare system.

Health shapes our quality of life, influencing not only how well we feel but also our ability to provide for ourselves and our loved ones and our capacity to contribute to society. The social determinants of health—socioeconomic and environmental factors such as race, ethnicity, citizenship or legal status, where we live and work, the types of jobs we have, and our income—affect our well-being.[7] Greg, a White Boston-area primary care physician whom I spoke with in 2013, shared how social determinants of health shape his immigrant patients' healthcare experience. In the second quote at the beginning of this chapter, he specifically identified nonmedical needs that directly affect their health care: housing issues, access to food, access to medications, social supports, and legal issues, especially around immigration status. As a healthcare provider, he cannot separate health care from these nonmedical needs when treating his patients. Sociologists Jo Phelan and Bruce Link argue that such factors are fundamental causes of health disparities in the United States.[8]

Having or lacking access to health coverage can make or break a person's ability to receive health care. Despite being home to world-class hospitals and healthcare innovations, the United States has the world's most expensive healthcare system.[9] Ironically, we get very few returns for those high costs. Americans have some of the worst health outcomes and are less likely to have health insurance than their peers in other Western countries.[10] While accessing quality care is not difficult for affluent Americans, it remains a huge financial burden for lower-and middle-income people, who struggle with rising premiums and co-pays and incur burdensome medical debt.[11] An estimated 26 million Americans were uninsured in the first half of 2024, a number that is disappointingly high.[12]

Quality health insurance and care are notably out of reach for the socially disadvantaged among us, especially people of color, who suffer from discrimination based on this country's persistent structural racism, and noncitizens, who have increasingly been excluded from health coverage and other social services because of their legal status.[13] Contemporary immigrants from Latin America, Asia, and Africa are racialized as people of color and routinely experience discrimination on the basis of their race and ethnicity and their documentation or legal status.[14] I refer to this intersection as racialized legal status because it highlights the ways structural racism intertwines with US immigration policy, subjecting noncitizens to unequal treatment under the law and in society. Similar racist and anti-immigrant exclusion has also been increasing in Western European countries that had generous social safety nets for their residents throughout the late 20th century.[15] Recent global recessions, sociopolitical conflicts, and climate change have sent non-European migrants toward the region, and these countries became more ethnoracially and religiously diverse. In response, debates over the reductions in public benefits that have been instituted since the 1990s became entangled with anti-immigrant, anti-Muslim, and White supremacist politics.[16] The increasingly overtly racist and xenophobic rhetoric that defines immigrants and some citizens of color as outsiders and criminals signifies the salience of racialized legal status for all those in this sizable category in the United States and other immigrant-receiving countries. Scholars have begun using this phrase to highlight how race, ethnicity, and documentation status affect social outcomes among immigrants of color and have spillover effects on citizens of color.[17]

According to the 2020 US census, the 21.2 million immigrants from Latin America—Mexico, the Caribbean, and Central and South America—constituted 53% of the country's foreign-born population.[18] Furthermore, both US- and foreign-born people who identify themselves as ethnically "Hispanic" made up 18.7% of the total population in 2020.[19] In the past decade, US policies on health and immigration have been dramatically transformed, as efforts to enable everyone living in this country to obtain health coverage were countered by simultaneous efforts to prevent immigrants from doing so. The 2010 Affordable Care Act (ACA), colloquially known as "Obamacare" because it was passed during the administration of President Barack Obama, was intended to extend health coverage to uninsured Americans.[20] But most immigrants remain excluded from its benefits because of long-standing restrictions based on documentation status in federal law. Moreover, the inhumane treatment of Latin American and other non-White migrants at the southern border under the administrations of Presidents Joseph Biden, Donald Trump, and Obama indicates the wholesale rejection that immigrants of color often encounter. Although more immigrants were deported from the United States under President Obama than under his successors, the election of Donald Trump ushered in harsher, zero-tolerance immigration policies that increased enforcement and further criminalized immigrants, especially those from Latin America.[21] At the same time, the Trump administration weakened Obamacare and changed the public charge designation to make it more difficult for lower-income immigrants to obtain lawful permanent residency.[22]

This book highlights the vital role of public policy in shaping and perpetuating unequal access to health care and other government benefits. I explore three important questions to assess the relationship between racialized legal status and changes in various policy realms as they have affected Latin American immigrants. First, how have recent health and immigration policy changes reconfigured their access to and lived experiences of health care? Second, how have differences in documentation status, race, ethnicity, and language affected their ability to obtain health coverage and navigate the healthcare system? Third, how has the intensified racialization of immigration and law enforcement influenced their healthcare decisions? Public policy facilitates racialized legal status discrimination through explicit discrimination based on documentation status and implicit discrimination based on race and ethnicity. For immigrants and citizens of color in the United States, the heightened disadvantage they encounter at the intersection of these two types of discrimination produces nuanced but significant forms of exclusion from public benefits, including health care and civic life.[23]

To explore these questions, I draw on interviews I conducted with 209 Brazilian, Dominican, and Salvadoran immigrants, healthcare providers, and immigrant and health advocacy organization employees in metropolitan Boston, Massachusetts, from 2012 to 2019. I aimed to examine the healthcare system from the perspectives of patients who rely on it to address their medical needs, medical professionals who provide care to those seeking it, and advocates who often work with patients to connect them with coverage and help them navigate the system. Historically a predominantly White city known for the virulent anti-Black racism of its segregated, White working-class neighborhoods, Boston is still perceived as one of the country's most racist and segregated cities.[24] But, the municipality became a majority-minority city in 2000, with a diverse population of immigrants, who constituted 28% of its population.[25] Seeking education and employment in Boston's robust service and knowledge-based economy, immigrants paid $10.6 billion in federal taxes and $4.5 billion in state and local taxes and generated $2.3 billion in business revenue for the state's economy in 2018.[26] In 2021, Boston voters chose Michelle Wu, the daughter of Taiwanese immigrants, as mayor, making her the first woman and the first person of color elected to preside over city government.[27]

Like many major US cities, Boston has a sizable population of people of Latin American birth and ancestry.[28] Unlike the Latinx population in cities such as Los Angeles, Houston, and Miami, Boston's Latinx population is not predominantly Mexican or even Spanish-speaking. Rather, it is composed mostly of Brazilians, Dominicans, and Salvadorans, reflecting the heterogeneity of ethnicities, races, documentation statuses, languages, and cultures under the "Latinx" umbrella.[29] Brazilians, whose primary language is Portuguese, are typically undocumented, come from middle-income backgrounds, and have physical features—lighter skin tones and straighter hair textures—that are racialized as White in the United States. Dominicans are usually lawful permanent residents (green card holders) or naturalized citizens, from lower-income backgrounds, and have physical features—medium- to dark-brown skin tones and curlier hair textures—that are racialized as Black. Some Salvadorans are eligible for temporary protected status, which entitles them to certain public benefits, although around 7% of Salvadorans are thought to be undocumented.[30] Many Salvadorans come from lower-income backgrounds and are racialized as Mestizo because they have Indigenous as well as European ancestry. Most research on people of Latin American origin homogenizes them or focuses primarily on Mexicans, Cubans, or Puerto Ricans without shedding light on Central or South Americans.[31] But Brazilians, Dominicans, and Salvadorans have distinct backgrounds and societal positions, as do those from other Caribbean and Central and South American countries. Including these understudied immigrants gives us a fuller understanding of how Latinx people's heterogeneity differentially influences their health care and social experiences over the course of a series of changes in public policy.

Boston has a national reputation as a politically liberal or progressive city, and it boasts some of the world's best hospitals and medical schools. Boston and other Massachusetts cities have recently been in the national spotlight because they have received a large influx of migrants escaping social unrest, violence, and political instability in Haiti, Venezuela, and Central America. While many arrived from the southern border, others were sent on buses and planes to the commonwealth and "immigrant-friendly" locales such as New York, Chicago, and Washington DC. These were political stunts orchestrated by Florida governor Ron DeSantis and Texas governor Greg Abbott to draw attention to the nation's "migration crisis."[32] The situation strained housing and other social support systems in these places. In response, Massachusetts governor Maura Healey declared a state of emergency for the commonwealth's shelter system, which is required to shelter families with children. The monthly cost to the state escalated to more than $45 million as of September 2023.[33] Massachusetts's national reputation as an immigrant-friendly state has arguably been a draw for migrants seeking refuge.[34] When state legislators developed its historic health reform in 2006, Massachusetts became the epicenter of inclusive and comprehensive health reform. *All* low-income residents were eligible for coverage, regardless of documentation status. The state's Republican governors cooperated with the Democrats who controlled the legislature to pass policies designed to reduce the proportion of residents without health coverage.[35] The success of the Massachusetts reform made it a model for the 2010 federal ACA.[36] There was one key difference between the two reforms, however: Obamacare extended coverage *only* to income-eligible citizens and certain documented noncitizens.[37]

Since ACA implementation in Massachusetts limited the scope of the state's original reform, this shift generated significant confusion regarding eligibility and made it more difficult for immigrants to (re)apply for coverage.[38] Part of this difficulty likely stems from the fact that nearly one in three state residents speaks a language other than English.[39] Then and now, Latinx immigrants, who are racialized as people of color and have limited English proficiency (LEP) and low incomes, are more likely to remain uninsured and have difficulty accessing health services.[40] Racialized legal status discrimination is a crucial reason people in this group remain disproportionately uninsured and have negative experiences with the healthcare system in Boston and across the United States. The intersectional discrimination produced through racialized legal status undermines the effectiveness of policies intended to improve health coverage and broaden access to social services for disadvantaged populations.

Examining the Effects of Racialized Legal Status on Healthcare Access

For this book, I interviewed immigrants, their healthcare providers, and employees of immigrant and health advocacy organizations in metropolitan Boston, eliciting their perspectives on the factors that shape immigrants' healthcare access (see Table I-1). In-depth interviews with the stakeholders who were most affected by policy changes enabled me to develop a comprehensive understanding of the concrete implications of racialized legal status for their ability to navigate the healthcare system. To assess the specific effects of major changes in health and immigration

Table I-1. Immigrants, Providers, and Advocates Interviewed in 2012–2013, 2015–2016, and 2019 (N = 209)

Stakeholder group	Pre-ACA 2012–2013	Post-ACA 2015–2016[a]	Post-2016 election: 2019[b]
Immigrants	n = 31	n = 39	n = 12
- Brazilians	21	15	8
- Dominicans	10	14	2
- Salvadorans	n/a	10	2
Healthcare providers at Boston Health Coalition	n = 19	n = 19	n = 14
- Physicians	5	6	5
- Medical interpreters	4	4	2
- Other medical staff	10	9	7
Immigrant/health organizations	n = 20	n = 25	n = 30
- Brazilian	6	4	7
- Dominican	2	4	2
- Salvadoran	n/a	2	2
- General immigrant organizations	3	5	9
- Health organizations	9	7	8
- City/state officials	0	3	2
Total	70	83	56

a. Salvadorans were added to the 2015–2016 sample amid political debates about TPS status renewal.
b. The 2019 immigrant sample is smaller due to recruitment difficulty in the sociopolitical climate.

policy at both the state and national levels, I conducted three rounds of interviews over nearly a decade.

Brazilians, Dominicans, and Salvadorans are among the largest immigrant groups in Boston. Despite their differing national origins, languages, and cultures, as well as their varied physical appearance and documentation status, they are racialized as Latinx in the United States. When I began the study in 2012, I focused on immigrants from Brazil and the Dominican Republic, but in 2015 the unprecedented influx of Central Americans prompted me to add Salvadorans. To give readers a better sense of how their appearance as immigrants of color shaped their lived experiences, I include physical descriptions of immigrant respondents when I quote or discuss them. Consequently, racialized legal status has shaped their lives to varying degrees. Table I-2 provides relevant demographic information on these groups.

Of the three groups, Dominicans have been in metropolitan Boston the longest. They began arriving in the 1960s after the assassination of the Dominican Republic's longtime dictator, Rafael Trujillo, which led to political instability, high unemployment, and low wages.[41] Many of those who arrived in the 1960s and 1970s were from urban, highly educated, and middle-class backgrounds. In contrast, those who arrived in the 1980s and 1990s tended to have rural and working-class origins.[42] The Dominican population has doubled since 2000 and currently constitutes 6% of Bostonians.[43] In terms of age, 58% of US-born Dominicans are children, while 81% of foreign-born Dominicans are adults between the ages of 25 and 64.[44] Many originally settled in Jamaica Plain, Mattapan, and Dorchester but have been displaced to suburbs such as Lynn due to gentrification and lack of affordable housing in Boston.[45] Many Dominicans have darker skin tones than members of some other Latinx groups and are typically racialized as Black.[46] Because of their length of time in the United States, most Dominicans have green cards or are naturalized citizens, making them the most advantaged and legally incorporated of the three groups with regard to documentation status.[47]

Salvadorans and other Central Americans began arriving in Boston in the 1980s, fleeing political upheaval, economic deprivation, and violence

Table I-2. Demographic Characteristics of Boston's Dominican, Salvadoran, and Brazilian Immigrants

Nationality	First arrival and reason	Estimated population size	Foreign-born	Speak English well	Educational level	Noncitizens	Median household income	Primary occupations	Uninsured
Dominican	1960s political instability	36,420	60%	24%	38% < high school 29% high school 33% some college	54%	$25,000–75,000	Landscaping Housecleaning Personal care/ support Transportation materials/ moving	8.7%
Salvadoran	1980s political instability	13,958	70%	28%	62% < high school	60%	$54,728	Office cleaning Housecleaning	14%
Brazilian	1980s political and economic instability	6,673	73%	47%	49% high school 35% college degree	51%	$66,435	Landscaping Housecleaning Construction	17%

Sources: Boston Planning and Development Agency (BPDA) 2016, 2017a, 2017b, 2019b, 2019c; Granberry and Agarwal 2021.

stemming from civil wars and US intervention in their countries.[48] Since then, Salvadorans from rural and lower socioeconomic backgrounds have continued migrating to the area, initially settling in Cambridge and Somerville. They now reside primarily in East Boston but have also moved to Chelsea and Everett as rents have risen in Boston. These neighboring cities, along with Lynn, where Dominicans have been moving, have some of the state's lowest median incomes and highest poverty rates.[49] In 2020, an estimated 13,958 Salvadorans lived in the Boston area, where they were the third-largest Latinx group after Puerto Ricans and Dominicans.[50] Their median age was 30, and the population was predominantly male. In terms of physical features, Salvadorans have a more Mestizo appearance than some other Latin Americans. While most speak Spanish, some are not literate in Spanish or speak Indigenous languages. Some fortunate Salvadorans arrived with temporary protected status (TPS), which shields them from deportation, grants work authorization, and allows limited access to certain federal benefits. But TPS does not provide a path to obtaining a green card or citizenship, and recipients must continually reapply for work authorization. Sociologist Cecilia Menjívar has referred to TPS as a "liminally legal" status that creates great precarity.[51] While an estimated 204,000 Salvadorans have this status, other Salvadorans account for 5% of undocumented immigrants nationally.[52] Romina, an undocumented 30-year-old Salvadoran with medium-brown skin tone and straight, shoulder-length black hair, spoke with me about the advantages and disadvantages of being in Boston and the United States in 2016: "There's much opportunity for all types of people to succeed. It's beautiful to be in a country where you can realize your dreams because we couldn't in our country. [But] there are lots of challenges and obstacles that prevent you from realizing your goals. . . . First, you need to study and learn the language. . . . Second, . . . if you don't have papers, you can't do anything."

Brazilians also began migrating to the Boston area in the 1980s amid economic and political instability at home.[53] Brazilians' ties to the Boston area began during World War II, when US engineers and technicians from local firms were posted in the state of Minas Gerais to mine and process the mica used to insulate radio tubes.[54] This connection later facilitated migration. Most Brazilians arriving in the 1980s came from cities and towns in Minas, although some hailed from São Paulo, Espirito Santo, and other parts of southeastern Brazil.[55] They were highly educated and from working- and middle-class families. By 2005, the Boston area was the top destination for Brazilian immigrants to the United States.[56] Their numbers trailed off before the Great Recession, as the Brazilian economy experienced a significant boom and some migrants in the United States returned to Brazil.[57] Recent political and economic instability since 2012, notably the election of Jair Bolsonaro and the coronavirus pandemic, has generated a renewed flow of middle-class professionals to the Boston area.[58] Originally, Brazilians settled in Brighton, Allston, Cambridge, and Somerville, where Portuguese immigrants were also clustered.[59] Later, Brazilians moved to smaller urban areas within a 30-mile radius of Boston, such as Everett, Malden, Framingham, Marlborough, and Hudson.[60] These declining manufacturing cities had more affordable housing, while the cost of living in Boston, Cambridge, and Somerville soared.[61] In 2018, Massachusetts had an estimated 111,224 Brazilians, second only to Florida.[62] Most of them live in Framingham, Natick, and Marlborough, on the western edge of the metropolitan area; another 6% live in and around Boston.[63] Almost one-fourth (24%) are self-employed and own businesses in landscaping, construction, and housecleaning, where Brazilians have created an ethnic niche.[64]

Racial stratification in Brazil privileges whiter or lighter Brazilians, and their higher socioeconomic status compared with Brown and Black Brazilians provides them with more financial resources and social capital for migration.[65] Consequently, most Brazilian immigrants racially self-classify and are perceived by Americans as White.[66] They tend to arrive with tourist visas and become undocumented by overstaying them. An estimated 178,000 Brazilian immigrant adults in the United States were undocumented in 2019.[67] That same year, Brazilians made up 20% of Massachusetts's unauthorized population.[68] Compared with other foreign-born immigrants, Brazilians are less likely to be naturalized citizens and are more likely to adjust their status to lawful permanent residency as immediate relatives of US citizens.[69] Despite the challenges of living in the United States without documents, many Brazilians were pleased with the Boston area. Jonas, an undocumented immigrant with light-brown skin and short, straight black hair who arrived with a tourist visa from Porto Alegre in 2000, expressed a common opinion in 2013: "Massachusetts is my home, I love this place. It is marvelous and blessed by God in terms of work, health; it's a real city. [But] you can get into trouble with the police. If you are undocumented, you will have problems. It's sad that when you want to cash a check, you're asked for an ID, but they won't accept your [Brazilian] passport. It's constraining and complicates things."

Unlike Dominicans and Salvadorans, Brazilians speak Portuguese rather than Spanish. Given the fluidity of racial classification in Brazil, Brazilian immigrants struggle with US ethnoracial categories, which have made it difficult for them to be accurately counted in the census.[70] While some identify as Latino, they are not Hispanic. Despite their heterogeneity, Brazilians, Dominicans, and Salvadorans are employed in traditional immigrant jobs, and their racialized legal status and limited English proficiency present significant barriers to social mobility. The demographic characteristics of the immigrants I interviewed for this book resembled those of their co-ethnics in the Boston area (see Table I-3).

While immigrants spoke directly about their personal challenges accessing coverage and care, healthcare providers working with immigrants from these and other countries yielded insights into how shifting Massachusetts and ACA policy regimes influenced their ability to provide care for immigrant patients. I was fortunate to interview a wide range of professionals, including physicians, medical interpreters, and social workers, at a public, safety-net healthcare network I call the Boston Health Coalition (BHC).[71] It has a reputation for providing quality care to underserved populations throughout the Boston area. The BHC is affiliated with local medical schools, provides hospitalization for patients with acute conditions, and operates ambulatory care offices that provide primary and specialty physical and mental health services. Its patients are racially and ethnically diverse; the majority are persons of color, and

Table I-3. Demographic Characteristics of Immigrants Interviewed in 2012–2013, 2015–2016, and 2019 (N = 82)

Demographics	2012–2013 immigrant sample (N = 31)		2015–2016 immigrant sample (N = 39)			2019 immigrant sample (N = 12)		
	Brazilians (n = 21)	Dominicans (n = 10)	Brazilians (n = 15)	Dominicans (n = 14)	Salvadorans (n = 10)	Brazilians (n = 8)	Dominicans (n = 2)	Salvadorans (n = 2)
Gender (# women)	12	5	8	10	6	5	2	2
Median age (years)	40	55	43	56	40	46	55	34
Average time in United States (years)	12	14	10	21	19	11.5	28	6
Average individual monthly income	$3,969	$480	$1,720	$843	$1,383	$3,017	$3,050	$1,380
Median individual monthly income	$2,560	$300	$2,000	$640	$1,350	$2,000	$3,050	$1,380
Employed at time of interview	16	6	11	8	8	6	2	2
Customary occupations	Hairstyling, childcare, cleaning, education	Childcare, cleaning	Childcare, cleaning, landscaping	Childcare, restaurant work	Childcare, clerical, restaurant work	Cleaning, nursing assistance	Dentistry, house cleaning	Clerical
Documentation status (at interview)[a]								
Undocumented	6	3	6		6	5		1
DACA						1		
Tourist visa (B-1)	2		1					
Religious visa (R-1)	1							

(continued)

Table I-3. (continued)

Demographics	2012–2013 immigrant sample (N=31)		2015–2016 immigrant sample (N=39)			2019 immigrant sample (N=12)		
	Brazilians (n=21)	Dominicans (n=10)	Brazilians (n=15)	Dominicans (n=14)	Salvadorans (n=10)	Brazilians (n=8)	Dominicans (n=2)	Salvadorans (n=2)
Student visa (F-1)	1		3					
Work visa (H-1A/B)			1					
Temporary protected status (TPS)	N/A	N/A	N/A	N/A	1			
Green card / lawful permanent resident	10	4	3	11	2			1
Naturalized citizens	1	3	1	3	1	2	2	
Health coverage type[b]								
Uninsured	1		2	2	3	1		
Health Safety Net	7	2	4	1	4			
MassHealth[c]	4	6	6	9	2	3		1
Commonwealth/ ConnectorCare	1				1			1
Private	8	2	3	2		4	2	

a. Blank spaces in the table for this variable indicate that no respondents had those statuses among the different immigrant groups. R-1 visas are for those in religious occupations who will temporarily volunteer with religious organizations. They are also very specialized.

b. Blank spaces in the table for this variable indicate that no respondents had those statuses among the different immigrant groups. The specific health coverage types listed are discussed in Chapter 2.

c. Undocumented immigrants with MassHealth coverage had MassHealth Limited, which covers only emergency services.

nearly half speak a language other than English. They typically belong to lower-income households; some have publicly funded and private health insurance, while others are uninsured.

Immigrant and health advocacy organization staff members described the sociopolitical climate that immigrants encountered in Boston, identifying other factors and policies that shaped immigrants' healthcare decisions. For example, despite continuous debate in the state legislature over the course of my interviews from 2012 through 2019, undocumented immigrants could not get Massachusetts driver's licenses, which made it difficult for them to access the health care they were entitled to under the state's inclusive policy.[72] Advocates' expert knowledge of health and immigration policies helped immigrants navigate healthcare and social service bureaucracies. Staff members of immigrant organizations often shared the national origins and ethnic backgrounds of their constituents. Their positionality shed light on their personal connections to the work they did and the marginalization they continued to experience because of their own racialized legal status. Other scholars have emphasized that such individuals serve as institutional gatekeepers, who can either assist or hinder marginalized groups' access to resources.[73] This study reveals the vital role advocates play in helping immigrants and others surmount numerous barriers in the health coverage enrollment process and navigate the healthcare system.

To recruit respondents, I posted multilingual flyers in Brazilian, Dominican, and Salvadoran neighborhoods; BHC healthcare facilities; and community centers. My attendance at civic meetings and volunteering with immigrant and health advocacy organizations also aided my recruitment. During the first year of the study, I participated in many events at the State House and used my social networks to learn about local advocacy organizations. Because of my proficiency in Portuguese and Spanish and previous experience of living and conducting research in Brazil and the Dominican Republic, I volunteered at some organizations to learn more about these communities' needs and challenges. I served as an interpreter at immigration clinics, helped individuals complete forms for social and community services, drafted and provided feedback on grants that some organizations submitted for funding, and attended health and other types of community fairs. Through my involvement in these grassroots activities, I was able to develop the sense of trust needed to recruit the initial respondents. I then relied on what qualitative researchers call purposive snowball sampling, typically used for vulnerable populations, to recruit additional immigrant respondents as well as providers and advocates who worked closely with them.[74] While this recruitment strategy was effective, given the intensifying racialized and anti-immigrant sociopolitical climate over the course of the study, it also produced more women than men in the study sample, which is common in human subjects research.[75]

Studies based on in-depth interviews rather than quantitative instruments such as surveys do not involve a large random sample, which means that their findings are not generalizable to entire populations. On the other hand, the findings presented in this book provide new insights into social processes that are often difficult to observe, especially among marginalized groups. The challenges that Latinx immigrants face and the discrimination they encounter while navigating our complex healthcare system are seldom documented but must be addressed to achieve the goal of universal access to health care. This study design reveals the complex intersections among city, state, and federal policies, as well as health, immigration, and welfare policies, which generate exclusion from and inequality within this system of public benefits.

To assess the influence of policy changes on immigrants' healthcare access over time, I interviewed respondents at three different periods— 2012–2013, 2015–2016, and 2019—that corresponded with significant health and immigration policy shifts at the state and federal levels. I began my first set of interviews in August 2012, six years after the Massachusetts health reform and before the ACA was implemented. At the same time, President Obama issued his executive order starting the Deferred Action for Childhood Arrivals (DACA) program, which granted temporary legal status and work permits for some undocumented immigrants whose parents had brought them to the United States as children.[76] In those interviews, providers and advocates expressed excitement about the upcoming implementation of the ACA in Massachusetts but had concerns about immigrants' ability to maintain coverage. I returned to Boston in 2015–2016 to conduct a second set of interviews to understand how that transition affected Latinx Bostonians' healthcare access. In those interviews, which coincided with the campaign for the Republican Party's 2016 presidential nomination, some people reported that immigrants were disenrolling from health and other social services out of fear of retribution under a Trump administration. Immediately after I finished collecting data, state legislators ended funding for the Health Safety Net program, through which immigrant and lower-income Latinx residents ineligible for ACA benefits could obtain preventive services. This policy change drastically reduced their healthcare access. After the 2016 election, the Trump administration's racialized rhetoric and policies directed against both US and foreign-born Latinx people intensified, and the 2017 federal Tax Cut and Jobs Act overturned the tax penalty associated with the ACA's individual mandate requiring health coverage. To understand the impact of these policy changes in Boston, I conducted a final set of interviews with stakeholders from April to November 2019. Despite my well-established connections to Brazilian, Dominican, and Salvadoran communities and organizations, I had a very difficult time recruiting immigrants for the final year of the study. The small number of immigrant respondents was a direct result of the intensely hostile climate they faced.

Although I sought new respondents in each year of the study, I reinterviewed some respondents throughout the study. Given concerns about the safety of immigrant respondents, however, I chose not to reinterview any of them. In the interviews I did conduct, most of which were with Brazilians, I did not collect any personal information that could potentially put them or their family members at risk of detention or deportation. I did reinterview 10 providers and 11 advocates. They spoke directly to the impact of both actual and threatened changes in health and immigration policies on the immigrant communities with which they worked.

In addition, I attended Latinx immigrant and healthcare-related community events each year to obtain additional insights into the local situation and issues under debate. These events included public hearings on proposals related to immigrants and health care at Boston City Hall and the State House, health coverage enrollment clinics, and immigrant legal clinics sponsored by advocacy organizations. I draw on my detailed notes about what I observed at such events throughout the book. I also used publicly available data to conduct policy analyses of changes in eligibility under the Massachusetts and ACA reforms, which are the basis for some of the tables and figures in the chapters. This mix of data has given me a unique opportunity to assess the multifaceted ways in which racialized legal status in policy, rhetoric, and social contexts shaped Latinx immigrants' healthcare experiences. Qualitative researchers refer to this as data triangulation, which gives us a more concrete, comprehensive, and multidimensional perspective on the social phenomena we are examining.[77] Furthermore, the data from interviews, qualitative observations, and publicly available policy material enabled me to trace themes that recurred across these sources.

Throughout this project, I was constantly aware of my positionality and often struggled with my contradictory positions of privilege and disadvantage. I am an African American cisgender woman. Because I was born in the United States, I know that even though I am racialized as Black, my citizenship is unlikely to be called into question. This provided a significant amount of privilege relative to many of the immigrants I interviewed, who experienced the precarity of their noncitizen status and uncertainty about what the future would hold as explicitly racist and xenophobic rhetoric gained traction in public discourse. Many encountered numerous challenges in their daily lives, especially when attempting to access health care. As a tenured professor, I have excellent (but expensive) health insurance through my job. My English fluency, high level of education, and expertise in health care gave me considerable agency to navigate this complicated system. I am also very fortunate to have been physically and mentally healthy throughout my life.

Yet, with parents who lived through Jim Crow segregation and an older sister who had lupus and was in and out of hospitals until she passed from lupus complications in 2001, I empathized with the stories of racialized exclusion and health challenges that immigrants shared with me. Fortunately, I was able to speak with respondents in their primary languages. My familiarity with their places of origin brought a level of connection and ease to our conversations about difficult or painful subjects. As a Black woman with lighter skin tone who is sometimes mistaken for Brazilian or Dominican, I enjoyed a level of acceptance that others might not have received. At times, community members asked me about my background, why I was doing this research, and what it would be used for. I explained that I hoped this study would help to improve health care for immigrants and other marginalized groups. Furthermore, I expressed my hope that findings might shed light on how and why racialized legal status—alongside English proficiency and socioeconomic status—matters, which might eventually contribute to making equitable health care accessible to all.

While I was quite privileged in my interactions with immigrant communities, I was conscious of my racial background in White spaces, particularly when I had to enter government and office buildings and go through security. I am mentally prepared to encounter these challenges as a Black woman. Because I have been navigating White and elite spaces for decades, I dress professionally and have both my driver's license and university ID easily accessible in case my presence is questioned. I developed amicable relationships with employees of advocacy organizations and healthcare providers who are passionate about making healthcare access more equitable, reforming immigration policy, and ending systemic racism. But I noticed that I was one of the few people of color at some events, particularly those involving state-level health and immigration policies. One crucial consequence of systemic racism is that those who are most directly affected by public policies often do not have access to the spaces where decisions are made. Until recently, too, physicians have been overwhelmingly White, which does not match their increasingly diverse patient population.[78]

In the chapters that follow, I discuss some of my observations that demonstrate how my positionality shaped particular aspects of the research. Many of those observations align with how racialized legal status influenced the healthcare access of Brazilian, Dominican, and Salvadoran immigrants in Boston and what implications their experiences might have for others struggling to access health coverage and services around the country.

A Brief Guide to the US Healthcare System

Because this book examines how Latin American immigrants navigate Boston's healthcare system, a brief guide to the US healthcare system may be helpful for those who have not encountered it firsthand or who, like many Americans, find it confusing. The United States is unique because, unlike other economically developed countries, it does not have a universal healthcare system, and Americans have worse health than people in many other countries despite the extremely high cost of care.[79] Some basic information on the development of the healthcare system, the structure of health insurance, healthcare costs, and the types of healthcare facilities that provide services is essential to understand how the system works—or rather, does *not* work—to provide quality care to everyone.

Origins and Development of the US Healthcare System

What we know as the current healthcare system, specifically with most care provided by medical professionals in hospitals and clinics, began in the late 19th century. Its development was marked by the increasing respectability and authority of physicians.[80] In the early 19th century, most doctors had relatively low status because most were trained through apprenticeships, and there were no agreed-upon standards of care. Receiving medical care at home was the norm, and few people were treated at hospitals, which were regarded as places where the poor went to die. Between 1875 to 1920, medical education was formalized and standardized, and professional organizations controlled access to the field. The primary place for receiving care gradually shifted from the home to physicians' offices and acute care hospitals. Despite these institutional changes, the fee-for-service model continued: physicians charged a fee for each office or hospital visit, treatment, or other service they provided, as did most hospitals. After the adoption of asepsis in hospitals and rising standards for medical licensing, the demand for services rose, and more patients with acute illnesses were treated in hospitals. At the same time, however, racial segregation meant that Black college graduates were seldom admitted to accredited medical schools, internships, and residencies. Consequently, institutions that served African Americans and the urban and rural poor were starved of funds and often closed because they could not afford to meet the new standards.

During the Progressive period and the Great Depression that followed, some reformers thought that strengthening public health measures and extending access to care would be more effective as well as less costly in preventing disease and treating illness. Their experiments included housing codes to decrease the prevalence and transmission of tuberculosis and baby wellness clinics to lower rates of infant mortality. Free clinics for the poor offered care without unduly burdening families and local governments. Group health plans for certain industries aimed to reduce workers' absences from their jobs. Unsurprisingly, many physicians opposed all these experiments and banded together through the American Medical Association (AMA) to prevent group health plans from reducing their autonomy and fees. Since 1912, organized medicine had been staunchly opposed to any form of health insurance, which might regulate their practice and limit their fees. At the time, physicians blocked a medical and accident insurance plan proposed by the trade unions representing railroad employees, who along with coal miners had the most dangerous jobs in the United States. During the Great Depression, when many more Americans were unable to afford medical care at all, the AMA considered whether voluntary insurance programs might be beneficial. The plans it endorsed, particularly the Blue Cross policies that groups of its members set up in each state, gave physicians sole authority over coverage decisions and generated significant profits for providers. By World War II, organized medicine had obtained "a high degree of control of the medical market and the relative stability of the structure of practice."[81]

As health care and health policy developed in the United States, it was not a single, unified system. Rather, it was more a set of arrangements negotiated by groups of powerful stakeholders—physicians and their professional associations, insurance companies, hospital and healthcare corporations, and pharmaceutical and medical device manufacturers—to ensure it served their distinct and often competing interests and guaranteed their profits. The paramount (and perhaps the only) goal they shared was to avoid empowering the nation-state to represent the needs of the population, which the stakeholders condemned as "socialized medicine" that they associated with communism. Consequently, the US healthcare system is a deliberate patchwork that was not intended to function as a rational, efficient, and cohesive system.

Sociologist Paul Starr traced the postwar development of US healthcare through three phases driven by expansion, equity, and cost containment. First, from 1945 to 1960, state governments allocated substantial funds to medical institutions without interrogating their organization or the quality of existing medical practices. Then, in the 1960s, the federal government established Medicaid and Medicare to provide insurance for lower-income and elderly individuals. The AMA vigorously opposed these publicly funded and federally administered programs, condemning them as illegitimate interference with individuals' freedom of choice and unwarranted regulation of physicians' practices and reinforcing the notion that socialized medicine is un-American.[82] Despite these new programs and the expansion of private medical insurance for some employees of corporations and government agencies, many Americans remained excluded from coverage. Payments to physicians and hospitals who cared for Medicaid and Medicare recipients without any regulation of what services were covered and what they could charge contributed to spiraling medical costs. This subsequently led to cost-control measures from the federal government, and these policies threatened to limit physician autonomy.

In the late 20th and early 21st centuries, healthcare costs paid by the government and by patients and their families continued to rise despite the varied measures adopted to limit them. The political power and organizational unity of physicians declined as other stakeholders in the healthcare system impinged on physicians' autonomy and authority.[83] Despite a physician surplus in the 1990s, there is currently a shortage of doctors, particularly in primary care.[84] The growing presence of large corporations in the healthcare system has created a hierarchy among physicians, with owners, administrators, and employees who come into conflict, as well as tensions between research and clinical practice. Patients face constantly increasing costs, plans that do not cover essential tests and treatments, and hospital closures and mergers that limit access to care.

Throughout its development, health care in the United States has been shaped by the exclusion and segregation of African Americans and other people of color, both as professionals and as patients.[85] The result is a separate and unequal healthcare system and a profession characterized by structural racism. White physicians and healthcare facilities treated White patients and excluded those who were not White. If Black patients and other patients of color were treated by White hospitals, even in life-threatening emergencies, they received substandard care and were discharged or sent to Black hospitals as soon as possible. Black physicians, who in many circumstances were the only doctors willing to treat Black patients, were categorically denied membership in the American Medical Association until the 1960s. Forming their own medical organizations, they fought for the improvement of healthcare facilities that served Black Americans, most of whom were too poor to pay the costs.[86] Many White Americans and those of other ethnoracial groups also lacked medical insurance or were unable to afford health care. Members of these groups, especially those with lower incomes, were vulnerable to exploitation. They sometimes "volunteered" to participate in medical experiments to receive much-needed medical care or "donated" their bodies for research and teaching in exchange for care during their final illness.[87] This exploitative exchange did not benefit the marginalized patients involved but served the interests of the White medical establishment and created lasting mistrust of the healthcare system among many African Americans and other communities of color. The racial and class disparities in access to quality health care remain with us today.

Documentation Status and Health Insurance

Without a national health insurance program, the United States relies on a mix of public and private programs.[88] The most familiar publicly supported programs are Medicaid and Medicare, which provide comprehensive health coverage to very low-income individuals and the elderly (over age 65) and disabled, respectively.[89] States administer Medicaid, which covers preventive, acute, and long-term care.[90] It is jointly financed by the federal and state governments. The federal government's contribution to the cost of Medicaid varies inversely with the average income of each state's residents. So, states with more impoverished people receive higher subsidies from the federal government than states whose residents have higher average incomes. To be eligible for Medicaid, individuals must have low income and be elderly, blind, disabled, pregnant, or the low-income parent of a dependent child. Before ACA implementation, the income cutoff for Medicaid eligibility for nondisabled adults was 64% of the federal poverty level, which limited the program to extremely poor individuals.[91] After the implementation of Obamacare, the income cutoff was 138% of the federal poverty level in states that decided to expand eligibility for Medicaid.[92]

Medicare is mostly funded by taxes from working individuals and consists of two types of coverage: Part A includes inpatient hospital care, limited nursing home services, and some home health services; Part B includes physician and other ambulatory services. Medicare requires co-payments (the amounts patients must pay for medical visits and prescription medications) and deductibles (the amounts patients must pay before insurance begins covering their bills). Moreover, it does not cover all types of health services. So, most Medicare recipients purchase private supplemental health plans to help pay for those expenses. The Medicare program is not considered financially sound because its expenses are increasing more quickly than its revenues. As the US population ages, the proportion of people who pay taxes on their earnings to support current retirees is declining. Eligibility for Medicare is limited to adults over age 65 and dependent children who were permanently disabled before they turned 19.

As federal programs, both Medicaid and Medicare limit eligibility primarily to citizens, long-term green card holders, asylees, and refugees. Immigrants who are undocumented but considered to have a Permanent Residence Under Color of Law (PRUCOL) classification are also covered. Although PRUCOL is an administrative classification rather than an immigration status, it carries eligibility for public benefits.[93] Short-term lawful permanent residents, visa holders, and most undocumented immigrants are excluded.[94] As in other policy areas, discussions of deservingness—who deserves to be or should be beneficiaries—centered on race, class, ability, income, age, and citizenship in the development of Medicaid and Medicare. The scholarship on deservingness has often argued and demonstrated that individuals who are White, women, children, working, and citizens are deemed more deserving of inclusion for public benefits than those who are not.[95] Ironically, despite their ineligibility for Medicaid and Medicare, which are funded through payroll taxes and the Medicare Trust Fund, respectively, unauthorized immigrants contributed an estimated $115 billion surplus to the Medicare Trust Fund from 2002 to 2009.[96] In fiscal year 2020, spending for Medicaid and Medicare accounted for 21% of the federal budget despite multiple efforts to contain the programs' costs.[97] Together, Medicaid and Medicare provided coverage for 36% of the US population in 2020.[98]

Privately funded coverage is administered through private health insurance companies that provide various arrays of services at differing costs depending on the premiums, co-pays, and deductibles subscribers are responsible for.[99] These health insurance companies have networks of affiliated providers whose services they will pay for at negotiated rates.[100] When patients see providers outside of those networks, the costs are not fully covered and thus are more expensive for patients. Premiums, co-pays, and deductibles vary, so that plans with high premiums tend to have lower co-pays and deductibles, while those with low premiums have higher out-of-pocket expenses.[101]

While documentation status does not explicitly limit access to private insurance plans, the high costs are especially prohibitive for noncitizens who are ineligible for Medicaid and Medicare. Research also suggests that when noncitizens do have private health insurance plans, they often pay more in premiums than the costs of the health services they access with their insurance.[102] Among the biggest sources of privately funded insurance in the United States are employers, who pay for a portion of their employees' premiums as a job-related benefit. Different employers provide different plans, which can affect continuity of care when individuals change employers. In 2021, 54% of those who were insured had employer-sponsored coverage.[103] But employers have been shifting the higher costs of premiums onto employees and reducing the health insurance benefits they offer.[104] Some individuals and families with employer-sponsored coverage still have difficulty in accessing services with their insurance.

Individuals who are ineligible for Medicaid or Medicare and do not have employer-sponsored coverage may purchase private plans through health insurance marketplaces or exchanges under the ACA, and they may qualify for publicly funded subsidies if their income is so low that they cannot afford private insurance. However, having private health insurance does not guarantee access to services, as high premiums, deductibles, co-pays, and other out-of-pocket costs are still financially out of reach for many. In fact, these necessary expenses have contributed to significant medical debt and bankruptcy even among those insured under the ACA.[105]

The ACA was successful in increasing access to health coverage for an estimated 31 million people and reducing the proportion of Americans who were uninsured to 8.8% by 2017.[106] The number and proportion of insured people have declined since then, as legislation intended to undermine the ACA limited the services it offers and removed the requirement that individuals obtain health insurance in 2017. Job losses related to the COVID pandemic resulted in an estimated 27 million people losing their employer-sponsored coverage.[107] As of mid-2024, nearly 8% of US adults were uninsured.[108] While accessing health services is possible without insurance, doing so is a huge challenge.

Previous laws had sought to make health care available to uninsured individuals. The Emergency Medical Treatment and Labor Act, which was passed in 1986, required hospitals receiving federal funds to stabilize patients experiencing life-threatening conditions and to admit those giving birth regardless of their ability to pay instead of refusing to treat them.[109] The Disproportionate Share Hospital program, also established in 1986, increased Medicaid payments to hospitals treating many Medicaid and uninsured patients and allowed hospitals to subsidize care for indigent patients, including unauthorized immigrants.[110] The national system of federally qualified health centers, popularly known as community health centers, was established in 1965 as part of President Lyndon Johnson's War on Poverty and became the principal source of primary health care for officially designated "medically underserved populations."[111] This category includes immigrants who are uninsured because of their documentation status. Community health centers receive federal funding to provide primary care and public health services and are considered part of the country's health safety net for low-income, uninsured, and rural individuals and families. By providing care to 1 in 10 Americans, they have played an important role in reducing ethnoracial and class disparities in health.[112]

Beyond understanding how health insurance works and its connection to federal policy, it is important to remember that this is a small part of the larger US healthcare system. Health insurance is important for determining how much patients pay. But employers and administrators working for health insurance, medical supply, and pharmaceutical companies as well as healthcare facilities play a crucial role in ensuring that payments are processed, medical supplies are delivered for patient care, prescription medications get developed and distributed to pharmacies, and health services are provided. This complex and incoherent system involves multiple stakeholders—corporations, nonprofit organizations, public agencies, and bureaucracies—and entails a myriad of relationships between government and private industry. While health (and immigration) policies are decided by congressional legislation, subject to review by the Supreme Court, and administered by the executive branch, healthcare-related (and other) companies have lobbyists that communicate their interests to lawmakers. Meeting the demands made by health insurance and pharmaceutical corporations was crucial for the design and ultimate passage of the ACA.[113] Individuals and families whose lives and well-being depend on health care are reduced to consumers and have significantly less power to shape healthcare policy.

Thus, health care in the United States is not an integrated "system" designed to serve the country's residents, but an incoherent array of programs, policies, and regulations that reflect the jockeying of stakeholders to gain as large a share of public and private expenditures for health care as possible. It is costly and inefficient, as well as notoriously difficult to navigate, and most Americans remain deeply dissatisfied by their experiences with health care.[114]

The Contradictory Consequences of Health Reforms for Immigrants

This book highlights how changes in health policy and the sociopolitical climate influenced Latinx immigrants' health coverage and access over time in Boston. Many books have separately analyzed the national implications of the Affordable Care Act, the impact of health and immigration policies on immigrants' healthcare experiences, and how documentation status shapes individuals' access to public benefits.[115] This book is unique in its in-depth exploration of individuals' challenges in obtaining coverage and care under the Massachusetts and ACA reforms. Furthermore, I underscore how the centrality of race, alongside documentation status, influences Latinx immigrants' engagement with advocates, providers, and institutions amid surveillance concerns that made them fearful of accessing care in Boston. In doing so, this book contributes to our understanding of the ways that explicit and implicit discrimination perpetuates racialized legal status inequality and undermines the goals of comprehensive healthcare reforms.

The first chapter outlines my theoretical framework of racialized legal status by tracing its origins in structural racism, the development of varying documentation statuses, the structure of US government, and different dimensions of US policy. I discuss the implications of racialized legal status for immigrants and citizens of color and outline the difficulties racialized legal status poses for those navigating vital institutions such as health care.

Chapters 2 through 4 analyze how racialized legal status negatively affected Latinx immigrants' access to and experiences with health care through successive policy changes at the state and federal levels. Chapter 2 explores the aftermath of the Massachusetts reform in 2012–2013. Originally passed in 2006, the reform was intended to extend access to coverage to every resident of the commonwealth. Yet, six years after implementation, coverage remained stratified by documentation status and constrained Latinx immigrants' health coverage options. Difficulties in understanding how public coverage worked and navigating the annual renewal process, coupled with the lack of language assistance during enrollment and at medical appointments, limited Latinx immigrants' use of the health services for which they were eligible.

Chapter 3 shows how racialized legal status discrimination further restricted Latinx immigrants' healthcare access after ACA implementation in 2015–2016. The ACA made it more difficult for foreign-born Latinx residents to obtain coverage than under the previous Massachusetts reform. The transition to Obamacare was marred by major problems in the state's system for determining eligibility, which led to many residents losing their coverage and experiencing disruptions in care.

Chapter 4 analyzes the devastating impact of the Trump administration's repeated efforts to hinder the ACA, coupled with its propagation of virulently racist anti-immigrant policies. Although state policymakers implemented legal protections to ensure that health reform could not be overturned, advocates and healthcare providers remained worried that the proposed public charge rule change set up a conflict for immigrants between receiving health benefits and prospects for lawful permanent residency. Stepped-up federal immigration enforcement sowed fear in Latinx communities, leading them to cancel medical appointments.[116] This sociopolitical climate intensified the racialized legal status discrimination that impeded immigrants' use of health services.

The conclusion discusses the study's contributions to current understandings of the social dimensions of health policy and considers the implications of these findings beyond Boston and Massachusetts. The extension of insurance coverage under comprehensive health reforms has not removed multiple barriers to health care, especially those associated with racialized legal status. Language-appropriate assistance is essential to enable immigrants with limited English proficiency to apply for coverage and navigate the system. They cannot be treated effectively by culturally insensitive or racist medical providers. Latinx immigrants' concerns about profiling, deportation, and potential denial of lawful permanent residency deter them from obtaining care. Their counterparts in other places encounter similar obstacles. The complex intersections among city, state, and federal polices, as well as among health, immigration, and welfare policies, generate inclusion or exclusion from public benefits based on income and ethnoracial background. In other parts of the country, some states' choice to not expand Medicaid under the ACA has left many income-eligible citizens and qualified immigrants without coverage and unable to benefit from preventive and specialty health services. Understanding and addressing racialized legal status discrimination in the healthcare system may yield significant improvements in healthcare access for marginalized and uninsured groups. Ultimately, policymakers must ascertain how these unintended negative consequences can be remedied and develop more inclusive policies that mitigate discrimination against people of color who are assumed to be noncitizens and feature community-based outreach and education programs to improve healthcare access.

CHAPTER 1

Racialized Legal Status and Healthcare Exclusion in Boston

I have definitely experienced discrimination, of us being abused and mistreated in jobs and hospitals for being Latino or an immigrant. They leave you waiting for hours until you're almost dead to treat you and they treat other [patients] before you. . . . Thank God I came with a green card. But we don't stop being immigrants or being less valued or rejected. No, because having papers to allow you legally in the country doesn't prevent everything, especially when talking about language. Discrimination has always existed and not only because of our skin color, [but also] from the moment we open our mouths.

—*Dania, Dominican immigrant interviewed in 2013*

I think that even people who immigrated with documentation, who are now citizens, . . . are feeling some mental health effects of the stuff that's going on. So even though they're not actually in any legal jeopardy, and don't have any real barriers [to] health insurance or employment, . . . the stigma and the rage against immigrants of color in particular, all immigrants really [affects them].

—*Madelyn, BHC provider interviewed in 2019*

Recently, public expressions of hostility to immigrants and of overt racism and White supremacy have again become commonplace in the United States. Politicians, pundits, and everyday Americans express support of militarized borders to prevent unauthorized entry; they also support pushing immigrants to "the back of the line" and requiring them to "get legal" before they receive any publicly provided or subsidized benefits, as well as banning discussion of anything related to systemic racial inequality in schools. These same people are quick to claim they are not racist. Yet race, immigration, and citizenship have been inextricably connected since the founding of the United States. The connections between these seemingly separate sociopolitical constructions remain pertinent today, as debates continue about who belongs—who has access to the rights and privileges of citizenship and is regarded as a "real" American. The quotations opening this chapter speak to the very real impact that the intersection of race, ethnicity, and legal status—now encapsulated in the concept of racialized legal status—has on the lives of contemporary immigrants. Dania, a Dominican immigrant I spoke with in 2013, shared how being Latino, having darker skin tone, and speaking English with an accent contributed to the discrimination that she and other immigrants experience. Having a green card does not remove or even decrease the likelihood of encountering anti-immigrant or racial discrimination. Rather, Dania emphasized that being perceived as non-White and foreign because of her skin color and way of speaking means that others treat her as if she does not belong here. For her, the intersection of these factors *undermines* the legal privileges she receives as a green card holder. She recognized that those who are perceived as legitimate Americans— that is, White Americans—are treated with more respect and dignity. In this chapter, I explain the theoretical framework of racialized legal status that I use to illuminate Latinx Bostonians' healthcare access throughout this book.

Because "racialized legal status," or "RLS," is a term that other scholars have used to describe this intersection between race, ethnicity, and documentation status, I begin by explaining the origins of this concept and its connections to our understandings of race and immigration. These socially constructed forms of difference have often been explored separately, although they intersect in daily life. Next, I outline my theoretical framework and show how racialized legal status operates at three levels in US society. At the macro level, the federal, state, and local laws and policies that govern society create and reify the ethnoracial and legal status categories that differentiate access to public benefits. At the same time, structural racism embedded in government, public policy, and major institutions perpetuates the unequal social positions and lived experiences of immigrants and citizens of color compared with those of White Americans. At the meso level, policy and government create the bureaucracies and institutions that administer public benefits to individuals. Employees of these institutions have some discretion in how firmly applicants must adhere to eligibility criteria and the rules to obtain services. Although those criteria appear to be neutral regarding applicants' race or legal status, the documentation they must submit is often more difficult for immigrants and citizens of color to produce. At the micro level, RLS may contribute to the discrimination people experience from law and immigration officials and others they encounter.

My racialized legal status framework builds on previous scholarship in three key ways. First, I argue and demonstrate that language, as a marker of race and ethnicity, is a legal basis of *racial* discrimination in US civil rights law that is separate from discrimination based on documentation status. Second, rather than focusing primarily on the impact of RLS on immigrants of color, I also highlight how structural and systemic racism undermines the privileges and benefits of citizenship and belonging for citizens of color. This point was brilliantly made by a BHC provider named Madelyn whom I interviewed in 2019. Her words, which are quoted along with Dania's at the beginning of this chapter, describe how the anti-immigrant sociopolitical climate under the Trump administration increased the vulnerability of naturalized citizens, particularly those of color, and affected their health and health care. For them and US-born citizens of color, legal citizenship does not protect them from discrimination associated with race, ethnicity, or their presumed otherness. Third, both language discrimination and the undermining of citizenship by race and ethnicity reflect the operation of RLS at the macro, meso, and micro levels in our society, in law and policy, in institutions such as healthcare facilities, and among individuals. My framework includes these key components, which have been less explored in previous RLS scholarship.

To show how racialized legal status shapes immigrants' ability to access health coverage and care in Greater Boston, I have selected especially clear and insightful statements made by people I interviewed. These quotations are exemplary in pointing to the negative, mutually reinforcing effects of discrimination based on documentation status, race, and ethnicity. These immigrants, medical professionals, and advocates, however, do not use abstract phrases like "racialized legal status," which is based in social theory, to explain what they have experienced and observed. The concept of RLS encompasses a range of experiences among individuals who belong to different social groups and helps us to understand how systemic, pervasive, and multifaceted this intersectional form of harmful discrimination is in the contemporary US. Deeply embedded structural racism and White supremacy continue to negatively affect the lived experiences of people of color, and being a noncitizen routinely results in systematic exclusion from institutions and activities that are essential for people to conduct their daily lives. Both have spillover effects that reverberate throughout society, exacerbating inequality. Naturalized citizens and their US-born children may be perceived and treated as if they are undocumented and thus without basic rights. Immigrants of color and their children may be misrecognized as Black Americans and treated by police and other authorities as though they are violent criminals. Black and Brown US-born citizens may be miscategorized as "illegal aliens" or "terrorists" and subjected to further denials of their rights. Perhaps the most egregious examples are when US-born Black or Brown persons are detained arbitrarily and held incommunicado because they cannot prove their citizenship—or when undocumented immigrants are detained and threatened with deportation when they testify as witnesses for the prosecution on behalf of those who are the victims of serious crimes in court. While these examples are extremes, they are increasingly common instances of racialized legal status discrimination. But RLS discrimination also occurs in a myriad of less visible but cumulatively damaging ways in many arenas—including in healthcare policies and settings that are intended to promote healing and enable people to thrive.

The Origins of Racialized Legal Status

Racialized legal status represents a nuanced form of discrimination and social stratification in the 21st century. Coined by education scholar Genevieve Negron-Gonzales, the phrase was initially used to describe how being Latinx and undocumented shaped youths' political awareness. She argued that this intersectional marginalization created a "hybridized sense of self" as simultaneously an insider and outsider: these young people feel culturally American from having been raised in the United States but are excluded from institutions and civic society because of their undocumented status.[1] Sociologists Asad Asad and Matthew Clair subsequently used the term to describe a type of social stratification in which race-neutral legal classifications stigmatize people of color— noncitizens and citizens alike—and contribute to health disparities.[2] Asad and Clair's concept built on a growing body of research that argues that individuals who are racialized as immigrants, especially those of Latin American descent, are stereotyped as undocumented and therefore criminalized.[3] Sociologist Tanya Golash-Boza and I also used the term to discuss parallels between the societal exclusion and segregation of African Americans in the early 20th century and the exclusion and segregation of immigrants and citizens of color in the contemporary United States.[4] We suggest that esteemed scholar W. E. B. Du Bois's theory of double consciousness could be applied to understand the "twoness" these groups experience as a consequence of being regarded as less than full members of the American family because of their race and ethnicity and despite their citizenship status.

Indeed, the link between race and migration has become a burgeoning area of research, which contends that people who are perceived as immigrants because of their race, ethnicity, or religion are stereotyped as undocumented or terrorists and subsequently criminalized.[5] The growing connection between race and migration, more specifically illegality, aligns with a convergence of federal immigration and criminal law referred to as "crimmigration": unauthorized immigration in itself is a criminal act. The enforcement of immigration law and criminal law closely resemble each other, and prosecuting immigration violations mimics criminal procedures.[6] Consequently, Latinx people, especially men, are targeted for more restrictive, violent, and militarized enforcement.[7] Research on the ties between policies and institutions connecting race and immigration has expanded recently, as their impact on immigrant communities of color has escalated. Pause to consider how racialized immigration profiling in the criminal legal system has promoted mass deportation and incarceration.[8] And residential segregation, gentrification, and unaffordable housing have perpetuated displacement and housing insecurity for people of color and immigrants, documented and undocumented alike. Collectively, this body of research has started to address a significant gap between studies of race and studies of immigration.

Theoretical and empirical scholarship on race has explored that concept as a social construction that justifies racism and perpetuates discrimination against individuals, within institutions and organizations, and throughout the broader society.[9] Within the prevailing racial hierarchy in the US, those who are categorized as White have significant social and economic advantages over people of color and wield disproportionate political power compared to everyone else. White supremacy is incorporated into a global system that remains profoundly shaped by colonialism and imperialism, making it very difficult to overturn even in the rest of the world, where Europeans and their descendants were always a small minority.[10] Race scholars have made important strides incorporating intersectional analyses to assess how race, gender, and other dimensions of power generate inequality and shape people's lived experiences.[11] Yet scholarship focused on race has still not sufficiently addressed the complex ways in which immigration and legal status affect people who are categorized in racial terms as they cross international borders.

At the same time, US scholarship on migration has primarily focused on developing theories to explain the more complete incorporation of early 20th European immigrants in contrast to the experiences of the mostly Black, Latin American, and Asian immigrants of the late 20th and early 21st centuries.[12] This body of work has not fully explored the impact of structural racism and US race relations on the incorporation of immigrants of color and their children.[13] Relatedly, research on citizenship has not analyzed how race and ethnicity alter what it means for people of color to have "papers" or obtain legal citizenship. This matter is crucial because race and ethnicity are significant, even determining, factors in US constitutional amendments, government policies, and Supreme Court cases establishing the terms of citizenship and the rights it confers.[14] Some scholars of citizenship emphasize the distinction between legal and sociocultural citizenship.[15] With *legal* citizenship, individuals are formally acknowledged as members of a society by the government. In contrast, *sociocultural* citizenship means that individuals are fully and unquestionably regarded as "Americans." Throughout the nation's history, race and other social constructions such as gender have defined the terms of both legal and sociocultural citizenship. Legal citizenship theoretically grants participation in the body politic through voting and access to public benefits to those qualified by income and age. The continuing lack of sociocultural citizenship, however, means that groups that were previously excluded from legal citizenship, such as African Americans, Asians, and immigrants of color, along with all women, are not shielded from pervasive forms of economic, social, and even political disadvantage and discrimination. Because structural racism is entrenched in US society, race affects who is considered a "legitimate" citizen, regardless of documentation status. Historically and today, some White Americans regard themselves as the only "real Americans," while they regard people of color—no matter their ethnicity or how long their ancestors have been in the country—as outsiders who not deserve the rights and privileges that Whiteness confers.[16] Consequently, some scholars have developed the concept of racialized citizenship, calling attention to racialized legal status as a relevant axis of social inequality that deserves more attention.[17] The 13 naturalized US citizens of Brazilian, Dominican, and Salvadoran heritage I interviewed felt that they would never be fully accepted because they are not White and either do not speak English or speak it with an accent. Their legal citizenship did not protect them when they were racially profiled and pulled over by police or detained for questioning by immigration authorities. Their stories and the experiences of many immigrants and citizens of color in the 21st-century United States reveal that racialized legal status perpetuates both explicit and implicit forms of discrimination associated with race and citizenship.

Racialized Legal Status at the Macro Level: The Policy Complications of Federalism

The federalist structure of the US government, which divides power between the nation and the states, shapes many aspects of making and implementing public policy.[18] At the macro level, racialized legal status is constructed in two main ways (Figure 1-1). First, the federal government uses policy to determine who is allowed to enter the country legally and creates the documentation status categories to which individuals are assigned.[19] Furthermore, federal government policies also shape the creation of the ethnoracial categories used on the Census, in government agencies, and in public discourse.[20] According to historian Natalia Molina, "Immigration laws are perhaps the most powerful and effective means of constructing and reordering the social order in the United States. . . . Moreover immigration laws can reproduce and reinforce pre-existing US racial hierarchies. . . . Thus, we must fully analyze the role of government and government actors if we want to completely understand how these various social orders came to be."[21]

Second, with regard to documentation status, federal policy positions those categories along a continuum, ranging from permanent residency, which includes eligibility for a green card and eventual naturalization, to undocumented status, which confers no durable rights and now carries substantial penalties.[22] The intersection of federal immigration policy with other policy domains, such as health care and welfare provision, contributes to the differential experience of racialized legal status through unequal benefits associated directly with legal status and indirectly with race and ethnicity given that most immigrants are racialized as people of color.[23] Since the 1970s, federal and state policies have allocated benefits based on documentation status. Over time, noncitizens' access to publicly provided and subsidized services has been restricted, stratifying the work of many vital social institutions.[24]

Regarding ethnoracial categories, the US government has explicitly and implicitly implemented and enforced policies that benefited individuals in the White racial group, usually at the expense of people of color since its founding.[25] For example, policies permitting the enslavement of and denial of citizenship to African Americans before the Civil War and sanctioning race-based segregation in housing, education, and other realms after the Civil War are linked to the various disparities that population still experiences. Other groups not defined as White, such as Native, Asian, and Latinx Americans, have also experienced abject exclusion because of federal policies that used race or ethnicity to determine who could immigrate to the country, naturalize as a citizen, or even receive public benefits.

Race influences the mindset of policymakers as they debate, write, and implement laws and policies.[26] With the establishment of the modern welfare state under President Franklin Roosevelt's New Deal, Black and Mexican Americans were routinely excluded while White immigrants were included.[27] Social Security and unemployment insurance programs excluded farmworkers and domestic workers, occupations in which many Black and Mexican Americans worked, and these groups did not benefit from those reforms until 1954.[28] New Deal housing policy excluded people of color from federally subsidized suburban developments and differentially color-coded neighborhoods based on racial criteria. Areas where African Americans and other people of color lived were deemed ineligible for mortgages, and their housing was devalued, condemning these properties to decay in spite of the high rents "slumlords" charged.[29] The consequences are still visible in racial residential segregation and the racial wealth gap today.[30] When it comes to state policies shaping access to public benefits, requirements are made more rigorous when Black and Latinx people—citizens or immigrants—are perceived as the potential beneficiaries because they are perceived as undeserving and prone to becoming dependent on welfare rather than relying on work.[31]

The most infamous policy realm where race has determined differential practices and outcomes is the criminal legal system, at both the state and federal levels. Drug use among people of color was punished harshly with long prison sentences followed by probation, while Whites were more often sent to treatment programs, even though Whites were more likely to be arrested for drug possession.[32] These racially biased patterns contributed to the disproportionate incarceration of Black and Latinx people.

At all governmental levels and across policy domains, racialized legal status differentially shapes resource allocation, indicated by arrows drawn from the "Resource Allocation Stratification" box in Figure 1-1 to the circles representing individual policy domains. I specifically include healthcare, immigration, welfare, and education policies, which have the greatest influence on immigrants' experiences. The overlapping policy domain circles demonstrate intersections between individual policy domains: (in)eligibility for healthcare benefits may (dis)qualify someone from welfare or education benefits, for example.[33]

The federal government has increasingly devolved responsibility for the administration and allocation of public benefits to state governments.[34] Consequently, subnational (state and local) governments can create policies that align with or contradict federal policies within their jurisdictions. This has had significant implications for immigrants and people of color when it comes to their eligibility for or successful enrollment in state and federal-level public benefits.

With regard to immigration policy, some subnational governments use state funds to provide benefits to federally ineligible immigrants. California extended Medicaid access to undocumented immigrants, Illinois extended Medicare access to older undocumented immigrants, and Massachusetts extended eligibility for state-funded health coverage to undocumented immigrants.[35] Other states pass more restrictive legislation. For example, Florida's SB-1718, as of July 1, 2023, permits racial profiling of anyone who looks "foreign" and criminalizes immigrants who are present in the state without required documents.[36] Some states allow cooperation between local law enforcement and federal immigration

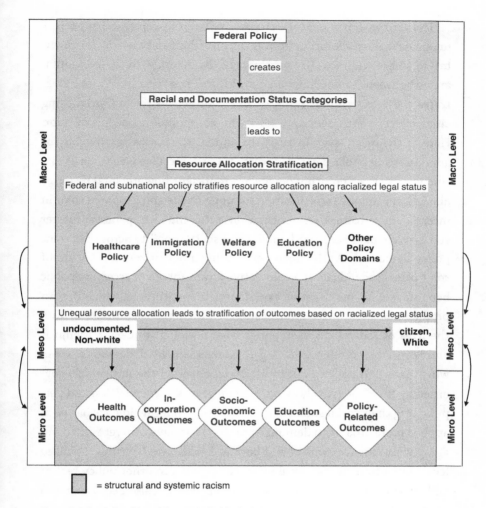

□ = structural and systemic racism

Figure 1-1. Racialized Legal Status in Public Policies

enforcement, while others do not, which means that one's jurisdiction makes the difference in determining whether a simple traffic stop can lead to detention and deportation.[37] This devolution has created what political scientist Monica Varsanyi and her colleagues refer to as a "multilayered jurisdictional patchwork," which catches immigrants in the crossfire of conflicting federal and subnational policies.[38]

The arrows drawn beneath the policy circles in Figure 1-1 represent unequal resource allocation from each policy domain based on documentation status and race. The next part of the figure, with the horizontal arrow between "undocumented, non-White" and "citizen, White," illustrates the direction that resource allocation moves toward, privileging citizens over noncitizens and those who are White over people of color. Here at the meso level, institutions and bureaucracies responsible for administering public benefits perpetuate such racialized legal status distinctions. Arrows pointing downward represent how unequal resource allocation generates stratification for noncitizens and people of color in intersecting outcomes. Documentation status and race operate as master statuses, shaping access to benefits and social mobility across different policy domains.[39] At the micro level, being a noncitizen and person of color places individuals at a cumulative disadvantage in accessing public benefits and having negative experiences in institutions, which in turn produces and reinforces stratification.[40] The deep reach of policy into the lives of individuals exemplifies what sociologists Cecilia Menjívar and Leisy Abrego refer to as "legal violence," or the dangerous ways in which laws and policies can inflict social harm on the individuals governed by them, negatively affecting immigrants' incorporation and perpetuating their social suffering.[41] The concept of legal violence has been applied more broadly to demonstrate that laws have concrete and damaging consequences within and beyond health care.[42] In the racialized legal status framework, "legal violence" extends to other policy realms and affects not only noncitizens but also people of color because racism is embedded in policies and their implementation.

Thus, while documentation status is crucially important within this racialized legal status framework, systemic and structural racism are embedded in the dynamic societal processes the framework depicts and indicated by the light gray background of Figure 1-1. Systemic racism refers to a range of racist practices that perpetuate the unequal allocation of economic and other resources along racial lines and that maintain White supremacy, privilege, and power.[43] Relatedly, structural racism accounts for how systemic racism operates, ramifies, and is reproduced across different types of institutions and time periods.[44] Sociologist Joseph Feagin argues that the United States has been racist since its founding and remains so today: "The US Constitution which embraced slavery and embedded the global racist order . . . remains the nation's legal, political, and . . . moral foundation."[45] Efforts to mitigate structural and systemic racism through constitutional amendments and congressional legislation have often been undermined by state and federal courts, including the US Supreme Court.[46] And in some cases, once legal and legislative changes created equal rights for marginalized Americans, the courts and Congress reversed those changes. Consequential recent examples include the 2013 *Shelby v. Holder* Supreme Court decision, which found that Section 4 of the 1965 Voting Rights Act was unconstitutional, and the 2023 *Students for Fair Admissions v. Harvard* Supreme Court decision banning race-conscious admissions in elite universities. The result is that laws and policies still have structural and systemic racism at their core, at times openly perpetuating White supremacy. Indeed, this is a key tenet of critical race theory, which is now being vilified as well as misinterpreted.[47] The arrows outside the figure pointing downward from the macro level to the meso level indicate how structural and systemic racism at the macro level may infiltrate bureaucratic institutions and organizations as laws and policies are implemented. Sociologist Victor Ray's theory of racialized organizations argues that governmental and related institutions are pervaded by processes that maintain racial hierarchies, even though they appear race-neutral, and distribute resources unequally along racial lines that benefit White citizens and disadvantage people of color.[48]

In the Boston area, immigrants experienced the consequences of racialized legal status when interacting with meso-level bureaucratic institutions and organizations to apply for health coverage and receive care. Advocates and BHC providers recognized and described how racialized legal status in federal and subnational policy affected the services immigrants could access. Without any promoting or even directed questions, these interviewees volunteered accounts of structural racism that shaped immigrants' experiences independently from their documentation status.

First, these advocates and providers thought that immigration policy had a racialized impact because most immigrants are people of color who are disadvantaged in US policy. Joshua, a health advocate I interviewed in 2019, spoke boldly about the connection he saw between White supremacy, racism, and immigration policy during the Trump administration's attempts to change the public charge rule:

> I think if we don't recognize the systemic White supremacy aspect of [immigration policy], we're ignoring a really key piece of what is really going on in the underbelly of these policies. . . . In fact, public charge policies . . . existed for over 100 years. . . . And it's always been about race and religion and class. . . . That's really important, you know, to understand the way that the race discussion in America has changed over time. I mean, today, what we see so clearly is that it's focused on people from Mexico, Central America, [and] to some extent, South America and the Middle East. . . . So, deeply embedded in the policy is this racialized element. Now, what's tricky about it from a legal perspective is that it's not necessarily facially racist. . . . The way that [legislators] do it is through subtext and focus on poverty, because in this country the link between poverty and race is so strong.

Joshua's analysis emphasizes that the race-neutral language on the surface of immigration policies conceals the racism that is silently but decisively incorporated in these laws and regulations. He ties the shifts in immigration policy to shifts in the ethnoracial demographics of immigrants over time, although many people are unable to recognize the White supremacy embedded in these policies because of their ostensible color blindness. The result is that race-neutral immigration policies have harmful consequences for immigrants of color.

The second way providers and advocates described the structural racism in macro-level policy was by pointing to the lack of sufficient language assistance for immigrants who apply for and use public benefits. Angelica, a language access attorney I spoke with in 2016, explained that access to assistance in people's primary language through competent interpreters is a civil right: "Title VI of the [1964] Civil Rights Act basically says that discrimination based on sex, age, national origin" is prohibited. "Now the established law is that your language . . . identifies you as being of a specific national origin," so discrimination on the basis of language is forbidden. "But if you look at this Civil Rights Act, it [does] not talk about language anywhere. It just talk[s] about national origin. The best thing that is most specific is [President Bill] Clinton's 2000 Executive Order 13166," called "Improving Access to Services for Persons with Limited English Proficiency," which sets standards for and enforces compliance with Title VI. Any program or activity that receives federal funds must provide proper language assistance to participants who need it. Not doing so is a violation of an individual's civil rights and represents a form of racial discrimination. Angelica works with and files complaints on behalf of immigrants who need language assistance in their interactions with federal bureaucracies. A key part of her job is to make sure Massachusetts state agencies that administer and provide federally funded or subsidized social services comply with Title VI, which is never easy but is especially complex when medical information and decisions about health care are involved. Thus, racialized legal status is at work in situations in which policies or the lack of policy enforcement allows practices that disadvantage people with limited English proficiency, the majority of whom are immigrants and citizens of color, in obtaining health coverage or services. In other words, language, specifically not speaking English or doing so with an accent, racializes individuals as being from another country or as a marker of not being "fully American."

Although the advocates and providers I interviewed in 2012–2013 and 2015–2016 noted that macro-level policies affected their constituents and patients, many observed that racialized legal status became more important during the 2016 campaign and the presidency of Donald Trump. Many believed that the explicitly racist and anti-immigrant rhetoric and policies had serious negative effects on individuals' engagement with healthcare institutions. Madelyn, a provider I interviewed in 2019 who is quoted at the beginning of this chapter, emphasized that racialized legal status influenced her immigrant patients' health regardless of their legal status. Being a naturalized citizen and a person of color made them vulnerable to the rage the president's virulent rhetoric expressed and promoted, intensifying the hostility they felt even in settings where they were entitled to receive services.

The immigrants I spoke with agreed that macro-level policies had a negative impact on their lives and recognized that their legal exclusion from benefits that citizens received was tied to their status under immigration law. Equally important, they typically connected racism with the ethnoracial discrimination they encountered in interactions with meso-level bureaucracies and officials and in micro-level interactions with other people. While immigrants realized that their documentation status posed structural barriers because of national policies, they recognized racism in interactions with other people more readily than they did the systemic racism embedded in macro-level policy and regulations. In what follows, I present their own perceptions of how their documentation status affected their lives. I discuss immigrants' perceptions of racism later in this chapter, when I turn to the meso- and micro-level manifestations of racialized legal status. At times, immigrants shifted pronouns in our conversations to express themselves and articulate their experiences more clearly.

Carlos, an undocumented Dominican immigrant I interviewed in 2013, arrived in Boston in 2002. His light-brown skin and short, black curly hair likely reinforced his being racialized as Latino. Carlos spoke openly about how his undocumented status shaped his experiences: "One goes through a lot when they arrive here. Without papers, it is difficult to get a job, rent a house or apartment, anything. If you don't have papers, you cannot get a job with a steady income, you have to live in the street or a shelter. You also can't get health insurance. They will treat you [in the hospital], but it's not equal. The first thing they ask for is your Social Security number. If you don't have it, they know you're an immigrant. You exist, but you don't [really]."

Each of the negative situations that Carlos described is directly connected to restrictive federal immigration laws, which limit or deny undocumented residents' access to public benefits; what civil rights laws call public accommodations, such as housing; and employment opportunities. He lacks health insurance because he cannot get a legitimate Social Security number. This consequence of Carlos's status as an unauthorized immigrant hinders his ability to meet his basic needs and to "exist" in the most ordinary ways that citizens and other legal residents do. This exclusion is inscribed in law and demonstrates the legal violence that Menjívar and Abrego describe as the dangerous consequence of immigration policy.[49]

Jazmin is an undocumented Salvadoran with medium-brown skin and long, dark, straight hair I interviewed in 2016. She discussed the myriad problems that her lack of legal status created: "Life has been very difficult. I don't have papers, I can't drive, work is hard to find." Her existence in the United States seemed precarious: "I feel I will experience more difficulty at any time." While Jazmin expressed gratitude for the assistance she receives from community members, she realized that it could not fundamentally alter her situation: "There are kind people who help, but they can't help us in respect to the laws. They can help with a car ride, but what we really need is to become legal in this country. We haven't received that help."[50]

Carlos and Jazmin were well aware of the ways their undocumented status penetrated their everyday reality, preventing them from conducting ordinary lives as many citizens and permanent residents are able to do. Yet naturalization does not protect many immigrants of color from the discrimination based on racialized legal status that is embedded in macro-level policies and regulations.

Yleana, a Dominican immigrant who was a naturalized citizen when I interviewed her in 2016, had arrived in the United States as a tourist during the 1960s and overstayed her visa. With medium-brown skin and short, loosely curled brown hair, she was likely perceived as a woman of color. Despite losing her legal status, she applied for a green card in the 1990s. But Yleana was detained by the federal Immigration and Naturalization Services (INS), the predecessor to Immigration and Customs Enforcement (ICE): "I was working in the factory and in came INS. When they approached me, they asked if I had papers and I [said I] was in the process. So, they took me to a detention center. Later when I applied for citizenship, I had to wait five years with residency [lawful permanent residency]. When the [citizenship] application asked if I had been detained, I had to say yes, even though I was not deported. I wasn't sure if I would have problems with my citizenship."

Yleana's experience occurred decades ago, but it exemplifies the vulnerability of documented noncitizens to immigration enforcement. Whether or not they "are in the process" of adjusting their status, noncitizens of all statuses face the prospect of detention and deportation in the very punitive post-9/11 surveillance system. Punitive macro-level immigration policy constantly intrudes into noncitizens' lives.

Racialized Legal Status at the Meso Level in Bureaucracies, Institutions, and Organizations

Racialized legal status is equally important for understanding individuals' engagement with the meso-level bureaucracies, institutions, and organizations that control access to services regulated and subsidized by the government. The complex processes of applying and demonstrating eligibility for benefits can be immensely challenging to navigate. In their research, Pamela Herd and Donald Moynihan describe the "administrative burdens" that arise when a person seeks public services.[51] They argue that these bureaucratic obstacles are "the product of deliberate choice occurring via political processes" and limitations on institutional capacity that are intended to deter people from obtaining services.[52] Requirements to submit proof of legal status or income to establish eligibility for benefits not only screen out those who do not qualify but also prevent some who do qualify for benefits from receiving them. Individuals or groups with less structural privilege in terms of race, income, and education face heavier administrative burdens than those who are more advantaged.[53]

These burdens often prevent people from signing up for health coverage. Herd and Moynihan demonstrate that the administrative burdens associated with the Affordable Care Act were especially formidable. States that opposed the ACA did not expand Medicaid and imposed stricter requirements to deter enrollment by those who were eligible for other parts of the reform, while states that expanded Medicaid did not have sufficient administrative capacity or support from the federal government during the disastrous rollout of Obamacare in 2013.[54] In practice, administrative burdens "quite literally determine who is and is not a member of society" and work to exclude those who are marginalized by their racialized legal status.[55] My interviews reveal that Latinx immigrants experienced heavy administrative burdens as noncitizens and people of color. Sociologist Victor Ray, in collaboration with Herd and Moynihan, introduced the concept of "racialized burdens" to account for how structural racism in public organizations generates racially unequal access to services.[56] Ray's previous theory of racialized organizations posits that government and associated institutions and bureaucracies operate via processes that maintain racial hierarchies.[57] Even when their rules and procedures seem race-neutral, institutions unequally distribute resources along racial lines, advantaging White citizens and disadvantaging both citizens and immigrants of color. Sociologist Alyasah Sewell contends that meso-level discrimination occurs in housing, as structural racism perpetuates residential segregation and concentrates people of color in unhealthy environments, which in turn negatively affect their health.[58]

I extend this analysis to the intersection of legal status with racialized burdens. Thus, I refer to administrative burdens at this intersection as "racialized legal status burdens." In the RLS framework, bureaucracies, institutions, and organizations that administer government-funded benefits as mandated by public policy, such as health and welfare, may generate overt anti-immigrant discrimination by not providing services to immigrants because of their legal status. In Figure 1-1, the bidirectional arrows outside of the figure between the meso and micro levels indicate how people's interactions with employees in meso-level settings may blur distinctions between these two levels. Though people may be receiving services in meso-level bureaucracies, institutions, and organizations, they often must engage in interpersonal communication with employees in those settings. Thus, the ways in which racialized legal status shapes people's experiences may occur in both directions, from the meso to the micro level and vice versa.

One way I observed this in my research was through lack of sufficient language assistance or enrollment materials for people with limited English proficiency (LEP). The fact that most public benefits applications are primarily available in English presents a nearly insurmountable racialized legal status burden for the estimated 25 million LEP individuals in the United States.[59] As Angelica pointed out, language access is a civil right protected by virtue of one's race or national origin under Title VI of the 1964 Civil Rights Act.[60] But it was often impossible for immigrants to obtain language assistance when seeking health or other social services. Kevin, a BHC provider I interviewed in 2012, explained that the inadequacy of language access was a major racialized legal status burden his patients encountered.

> I have a bunch of patients who feel like, because of the wait time [on hold] or lack of people even picking up the phone and then language problems once they do, that they have to physically show up at the office to get any business done, like if they wanted to schedule an appointment, get a refill, or you name it. They might call and hope that people at our front desk, we might have two of eight who speak Portuguese, but maybe they hang up. So, when they come [to the office], they know who speaks Portuguese, they go up to them and talk to them about it.

Kevin's patients and others with LEP must go to the office in person to schedule services, not just to see their physician. Kevin's quote aptly demonstrates how insufficient language access at the meso level influences his patients' micro-level interactions with providers at his clinic. Given patients' already busy schedules, this burden deters them from seeking and obtaining care, especially if they do not have access to reliable transportation. The extra time and effort required compounds the existing racialized legal status burdens immigrants experience in labor-intensive application and renewal processes.[61]

I heard a similar account about the impact of RLS through language from immigrant respondents. Dania, the Dominican whose reflections on the discrimination she has experienced are quoted at the beginning of this chapter, recounted her own experiences: "It's hard, so many tears have been shed, crying from going to the hospital and no one understanding what I was saying. I couldn't even ask for anything to eat." Dania knows that being racialized as non-White and speaking Spanish rather than English are serious disadvantages even though she has a green card. Dania was emotionally distressed as she described this discrimination and her difficulty communicating with providers. I felt upset as well, imagining how I would feel if I were sick and could not tell anyone what I needed.

Leonel, a Salvadoran I interviewed in 2016, felt that race affected how patients were prioritized for treatment: "So, many times you go to the hospital and they [staff/providers] look at your skin color and leave you waiting one, three, or four hours waiting to be seen. And you see other people come and get treated more quickly. But then you go and ask why that happened and you're told 'that person has more priority' or something like that." With medium dark-brown skin, black eyes, and short black hair, Leonel felt that his skin color resulted in longer wait times.

Staff in meso-level settings may be implicitly biased against immigrants in their interactions with patients. Lack of language access and unequal treatment, as well as the frustration and mistrust they generate, deter immigrants from seeking and obtaining care and contribute to their ill health relative to that of White Americans whose primary language is English.[62] These experiences are very common, showing that RLS is entrenched in both macro-level policies and meso-level settings where Latinx immigrants seek health and other social services.

In 2019, as racialized anti-immigrant sentiment peaked, advocates and immigrants emphasized that insufficient medical interpretation services exacerbated immigrants' health problems. Josefina, a Dominican advocate I interviewed in 2019, discussed what she viewed as intentional RLS discrimination against Latinx people in medical facilities: "'Oh, we don't like or deal with Latinos here.' So, there's segregation in every sense. Even when going to the hospital, you can't find someone who speaks Spanish, and they don't try to find anyone who does to do the interpretation because they don't want Hispanics there. At least, that's the message we receive: 'learn English or leave.'"

In addition to experiencing mistreatment from providers, immigrants feared seeking services amid the worsening climate of the Trump administration. Alexandre, a Brazilian naturalized US citizen with Indigenous features of dark-brown skin and medium-length, curly black hair, whom I interviewed in 2019, shared: "There are many immigrants from Brazil and other countries that are afraid to go to the hospitals. Because you know that President Trump, I don't know if it is the president or Congress, [but] if you want to apply for your green card or citizenship one day, they [the government] will see if you got medical attention or anything else [other public benefit]. And that could be an impediment [to legalizing status]. So, that's why many times people are not going to the doctor or are afraid to go." Though Alexandre did not specifically mention race, the Trump administration's rhetoric portrayed unwelcome immigrants as non-White. Such connections made Brazilians and other immigrants afraid to obtain treatment.[63] Alexandre's reference to the misconception that getting care could jeopardize immigrants' prospects for legalizing their status in the US is another example of how racialized legal status in macro-level policy shapes immigrants' engagement with meso-level institutions.

Racialized Legal Status at the Micro Level in Everyday Life

Racialized legal status affects people in their everyday interactions with others, beyond its impacts at the macro and meso levels. Figure 1-2 shows how RLS influences people's experiences at both the meso and micro levels. Along the y-axis, I have listed "more racially privileged" at the top and "least racially privileged" at the bottom to indicate how the physical features—like skin tone, eye color, or hair texture—associated with one's presumed race or ethnicity can be an advantage or disadvantage in society. In the past and present, individuals in the White racial group have been more privileged while people of color have been less privileged. My use of "more/less racially privileged" instead of specific ethnoracial categories avoids replicating the Black-White binary in focusing on the Black-White differences to the exclusion of other groups in US racial discourse and also better accounts for the immense diversity among the US population. Many groups that share a national origin are internally diverse in ancestry and appearance. For example, among Latinx people, some lighter-skinned individuals identify as White and are regarded that way by others, while those with darker skin tone identify as and are perceived and treated by others as Black. Those with mixed European and Indigenous ancestry who were classified as Mestizo at home may be racialized in inconsistent ways in the United States. Many studies have shown that these differences contribute to disparate socioeconomic and health statuses among Latinx people of various ethnicities.[64]

Along the x-axis in Figure 1-2, I have listed the range of the most common documentation statuses, from undocumented to US-born citizens. The statuses most vulnerable to legal exclusion and deportation are on the left, and the least vulnerable statuses are positioned toward the right.[65] Starting on the far right, US-born citizens are most privileged, as in theory they can access benefits if they are eligible by income or age, can vote (in some states, only if they are not convicted felons), and cannot be deported for minor criminal offenses. While naturalized citizens have similar rights as US-born citizens, misrepresentation on naturalization applications or membership in certain organizations can lead to the revocation of their citizenship and deportation.[66] Noncitizens—everyone to the left on the continuum—do not have the same privileges and are deportable for minor offenses or for being a "public charge."[67]

Among noncitizens, lawful permanent residents (LPRs, or green card holders) are most privileged. LPRs can apply for citizenship after three to five years.[68] Nonetheless, the 1996 Personal Responsibility and Work Opportunity Act, called "welfare reform," distinguished among LPRs based on length of residence, establishing a five-year residency bar on their eligibility for public benefits.[69] Refugee and asylee status are granted to individuals unable to live in their home country because of sociopolitical

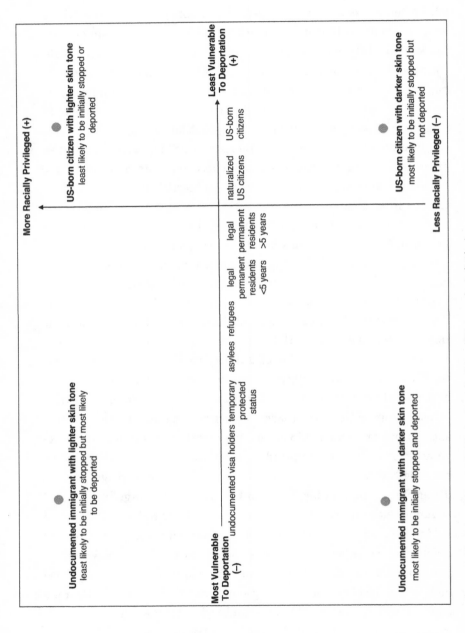

Figure 1-2. The Consequences of Differing Racialized Legal Statuses for Individuals

conflicts or persecution based on race, religion, nationality, or membership in certain groups.[70] Refugees apply before arriving, whereas asylees apply after fleeing imminent danger and arriving on US territory. Gaining asylum after entering this country is more difficult than receiving refugee status prior to arrival, which is why refugees are placed to the right of asylees.[71] Both refugees and asylees may apply for LPR status and eventually citizenship. They can receive federal benefits during their first seven years of residence.[72]

To the left of asylees are those with temporary protected status (TPS). Recipients enter with legal status for a period of six to eighteen months, which can be extended.[73] Although TPS recipients cannot be detained or deported simply for being in the United States, this status provides no path to LPR status or citizenship. TPS holders can become undocumented if they fail to renew their paperwork or if the president of the United States ends their home country's TPS designation, leaving them in "liminal legality."[74] To the left of TPS recipients are visa holders who must return home when their visas expire unless they renew their visas or obtain LPR status.[75] Otherwise, they become undocumented and are deportable.[76] Finally, undocumented immigrants are furthest left and most vulnerable to detention and deportation.[77]

Movement to the right along the x-axis brings individuals closer to legal citizenship and related privileges. Most important, it decreases their deportability. Leftward movement decreases benefits and increases deportability. Those with undocumented, visa, asylee, or refugee status must first obtain LPR status; only after three to five years as LPRs can they apply for citizenship. Naturalization remains a costly and burdensome bureaucratic process.[78] In the absence of comprehensive immigration reform, many noncitizens will remain in their current position or lose it and become increasingly vulnerable.[79]

Figure 1-2 illustrates how racialized legal status functions at the micro and meso levels in shaping a person's likelihood of experiencing interpersonal discrimination or being racially profiled by law or immigration enforcement and subsequently detained, arrested, and deported. US-born citizens with lighter skin tone (in the upper right quadrant) are least likely to be profiled and stopped by enforcement officials and are not subject to deportation. Undocumented immigrants with lighter skin tone (in the upper left quadrant) are less likely to be stopped based on their perceived racial background, but if they are stopped and enforcement officials discover their undocumented status, they are likely to be deported. Those who have darker skin tone (in the bottom right and left quadrants) are significantly more likely to be stopped by enforcement officials. For example, Black and Latinx men, regardless of legal status, are significantly more likely to be profiled and detained than individuals racialized as White.[80] For the darker-skinned citizen who is profiled, that encounter with law or immigrant enforcement will not lead to deportation, although it could lead to arrest, incarceration, and even death in some tragic cases.[81] For the undocumented immigrant with darker skin tone, being stopped is more likely to lead to detention, deportation, and possibly death. Documented immigrants who are noncitizens, however, are similarly likely to be detained and deported.[82] A 1996 immigration law actually made all noncitizens subject to detention and deportation, as arrests trigger the removal process.[83] Although Black and Latinx citizens and undocumented immigrants may have different final outcomes, it is important to note that many of the private corporations that run prisons also run detention centers.[84] So it is very likely that both groups would be caught in the prison/detention industrial complex. Whereas citizens might be deemed felons and lose some of their rights, undocumented immigrants would be expelled from the country.[85] This example demonstrates the intersectional power of racialized legal status in shaping individuals' lives and contributing to the differential outcomes of interactions with police, immigration enforcement, and other agents of the state in everyday life.

Among the immigrants I interviewed, RLS discrimination occurred in daily interactions with official representatives and employees of the government. Despite their different nationalities and legal statuses in the US, immigrants had negative experiences with police and immigration officers. When raids or threats of raids were shared within the community, people would stay home and not take their children to school or go to doctor's appointments. Many felt that being presumed to be undocumented or an immigrant because of their physical features might lead to ethnoracial profiling. Benjamin, a Salvadoran with medium-brown skin and short, straight black hair whom I interviewed in 2016, talked about this constant fear of being targeted: "I have noticed since I came 14 years ago . . . that the biggest challenge you have to overcome is fear, fear of leaving your home and going out. I think the authorities are going out and targeting people based on their skin color or race. . . . You can be detained for anything. You can't complain about your rights because many times, the police abuse their power, and you can't say anything to anyone about it. They always view us as less than." Benjamin has learned that his appearance makes him likely to be targeted by authorities even though he is documented. He regards race or skin color as a major factor in determining who is detained and deported. The vulnerability he felt was palpable as he spoke about being viewed as inferior and subject to abuse at the hands of the police. Research has shown that the constant stress of living in heavily surveilled and aggressively policed neighborhoods can take a toll on mental and physical health.[86] The added risk of being arbitrarily detained and deported can only make that worse.

Some immigrants I spoke with told me about many negative encounters they had with other people who were prejudiced against immigrants and people of color. Andrea, a Dominican with dark-brown skin, brown eyes, and shoulder-length, straight black hair whom I spoke with in 2016, directly connected her experiences of racism with being an immigrant: "In reality, I would say that racism is marked. Still there are people who believe that Latinos, that immigrants do not have the same human rights as Whites. But why? Still there are people who think that, and they express it, and it manifests itself in their attitudes." Notice that Andrea used the terms "Latinos" and "immigrants" interchangeably. Despite being a naturalized US citizen, she clearly recognized the link between the two, not only for herself but in the minds and actions of hostile White and US-born people. Andrea explained that the mistreatment of Latinos and immigrants is rooted in racism and xenophobia, clearly connecting the social constructions of race, ethnicity, and legal status.

Most immigrants I interviewed felt that they were not seen as legitimate members of US society, including the 13 naturalized US citizens of Brazilian, Dominican, and Salvadoran heritage whom I interviewed. Regardless of variations in their physical appearance and legal status, most felt they would never fully belong because they are not White by US standards and do not speak English or speak it with an accent.[87] They believed that their legal citizenship would not protect them from being racially profiled by police or detained for questioning by immigration officials. For these immigrants, physical appearance, nationality, and language were visible markers of their racialized legal status that would always make them outsiders in the eyes of White Americans. In 2016, Charles, a naturalized US citizen of Brazilian heritage with dark-brown skin and short, loosely curled black hair, told me: "Whether I like it or not, they [Americans] will see me as an immigrant. They don't see me as an American. Even with my citizenship, I will never be, in the minds of Americans, a real American. They'll never see us as Americans. No immigrants! That's what Donald Trump says and it's absurd that people listen to him." The conflation of Americanness with Whiteness and speaking unaccented English language was reported in interviews with immigrants throughout the study. I interviewed Charles in 2016, when Trump's campaign challenged the legitimacy of then-president Barack Obama's US citizenship and derided immigrants and citizens of color. These sentiments increased during Trump's presidency.

When I interviewed Gloria, a BHC provider, in 2019, she emphasized that Trump's rhetoric had directly affected her Latinx immigrant patients: "They feel more unsafe in terms of society largely due to the quality of the language they speak and their race," because "now there is freedom" to express anti-immigrant, racist animus toward them. One of Gloria's Salvadoran patients quit her job at a laundromat after her longtime coworker began taunting her, repeating Trump's contemptuous words about Mexicans and, by association, Salvadorans. Because Gloria's patient was deemed to have left her job "voluntarily" despite the constant harassment, she could not collect workers' compensation. These experiences had devastating health, financial, and social impacts on Gloria's patients. Accounts like these from immigrants, advocates, and providers throughout the project revealed how racialized legal status was manifested in Latinx immigrants' direct encounters with discrimination by enforcement officials and ordinary people in their everyday lives.

Conclusion

Racialized legal status pervades all levels of US society and is evident in macro-level government policies and laws, meso-level health and social service institutions and bureaucracies, and micro-level interpersonal interactions. First, policy operating at multiple levels of government includes or excludes immigrants based on their documentation status and negatively affects immigrants and citizens of color through structural racism embedded in the government. Second, RLS exacerbates the administrative burdens and significantly increases the time and effort it takes to apply for health coverage, navigate the complex healthcare system, and engage with bureaucrats and providers despite policies that aim to improve healthcare access. Third, micro-level experiences of interpersonal discrimination and exclusion shape healthcare access, general well-being, and individuals' lived experiences. Cumulatively, racialized legal status acts as a major deterrent to seeking health and other social services for immigrants and citizens of color. People's racialized legal status can heighten their experiences of implicit and explicit exclusion. In the chapters that follow, I demonstrate how racialized legal status shaped Latinx immigrants' healthcare experiences in Boston amid policy shifts in 2012–2013, 2015–2016, and 2019.

CHAPTER 2

Included in Coverage but Excluded from Use (2012–2013)

You hear prejudiced comments like "I can't stand these immigrants without papers taking jobs from Americans," which is a big lie. But you hear discriminatory things like "Ah, they don't pay taxes, they live off the government, have children to make money." . . . Now that I have my papers, I feel more secure and it's different. But when you're illegal, it's so difficult, you have to subject yourself to certain things that you don't want to. But what are you going to do?

—*Pedro, Brazilian immigrant interviewed in 2013*

They [some immigrants] are not getting preventative care. They're relatively healthy but they're not really being seen by a doctor. . . . There's also this problem that people are actually working full-time. They're really scared that if they go above a certain level of income, they're going to lose their ability to get assistance or subsidized health care.

—*Bianca, immigrant advocate interviewed in 2012*

As the first state to pass comprehensive health reform in 2006, Massachusetts had the country's lowest proportion of uninsured people by 2010. Just 4% lacked health coverage, while the national average was 16%.[1] One remarkable aspect of that reform was its inclusion of noncitizen residents of the state, who were allowed to apply for and receive coverage regardless of whether or not they were documented. And if their income was low enough, they qualified for publicly funded care. While other states were passing more restrictive immigration-related policies and reducing immigrants' healthcare access, Massachusetts was a model for nearly universal coverage. In 2012–2013, as I traveled around Boston speaking with immigrants, healthcare providers, and advocates, I sought to understand the on-the-ground reality that immigrants encountered when applying for coverage and navigating the healthcare system.[2]

What emerged from my 70 interviews with Brazilian and Dominican immigrants, providers, and advocates, along with my attendance at numerous public meetings, was a far more complicated picture. Language barriers, lack of knowledge about health coverage and the unusual concept of a primary care physician, and difficulties inherent in the (re)enrollment process posed significant challenges for immigrants who wanted and needed health care. Some respondents even said that it was harder for immigrants to get coverage after the landmark 2006 reform than before.

Beyond the shifting health policy landscape, the prevalence of local raids by Immigration and Customs Enforcement (ICE), cooperation between local police and ICE agents, and concerns that obtaining and using health coverage could damage their prospects for being granted green cards generated significant fear among immigrants. These factors decisively affected their healthcare decisions. Although income-eligible immigrants of any status living in Massachusetts could apply for and receive coverage in the commonwealth, various structural barriers impeded their ability to enroll and then get the care they needed.[3] Examples of these structural barriers included complicated enrollment procedures as well as language and cultural differences between patients and providers that hindered positive relationships conducive to quality health care. These obstacles reflect the intersectional discrimination Latinx immigrants encountered because of their racialized legal status. In this highly politicized context, members of marginalized social groups were disproportionately harmed.

This chapter explores the racialized legal status discrimination that Latinx immigrants experienced in navigating the healthcare system in 2012–2013.[4] Respondents from each stakeholder group felt that immigrants had sufficient access to health coverage under the Massachusetts reform but recognized that their access was stratified, because the legislation consigned many immigrants to an inferior level of coverage. Moreover, access to coverage did not guarantee that people were able to use their coverage to obtain health services. Many encountered difficulties understanding how their coverage worked and where it could be used, as well as problems with the requirement to renew it each year. The lack of enrollment and informational materials in Portuguese, Spanish, and other languages, along with the shortage of medical interpreters and culturally sensitive healthcare providers, presented additional structural barriers. These problems, coupled with the increase in racialized immigration enforcement in Boston and nationally, deterred both US and foreign-born Latinx residents from obtaining health coverage and using health services despite their eligibility. Their experiences highlight the complexity of the US healthcare system under Massachusetts's comprehensive health reform and show that the reach of the federal government into the state through racialized immigration enforcement limited the inclusivity that was Massachusetts legislators' goal.

To illuminate what navigating the Boston healthcare system was like for immigrants, the chapter begins by explaining the health and immigration policy context at the local and national levels that shaped the healthcare system leading up to 2012, when I began the research for this book. Specifically, I provide valuable background about the historic Massachusetts health reform and the 2010 federal Affordable Care Act amid their overlap with increasingly more restrictive federal immigration policies. Next, I examine Brazilians' and Dominicans' healthcare experiences in their home countries, the adaptation issues they faced in the United States, and their work and personal lives in Boston, all of which shaped their experiences in the US healthcare system. My conversations with providers and advocates shed light on the major health problems of their immigrant patients and constituents, which informed why and when they needed health care. Finally, I delve into how Brazilians' and Dominicans' health profiles shaped their healthcare encounters when they tried to apply for coverage. All but 2 of the 31 Brazilian and Dominican immigrants I interviewed had health coverage and felt that it met their needs, but many struggled to understand what the coverage provided and where it could be used. These individuals' formal access to health coverage made them a privileged group, because Latin American immigrants then and now are more likely to remain uninsured, even in Massachusetts.[5] Nationally, most Latinx immigrants and citizens are less likely than people of other ethnoracial groups to have health coverage.[6] As of 2022, among the uninsured population, nearly one in five is of Hispanic ancestry.[7]

Examining these respondents' experiences with the commonwealth's "best-case" healthcare system reveals that racialized legal status discrimination is pervasive at each stage of the process, from applying for coverage through scheduling medical appointments and interacting with providers. Consequently, Latinx Bostonians do not always receive the health care they desperately need. Unless indicated otherwise, the quotations in this chapter come from interviews I conducted in 2012–2013, when Democrat Thomas Menino was the mayor of Boston, Democrat Deval Patrick was the governor of Massachusetts, and Democrat Barack Obama was the president of the United States.

The Massachusetts and National Health Policy Landscape Before 2012

Both the Massachusetts and federal ACA reforms were intended to extend healthcare coverage to more people and to limit the rising costs of health care. But only the Massachusetts reform offered *any* coverage to undocumented immigrants. Given the differences between the Massachusetts and ACA reforms, as well as the complexities of each, I begin by tracing relevant policy changes from 2006 to 2012–2013, when I conducted the first round of interviews. At this time, the Massachusetts reform had been implemented six years earlier; Obamacare had been enacted (in 2010) but had not yet been implemented.

Massachusetts Health Reform

Massachusetts passed and implemented comprehensive health reform (also known as Chapter 58) under Republican Governor Mitt Romney in 2006. The goal of the legislation was to extend coverage to more state residents and to contain healthcare costs. By 2011, the proportion of state residents who were uninsured had fallen to 3.1%, compared to 15% at the national level before ACA implementation.[8] Under Chapter 58, all income-eligible Massachusetts residents could apply for and receive some type of state-funded health coverage regardless of documentation status. Nevertheless, the legislative process of including immigrants in the program was shrouded in secrecy to avoid controversy. According to Edward, a health advocate I interviewed in 2013, "It was done very quietly because it's an explosive issue politically once it becomes public." Despite the inclusion of immigrants in the reform, distinctions in documentation status and income shaped eligibility for coverage and access to care.[9] Citizens and long-term green card holders as well as higher-income individuals had access to more robust coverage than noncitizens and those with lower incomes.[10] Sociologist Donald Light refers to this stratification in coverage as "categorical inequality."[11] Those covered by the Health Safety Net (HSN), who are primarily low-income and undocumented immigrants, could receive treatment only at designated facilities. MassHealth, which provides fairly comprehensive coverage, can be used anywhere that Medicaid is accepted. But healthcare providers in private practices can opt out of seeing Medicaid patients because of its low reimbursement rates.[12] Individuals with private insurance plans, which are partially subsidized or unsubsidized, generally have access to a larger group of providers who accept their coverage.

Table 2-1 shows simplified coverage options for adults ages 21 to 64 from left to right for: (1) Massachusetts under the Chapter 58 reform; (2) Massachusetts under the ACA; and (3) states that expanded Medicaid under the ACA. The first column lists the documentation status categories from top to bottom, starting with undocumented and ending with US-born citizens. This is not the full range of statuses that exist, and ex-

Table 2-1. Immigrants' Documentation Status and Health Coverage in Massachusetts After State Reform and in States Where Medicaid Was Expanded After Affordable Care Act Implementation

Adult (Ages 21–64) Coverage Based on Documentation Status	Massachusetts: Chapter 58 (Pre-ACA)	Massachusetts: Post-ACA Implementation	ACA in Expansion States
Undocumented	Yes: HSN[b], MassHealth Limited, could purchase coverage through exchange	Yes: HSN	
	No: exchange subsidies	No: exchange subsidies, cannot purchase coverage through exchange	No coverage
Undocumented Deferred Action for Childhood Arrival (DACA) recipients (Dreamers)[a]	Yes: HSN	Yes: HSN, MassHealth Family Assistance	No coverage
	No: exchange subsidies	No: exchange subsidies, cannot purchase coverage through exchange	
Certain non-immigrant visas: student, work, etc.	Yes: HSN, MassHealth Limited, could purchase coverage through exchange	Yes: HSN, MassHealth Limited, can purchase coverage through exchange, ConnectorCare	Yes: purchase coverage through exchange
	No: MassHealth Standard, CommonwealthCare	No: MassHealth Standard	No: ineligible for Medicaid
Temporary protected status (TPS)	Yes: HSN, MassHealth Limited, could purchase coverage through exchange, Commonwealth Care	Yes: HSN, MassHealth Limited, can purchase coverage through exchange, ConnectorCare	Yes: purchase coverage through exchange
	No: MassHealth Standard	No: MassHealth Standard	No: ineligible for Medicaid
Asylees, refugees	Eligible for all if income eligible	Eligible for all if income eligible	Eligible for all if income eligible
Lawful permanent residents (< 5 years in the United States)	Yes: HSN, Commonwealth Care, could purchase coverage through and receive subsidies for exchange	Yes: HSN, Connector-Care, can purchase coverage through and receive subsidies for exchange	Yes: can purchase coverage through and receive subsidies for exchange
	No: MassHealth Standard	No: MassHealth Standard	No: Medicaid
Lawful permanent residents (5+ years in the United States), naturalized and US-born citizens	Eligible for all if income eligible	Eligible for all if income eligible	Eligible for all if income eligible

a. DACA did not exist when the 2006 Massachusetts reform was enacted.
b. "HSN" stands for Health Safety Net.

ceptions are made under some documentation status categories.[13] For example, undocumented pregnant women are eligible for emergency Medicaid to cover prenatal care and childbirth. Moreover, the terms related to documentation status that are used to determine eligibility may differ among immigration policy, welfare policy, and health policy.[14] These and other inconsistencies create confusion about who is eligible for what depending on their circumstances and the public benefit involved.

Coverage options for residents under the Massachusetts reform are shown in column 2 of Table 2-1.[15] The *state-funded* Health Safety Net program allowed low-income residents of any documentation status to obtain preventive and some specialty care at designated facilities. Although not formally considered insurance, HSN provides robust access to most healthcare services.[16] The next coverage option, which was available to low-income, long-term lawful permanent residents (LPRs) and citizens, was the state's version of the federal Medicaid program, called MassHealth.[17] The state also developed a *state-funded* coverage option, called Commonwealth Care, for short-term LPRs, who were ineligible for MassHealth, to obtain subsidized private insurance through the Massachusetts health exchange.[18] Income-eligible residents who held student and work visas could apply for HSN and coverage through the health exchange but were not eligible for MassHealth and Commonwealth Care. Income-eligible temporary protected status (TPS) recipients could apply for HSN, Commonwealth Care, and coverage through the health exchange, but were ineligible for MassHealth. All forms of coverage were available to income-eligible refugees, asylees, long-term LPRs, and citizens. The dark gray boxes represent individuals eligible for all options. Lighter gray boxes represent those with fewer options based on documentation status.

Figuring out what options were available to whom was daunting. Quinn, a health advocate I interviewed in 2019, told me: "Some low-income immigrants can be eligible for Health Safety Net, for Connector-Care, and for limited forms of MassHealth. Perhaps someone isn't quite sure of all the different kinds of overlaps. But it can sometimes be overwhelming." The multiplicity of options shown in Table 2-1 indicates a patchwork of health coverage, which creates gaps that left many people excluded from coverage, particularly those who were neither children nor elderly, had very low incomes, or were not beneficiaries of employer-sponsored insurance plans.[19] The aim of the Massachusetts reform—and later the ACA—was to extend coverage and fill some of those gaps. Although fewer people are uninsured, some remain excluded or have only partial coverage. Those who are uninsured or underinsured continue to have high co-pays and deductibles, which makes health care expensive both in and beyond Boston.[20]

Obamacare Becomes the Law of the Land

The commonwealth's success in expanding access to coverage was so remarkable that the program served as the model for the Affordable Care Act, which was passed by Congress in 2010. But documentation status and income distinctions continued to have important implications for noncitizen immigrants and low-income residents of Massachusetts amid changes related to the implementation of Obamacare in late 2013. Column 4 in Table 2-1 shows the coverage options available under Obamacare for states that expanded Medicaid.

One key difference between the state and federal reforms had an impact on coverage options for noncitizens living in Massachusetts. The Massachusetts reform made *all* income-eligible residents qualified for some form of coverage. But the ACA extended coverage only to citizens and some documented noncitizens, because in 1996 the Illegal Immigration Reform and Immigrant Responsibility Act (IIRIRA) and the Personal Responsibility and Work Opportunity Act (PRWORA) limited public benefits for immigrants. Although these laws regarding immigration and welfare reform were passed nearly 15 years earlier, Obamacare complied with those restrictions and added new verification requirements that further limited immigrants' access to ACA benefits.[21] Thus, ACA implementation in Massachusetts narrowed the scope of the state's programs. This policy shift affected some immigrants' ability to reapply for coverage.

State legislators revised the 2006 legislation to keep programs intact and ensure that the state could receive federal funds available under the

ACA (Table 2-1, column 3). For income-eligible undocumented immigrants and those who had green cards for less than five years, eligibility for state-funded programs such as Health Safety Net and Commonwealth Care did not change. Massachusetts reduced HSN funding, however, as low-income and middle-income LPRs with that status for at least five years, refugees, asylees, and citizen residents were shifted to Medicaid. Thus, an unintended consequence of this shift in income eligibility under Obamacare's Medicaid expansion was that HSN primarily covered undocumented immigrants. Since I concluded my 2013 interviews in July and preparation for ACA implementation began in late 2013, I discuss more of the challenges associated with implementation in Chapter 3.

Nationally, the ACA generated stratification in coverage based on where people lived because the US Supreme Court ruled that states had the right to decide whether to participate in the Medicaid expansion. Some states moved forward with this provision of the ACA, while others did not.[22] Many citizens were entirely excluded based on their income level, even though they would have been eligible for Medicaid had their states chosen to expand it. Consequently, the proportion of uninsured individuals declined among "legally eligible" residents in states that expanded Medicaid and stagnated in states that did not.[23]

Even in states that did expand Medicaid, coverage for immigrants remained limited because undocumented immigrants, visa holders, TPS recipients, and LPRs with less than five years' residency were ineligible for the program (Table 2-1, column 4).[24] In all states, student and work visa holders and income-eligible LPRs with less than five years of residency could purchase coverage in the exchanges.[25] Income-eligible asylees, refugees, LPRs with more than five years' residency, and citizens were eligible for all provisions. Thus, access to ACA provisions was stratified by state of residence, income, and documentation status.

Immigration Policy Is Welfare and Health Policy, Too

As discussed in Chapter 1, a key reason that a person's legal status determines their eligibility for the ACA is the intersection between immigration and health policy (see Figure 1-1). In recent decades, the most consequential federal policies shaping immigrants' access to, or exclusion from, programs such as Medicaid and Special Supplemental Nutrition for Women, Infants, and Children (WIC) were two pieces of federal legislation signed into law in 1996 under President Bill Clinton. The first was the Personal Responsibility and Work Opportunity Reconciliation Act, known as "welfare reform," which made LPRs and green card holders ineligible for public benefits for a five-year period after they attained this status.[26] The legislation also allowed states to determine immigrants' eligibility for state-funded public benefits.[27] The second was the Illegal Immigration Reform and Immigrant Responsibility Act, which tightened border security, intensified enforcement within the United States, criminalized the use of fraudulent immigration documents, and made all noncitizens deportable for minor offenses or for being a "public charge."[28] Together, these two reforms dramatically curtailed immigrants' access to public benefits and made them more easily deportable. The PRWORA rendered many immigrants ineligible for healthcare provisions under Obamacare. In Massachusetts, legislators had to work around these exclusions to minimize the number of immigrants residing in the state who had access to coverage under Chapter 58 but could lose it under Obamacare. This case illustrates an important way that documentation status is embedded in other policy realms and has profound effects on noncitizens' lives.

Most aspects of immigration policy, such as who is allowed to enter the country, are determined at the federal level. But subnational governments can make decisions about other aspects of immigration policy, such as permitting or forbidding state law enforcement authorities to share information with ICE about arrested individuals. Another example of the federal–state divide on immigration-related issues is the exclusion or inclusion of immigrants for state-funded public benefits. Although the ACA has legal status restrictions for federally funded Medicaid and Medicare programs, states can use their own funds to provide coverage for federally ineligible immigrants, as Massachusetts and some other states have done.

Around the same time that Massachusetts implemented its own health reform, the federal Secure Communities (S-Comm) pilot program was introduced in Suffolk County, which contains the City of Boston.[29] Under the program, the fingerprints of individuals booked by local police were sent to the Federal Bureau of Investigation to be checked against immigration databases kept by the Department of Homeland Security (DHS). When a match was found, DHS officials could issue a detainer and request that police hold the individual until federal agents could pick the person up.[30] In 2011, before I began conducting research for this book, Governor Deval Patrick and Mayor Tom Menino, urged by local immigration advocates, objected to the state's participation in the program. They expressed concern that immigrants who had never been charged with a crime would be deported and that ethnoracial profiling might target all those perceived as foreigners regardless of their citizenship or documentation status.[31] But that objection did not prevent the Obama administration from enforcing the program in Massachusetts and expanding it nationally in 2013.[32] Increased immigration enforcement under S-Comm contributed to raids in Greater Boston that made immigrants afraid to seek healthcare and other services. Immigration enforcement had a direct, detrimental impact on immigrants' health and healthcare access.

2013 Boston Marathon Bombing and Implications for Local Immigrants

In April 2013, while I was conducting the first round of interviews, the Boston Marathon was bombed by two immigrants.[33] This traumatic and widely publicized event had significant implications for Boston-area immigrants. The two perpetrators, the brothers Tamerlan and Dzhokhar Tsarnaev, had come to the United States from Kyrgyzstan with their parents, and their family background was Muslim. Originally arriving on tourist visas, both received asylum status and eventually green cards. Though Dzhokhar became a naturalized citizen in September 2012, Tamerlan was denied citizenship because of a conviction for domestic violence.[34]

The case generated intense debate over the standards for entering the country and obtaining green cards and citizenship. Nationally, the bombing played a key role in ending bipartisan support for the proposed Border Security, Economic Opportunity, and Immigration Modernization Act of 2013. This comprehensive legislation, which was designed to address many gaps and contradictions in existing laws, included a path to citizenship for qualified undocumented immigrants.[35] Recognizing that a congressional consensus on reforming immigration policy was impossible to achieve, the Obama administration sought to prioritize the deportation of those convicted of violent crimes rather than those who were simply undocumented. When the Secure Communities program was replaced with the Priority Enforcement Program in 2014, it became easier for some undocumented immigrants to remain in the country.

In Massachusetts, legislators were unable to pass laws granting driver's licenses to undocumented immigrants, allowing in-state college tuition rates for undocumented immigrant students, and limiting cooperation between ICE and local law enforcement.[36] This was the case under two successive governors, Republican Mitt Romney and Democrat Deval Patrick.

The state's lack of inclusive immigration policies led some advocates I interviewed to describe Massachusetts as less progressive on immigration than other states. According to Cyrus, an immigrant advocate I interviewed in 2019, "I think if you take a national view of things, people think of Massachusetts as this very blue state." But "the state legislature's approach to immigrants here is really, at times, hostile." He specifically cited the state's decision to cut some immigrants' health coverage and place them in less expensive plans to balance the state's budget in 2009.[37] Cyrus felt this was a clear example of how immigrants' essential needs are put on the state's chopping block in times of fiscal distress.

The anti-immigrant backlash that followed the Boston Marathon bombing, coupled with the immigration and health policy landscape, significantly shaped the social context in which I interviewed respondents from 2012 to 2013. I now turn to how Massachusetts' health reform and the national policy context influenced Boston immigrants' healthcare access.

Health Migrations: How Health Care at Home Affects Health Care Here

When speaking with immigrants about their overall health and health-care experiences in the United States, many referred to their experiences in their home countries. While some mentioned feeling healthier before they migrated, others compared their medical encounters in Brazil or the Dominican Republic (DR) with their experiences here. From my conversations with immigrants as well as with healthcare providers, I realized that home provides a crucial reference point, shaping how immigrants manage their health and navigate health care in the United States. Research on the transnational linkages that migrants maintain between "here" and "there" demonstrates that immigrants make sense of the racial dynamics, gender relations, religious practices, and other aspects of the social environment in the United States by relying on frameworks from their home countries.[38] Thus, in order to understand how race, ethnicity, and class, in addition to documentation status, shape immigrants' healthcare experiences, I begin by exploring my immigrant respondents' exposure to the Brazilian and Dominican healthcare systems before they migrated.

Premigration Racial Identification, Health, and Health Care

Brazilian and Dominican respondents had very different experiences with health care before they came to the United States, which likely stemmed from their socioeconomic backgrounds and their countries' economic situations.[39] Because socioeconomic status is correlated with race and skin color in Brazil and the Dominican Republic, it is likely that being classified as White, racially mixed, or Black differentially influenced these respondents' experiences with the healthcare system at home. In terms of racial classification before they migrated, most Brazilian respondents (13 of 21) defined themselves as White and some (5 of 21), as Pardo, while half of Dominicans (5 of 10) identified as Moreno.[40] Both the Pardo and Moreno categories refer to individuals of mixed racial background—generally European and Black or Indigenous—in Brazil and the Dominican Republic, respectively.[41] Interestingly, two Brazilians called themselves Amarelo, or Yellow. Although this Brazilian census term is intended for those of Asian ancestry, some Brazilians use it because they feel their skin tone is closer to Yellow than to White or Pardo. Most Brazilians' physical features—fair skin, light or medium-brown eyes, and long, straight light or dark hair—mean they are considered White in Brazil and, in some but not all cases, in the United States as well. Despite the substantial presence of people of African descent in the Dominican Republic, only one Dominican respondent identified as Black before migrating. The tendency to avoid being classified as Black is a response to the strong anti-Black sentiment in the country.[42] Most Dominicans' physical features are closer to my own—light- to dark-brown skin with dark eyes and curly dark hair—and would be considered Moreno in the DR but are classified as Black in the United States.

With regard to socioeconomic status, most Brazilians had completed some college or postgraduate education and reported coming from families that were in the lower-middle or middle class.[43] Among Dominicans, most had completed primary education and reported coming from lower-income backgrounds.[44] While both countries' economies have struggled in recent years, in the early 2000s Brazil, under the leadership of President Luiz Inácio Lula da Silva (commonly called Lula), was considered a highly successful emerging market and underwent significant social reforms that reduced poverty and implemented a publicly funded health coverage option.[45] The economic outlook in Brazil had improved so much that Brazilian migrants, many of whom were facing difficulties in the United States from its increasingly restrictive immigration policies, returned home in large numbers to invest in real estate and business ventures.[46] Brazil's economic boom halted a few years after the Great Recession hit in 2008, and a conservative backlash precipitated political controversies affecting Lula; his successor, Dilma Rouseff; and their Workers' Party.[47] Brazil's economy continued to spiral downward, leading to a more recent exodus of Brazilians to the Boston area starting in 2018.[48]

Like Brazil, the Dominican Republic has experienced economic and political instability. Whereas the Dominicans who arrived in the United

States after the fall of the Trujillo regime in the 1960s tended to be middle-class, subsequent immigrants came from working-class backgrounds.[49] The DR's economy has improved and significant poverty reduction has occurred recently, despite the challenges of multiple hurricanes and COVID-19.[50] Consequently, the growth in Boston's Dominican community is due to natural increase rather than newer migrant flows.

Most of the Brazilians and Dominicans I interviewed in 2012–2013 reported that their premigration physical health was excellent or very good.[51] But 13 out of 20 Brazilians, compared with only 2 out of 10 Dominicans, had health coverage before migrating. Among Brazilians with coverage, the majority had private plans. Thus, many more Brazilians than Dominicans reported having a regular medical provider before migrating.

Members of both groups described and evaluated their experiences with the healthcare system at home. Those who were White and had middle-class status had better access and more positive experiences than those who were non-White and working-class or poor. Patricia, a 36-year-old White Brazilian immigrant from a middle-class family, reported: "When I lived there, I never had any problems with the healthcare system. I was always seen and had everything I needed. I had a few minor health problems with my stomach, but nothing major. I went to the ER a few times, but I didn't need much medical attention. I thought the healthcare system functioned [well], at least for us with our insurance plan." At the time I interviewed Patricia, she and her husband were in the United States on religious visas and in the process of applying for green cards. They already had two children, and Patricia was pregnant with their third. Later in our interview, she said that she maintained her health coverage in Brazil, and she and her family had medical appointments whenever they visited.

In contrast, Marcos, a 45-year-old White Brazilian immigrant from an upper-middle-class family on a work visa, criticized Brazil's healthcare system because socioeconomic class determined whether people had public or private coverage and what medical treatment was available to them. "The Brazilian healthcare system, for someone without private health insurance, is a system of long lines. There is inadequate medical attention. Medical providers don't treat patients with public coverage the same as those with private insurance. . . . Because there are doctors in my family, I got the medical attention I wanted, privileged access to health care." As a law school professor at a Boston-area university, Marcos was also privileged to have high-quality private health insurance in the United States.

Carlos, a 35-year-old undocumented Dominican immigrant with medium-brown skin tone, black eyes, and short curly hair, had limited encounters with the healthcare system at home because of his family's low socioeconomic position. He began with an ironic declaration: "In DR, there is health insurance. The health insurance there is money. If you go to the hospital with pain or any medical problem, they won't treat you if you don't have money, they won't give you an injection. . . . To get any treatment, you must sign a form indicating who's responsible for the payments."

Immigrants' premigration socioeconomic status and healthcare experiences also affect their health literacy. The US Department of Health and Human Services defines health literacy as "the degree to which individuals have the capacity to obtain, process, and understand basic health information needed to make appropriate health decisions."[52] High health literacy helps people navigate the system, while low health literacy makes it difficult or impossible. Race, income, gender, and educational level are correlated with health literacy. Due to restrictive policies limiting access for noncitizens, legal status can also shape health literacy. In the United States, adult White women under age 35 with a graduate degree and an annual household income of $200,000+ have the highest level of health literacy.[53] Education level, income, and occupation are also associated with health literacy in Brazil and the Dominican Republic.[54] Brazilian respondents' premigration familiarity with health care, which is related to their race and class status, gave them an advantage over Dominicans in the Boston healthcare system. Greg, a BHC primary care physician, said that Brazilian patients were unusually adept at navigating the system. They "have a high level of knowledge of medical care in general, health care in general, how it works. It's not atypical that some patients will have worked in pharmacies or as physical therapists . . . in Brazil. On the other hand, many of my other immigrant populations have a lower level of education and would not have that same kind of professional experience."

Immigrants' premigration healthcare and socioeconomic status provides a vital reference point as immigrants approach the US healthcare system. Scholars have found that immigrants' premigration socioeconomic position shapes their incorporation and ability to adjust their legal status in host countries.[55] But researchers have seldom examined the implications of migrants' premigration healthcare experiences for their encounters in the US system. Just as more Brazilians than Dominicans had private coverage and middle-class socioeconomic status before migrating, more Brazilians had private coverage in the United States.[56] In order to understand immigrants' experiences in the US healthcare system, immigration and health researchers should consider how their premigration social background influences their postmigration health care.

Deteriorating Health: The Not-So-Good Thing About Becoming "American"

Most of the Brazilians and Dominicans I spoke with had migrated to Boston for better economic opportunities, and they were surprised to find that living in the United States would make their health decline over time. A substantial body of research has established that, due to selective migration, immigrants typically have better health than their nonmigrant counterparts at home and better health than most Americans upon their arrival.[57] Over time, however, they lose that health advantage as adaptation to the norms and stresses of American life takes a physical and psychological toll.[58] Living in the United States makes people sick. The causes include our sedentary lifestyle, the nutritional deficiencies that result from eating highly processed foods, and the fast-paced, workaholic way of life that leads to sleep problems. There is also the fact that access to affordable and comprehensive health coverage and care are generally out of reach for the broader population.[59] For immigrants who are perceived as people of color, the extra stresses of dealing with racism and the stigma of being an immigrant—and, especially, the anxiety that accompanies being undocumented in a hostile sociopolitical climate—are harmful to their health.[60] Sociologist Meredith Van Natta finds that Latinx noncitizens living in politically red, purple, and blue states suffer health consequences due to federal restrictions limiting their access to public health coverage and federal immigration enforcement that makes them fearful of seeking health services.[61] The result: immigrants seek treatment primarily in life-or-death situations.

Although most Brazilians self-classified as White and most Dominicans self-classified as Moreno in their home countries, some identified themselves in ethnoracial terms as Latino or Hispanic at the time of our interviews.[62] Because Portuguese is Brazil's national language, no Brazilian immigrants described themselves as Hispanic when that category was separate from Latino, but 8 out of 21 Brazilians classified as Latino. Interestingly, 5 of 10 Dominicans self-classified as Hispanic while 3 self-classified as Latino. No Dominicans classified themselves as White or Black even though most had physical features similar to my own, which are racialized as Black in the United States. Conversely, 3 Brazilians self-classified as Black and 6 Brazilians as White.[63] These ethnoracial profiles of the 2012–2013 immigrant respondents are important to keep in mind as we consider their health and healthcare experiences after migration.

Many Brazilians and Dominicans who felt they had arrived with good health said that in the United States, the faster pace, harsher climate, and physically taxing, low-paid jobs without benefits, coupled with the difficulties of adjusting to the dominant culture, compromised their well-being. Daiane, a 40-year-old Brazilian immigrant with a green card, recounted: "Here, it is a lot of stress because of the language, and you don't want to do anything wrong because you are an illegal immigrant." Despite having brown skin tone and dark eyes and hair, Daiane self-classified as White in Brazil and as "Other: Pardo" in the United States.

Not speaking English fluently was a big hurdle for 12 of the 31 immigrants I interviewed.[64] Some had not learned English, while others rated their English proficiency as good or average. Limited English proficiency impeded the socioeconomic mobility of Dominicans who arrived with green cards and of undocumented Brazilians. Regardless of their premigration educational level or occupation, inadequate English language skills limited the types of jobs open to them.[65] Consequently, many were employed in service occupations as house cleaners, restaurant workers, construction workers, landscapers, childcare providers, and in hair salons or barbershops, as are Latin American immigrants nationwide.[66] Despite having lived in this country for an average of 14 years, many of those I interviewed worked in the same physically demanding jobs they found when they first arrived.

Because of the high cost of living in metropolitan Boston, many of the immigrants I spoke with worked long hours in multiple jobs yet still did not earn enough to make ends meet. High rents and lack of affordable housing due to gentrification forced some immigrants to live in cramped conditions, with 10 people in a two or three-bedroom apartment. Those from modest backgrounds who had to pay off debts for their journeys here and those who sent remittances home to support relatives or invest in their future treated their demanding work schedules as a necessary evil. They had little time left to cook nutritious meals, get enough sleep, or attend medical appointments.

Samantha, a Dominican immigrant advocate, pointed out that these conditions damage immigrants' health:

When a person comes as an immigrant without documents, or even with documents, their status does not matter, in order to survive in this country, you have to work at least 12 hours a day because the salary is not enough to support a family. Imagine being in a situation where almost all of your income goes towards living expenses. Health insurance isn't available because you can't afford it. And often people without documents, aside from not having access, are afraid to go to the doctor. So they use over-the-counter medications. It's been proven that people come here with good health and after five years, they start having health problems—including myself, as I am overweight. You don't have a relaxed life, you live to work all the time, it does not matter what type of job you hold. You have to work to survive.

Brazilian and Dominican immigrants described the difficulties of adapting not only to the cold New England winters but also to the coldness that Americans exhibited in interpersonal interactions. Well before the coronavirus pandemic made "social distancing" a common phrase, Brazilians and Dominicans often described Americans as socially distant. Brazilians said Americans lacked *calor humana*, human warmth. Being teased, chastised, or berated for not speaking English or doing so with a foreign accent strained the limited interactions that Brazilians and Dominicans had with non-Latinx Americans. Natalia, a 44-year-old undocumented White Brazilian immigrant who arrived with a tourist visa, recounted: "I practically understand 100 percent of what people say, but the difficulty is if they understand me. I need to be around people who have patience and won't discriminate against immigrants, or at least be more flexible about English fluency." Her ambivalence about American society is clear in what she said next: "This isn't my country. I love [it] here. But there are difficult barriers. . . . In reality, I am not living here, I am just passing time."

Despite the acculturative stressors that immigrants experienced, 23 of the 31 Brazilian and Dominican immigrants I spoke with in 2012–2013 rated their health in the United States as good or excellent.[67] Of the others, 2 Brazilians and 4 Dominicans rated their health as average; no Brazilians and 2 Dominicans rated their health as bad. Brazilians were more likely to say their health had improved since their arrival, and Dominicans were more likely to say it had declined. Surprisingly, Jessica, a 40-year-old undocumented Black and Latina immigrant from Brazil, said she became more physically active and ate a better diet in the United States. The majority had health coverage (29 of 31) and a regular medical provider (30 of 31) who they felt could address their needs. At the same time, a considerable number had developed ailments such as diabetes, high blood pressure, and musculoskeletal problems. Nearly half (10 of 21) Brazilians and almost all (9 of 10) Dominicans had been diagnosed with those major health conditions in the United States. This significant difference between the two groups could be related both to their different premigration socioeconomic statuses and to their different racialized legal statuses in the United States. Interestingly, immigrants rarely made explicit connections between their occupations and their health.

In contrast, immigrant advocates and BHC providers with Brazilian and Dominican patients regarded these health conditions, along with obesity and chronic pain, as caused directly or indirectly by their occupations and the stresses of their precarious situation. Olivia, a BHC provider, explained: "The work situation of a lot of them is really what stands out to me. I think a lot of them are working under conditions that are affecting their health and they need to continue doing that to support their family. They're hard jobs, manual labor and long hours. They have a couple of full-time jobs, finishing early in the morning and doing cleaning in one place and going to another job way up to midnight. They just keep going."

Seven immigrants—four Dominicans and three Brazilians—reported having been diagnosed with mental health conditions. I heard from Brazilian immigrants, providers, and advocates that a number of Brazilians had died by suicide within the previous year. Moreover, BHC providers and immigrant advocates mentioned that alcoholism and substance abuse were coping mechanisms used by those who were emotionally distressed. Many attributed suicide, depression, and anxiety to the difficulties of living without documents, being separated from family, and racial profiling by police and immigration enforcement. My conversation with Pedro, the 39-year-old documented Brazilian quoted at the beginning of the chapter, revealed the mental toll taken by the dilemmas immigrants face, which were compounded by the increasingly hostile sociopolitical climate:

> Being undocumented is a problem. I am anxious, depressed because of my situation. The problem of being illegal is sad. . . . You lose those family ties and start to feel that you are not here, you are not there. You live in doubt and don't know where you belong. You want to return, but you want to stay. This is sad and I feel this way today. . . . Although your life improves, you are paying the price by not returning. [Now] they are trying to take everything you have, your driver's license, your rights, they're

cutting out everything. You think to yourself, is it worth the trouble, but I want to grow.

Pedro, who has light-brown skin tone with dark curly hair and identifies as Latino, was in a morose mood and said several times that he needed therapy for his depression. Researchers are supposed to remain "objective," but at the end of this interview, I felt compelled to share information about the mental health resources that advocates and providers I had spoken with said were available. Long after this interview, I continued to think about Pedro, hoping that he had found the help he so desperately needed.

BHC providers thought that these mental health conditions were connected to traumas that immigrants had experienced at home or because of family separation. Some BHC providers, especially social workers, said that the children of immigrants were often vulnerable to these ailments as well, acquiring them from their parents and the acculturative tensions they experienced while navigating the school system. Research shows that premigration trauma, family separation, and acculturation among immigrant adults and their children are associated with higher levels of depression, anxiety, and other psychological disorders.[68] The range of physical and mental conditions that immigrants have amply demonstrates their need for health care. While most of the immigrants I interviewed had coverage, the process of enrolling, using, and keeping coverage was so complicated that it could not be managed without the assistance of knowledgeable advocates.

How Immigrants Got and Kept Coverage Under the State Health Reform

Earlier, I outlined the Massachusetts health reform and explained the various coverage options that were available to all income-eligible state residents. Members of all stakeholder groups expressed positive views of this inclusive coverage, and many immigrants felt fortunate to live in a state where it was available. Being eligible to apply for coverage did not guarantee it would be granted, however, and having coverage did not ensure access to care. The numerous administrative burdens imposed on residents seeking fully or partially subsidized coverage created difficulties at every step of the process. Despite my advanced degree and my expertise in health policy, I found the system difficult to understand and explain. Here I rely on the insights of my respondents to walk us through the process of applying for coverage under the Massachusetts reform. Documentation status, income level, and limited English proficiency made this process more complicated for immigrants, people of color, and individuals with lower socioeconomic status than for other more structurally privileged residents of the commonwealth. Such factors demonstrate the importance of health literacy and amplify the impact of racialized legal status in accessing essential services. Applying for and using health coverage under the Massachusetts reform represented a clear example of the embeddedness of racialized legal status in the health insurance and healthcare system, which persistently disadvantaged the state's most marginalized residents despite the reform's intent to extend coverage to everyone.

Applying for "Health Care for All"

In my interviews, I asked immigrants what they knew about the healthcare system in Massachusetts or the United States. Although all 31 of them knew where to go if they had a medical problem, most said they knew little about how to navigate the system. Only a handful were aware of the state's health reform, which had passed six years before, or about the Affordable Care Act, which had just passed and would soon be implemented. One of the better-informed immigrants, Marcos, the White Brazilian law school professor quoted earlier, thought that, although medical treatment in the United States is better than in Brazil, the healthcare system is more bureaucratic and less universal. Massachusetts had reformed a system he characterized as "unjust," but it was still not equal for everyone. Other immigrants who had heard of the reforms were unsure whether they were eligible for coverage and about how these policies might affect their existing medical debt. Pedro, the undocumented Brazilian who shared his mental health struggles, said he had incurred high medical expenses after an accident because "I didn't have FreeCare. I could have applied for FreeCare, but the hospital didn't tell me" about it. When "the 911 bill" for the emergency came, "I was unable to pay. . . . I kept receiving these bills for years and years." Although the comprehensive state health coverage known as FreeCare was renamed the Health Safety Net after the 2006 reform, many immigrants still referred to HSN coverage as FreeCare in our interviews. Like Pedro, some immigrants ended up without coverage and with large medical bills and debts because no one informed them that they were eligible for HSN. The same thing also happened to citizens who were not aware of the reform or their eligibility for coverage.[69]

For some immigrant respondents, language barriers and the lack of information about the reform limited their ability to apply for coverage. Francisca, a 35-year-old undocumented White Brazilian, remarked that figuring out how the system works "is a pain":

> I have been able to apply for coverage here and get access to information, but I had to seek it out. But there are many Brazilians who don't know and end up living more difficult lives. The friend who hosted me when I arrived has been here for 10 years and hasn't been to the doctor because it was written in her policy that she only had access to emergency care. She never looked into or asked about her plan, Health Safety Net, which would have allowed her to see a doctor. . . . She's afraid because she's undocumented and thinks she could be arrested.

Francisca held the government responsible for not letting immigrants know how to apply for and use the coverage it offered. Its failure to do so proactively disentitled eligible individuals from receiving care.

In an attempt to understand the application process, I put myself in the position of my respondents and looked online for information about how to sign up for coverage in Massachusetts in 2012. After several internet searches, I landed on the MA.gov website, which had a link to an application that could be downloaded and printed.[70] After completion, it was to be mailed to the Massachusetts Health Connector, where employees would review applications and sort applicants into state or federally subsidized coverage options (presented in Figure 2-1).

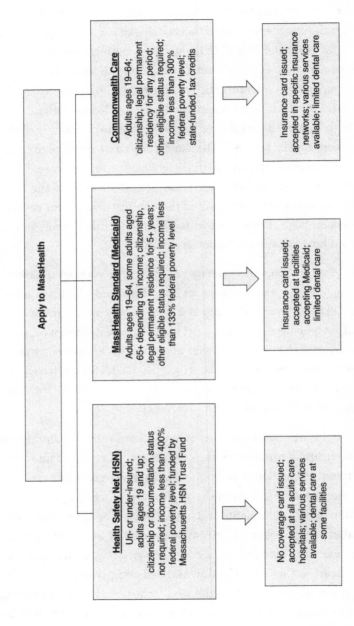

Figure 2-1. Public Options Under the Massachusetts Health Reform for Adults (Ages 19–64)

Depending on income level and documentation status, some applicants may have been eligible for and received multiple types of coverage. For example, a 30-year-old citizen with an income of less than 133% of the federal poverty level may have received both Health Safety Net and standard Medicaid (MassHealth Standard in Massachusetts) to cover healthcare services and related costs. The eligibility requirements for the state-funded Health Safety Net program, which is open to undocumented immigrants, are listed in the left-hand column.[71] The middle column indicates the eligibility requirements for the federally funded MassHealth program, which is limited to low-income citizens, long-term green card holders, and refugees and asylees.[72] The right-hand column gives the eligibility requirements for the state-funded Commonwealth Care program, which provided subsidized private coverage for low- to middle-income adult citizens and green card holders. Commonwealth Care recipients could receive subsidies to purchase plans from private health insurance companies. Such plans would be accepted at healthcare facilities allowed within the insurance provider's network.[73] Typically, those coverage options were available only until people turned 65.

At age 65, citizens and long-term green card holders are eligible to apply for Medicare, and Health Safety Net remains open to lower-income undocumented immigrants in Massachusetts. Although many of those who are undocumented have worked, paid taxes, and contributed to Social Security and Medicare for years or decades, they are excluded from receiving any of these benefits when they reach the age of eligibility.[74] Those who are unable to continue working are often impoverished and do not always have health coverage, even in Massachusetts.

The complexity of these options and their differing criteria for eligibility were enough to discourage some people from applying. The enrollment process represented a clear example of how racialized legal status operated at the meso level to shape individuals' experiences with bureaucratic institutions. Lack of English proficiency and documentation status added to the administrative burdens that applicants experienced in preparing their materials. The application form consisted of a few pages in English, in a very small print, requesting essential information about documentation status, state of residence, and income. Applicants were required to submit proof that they met the criteria, with a list of acceptable documents: copies of a US passport or green card for documentation status; a Massachusetts driver's license, apartment lease, or utility bill for state of residence; and a pay stub or W-2 form for income. After the sorting process, which could take weeks or even months, applicants would receive a letter in the mail indicating what coverage option, if any, they were eligible for and the necessary next steps for finalizing their coverage.

According to people I interviewed, the correspondence applicants received from the state was confusing and deterred some from pursuing coverage. Although some immigrants received letters confirming their coverage type and medical plan, others were denied coverage from MassHealth and had to look for coverage through the state health exchange. Evelyn, a BHC administrator, explained that those who are ineligible for MassHealth must apply for it anyway to get Health Safely Net: "There is no separate application. And in the process, you are actually denied MassHealth and Medicaid. But if you flip over the letter, it says you're eligible for Health Safety Net. And there is a certain number or percentage of folks who read that [first page] and don't read the other side because all they see is '*denied*.'" Once deemed ineligible for HSN because of their income level, undocumented immigrants could have used Massachusetts's state health exchange to research and apply for private coverage. But this option disappeared after the state began preparing for ACA implementation in late 2013 due to stricter federal requirements for documentation status.

Applicants with limited English proficiency struggled with the application and follow-up materials, given the absence of information about how to obtain assistance in other languages. Providers and advocates attested to the language barrier their patients and clients faced in applying for coverage. Unless they were connected to social networks where they could find out about organizations that provided assistance, they were out of luck. In gaining access to health coverage and care, as in other aspects of life, whom you know and what they know makes a crucial difference.[75] Medical interpreters and health advocates stressed the importance of social networks for connecting immigrants with language-appropriate assistance at local organizations and healthcare facilities. BHC providers praised a health insurance helpline at a local health advocacy organization for helping immigrant "healthcare consumers" navigate the complicated application process. I interviewed numerous helpline counselors and staff about their collaboration with the Massachusetts Health Connector. Edward, a health advocate who was quoted earlier, explained that his organization receives

> hundreds of calls a day in English, Spanish and Portuguese, and in fact more than half of our calls are not in English. We have native speakers in Spanish and Brazilian Portuguese who help people navigate the system and figure out to how enroll, what are the complicated rules, including immigration status and how that affects your application. We fill out applications over the phone; we're the only place in the state you can fill out an application over the phone. We have custom software that we developed. We can basically do the questionnaire in six minutes. Then we fill out the form and mail it to them, they sign it and mail it back to us. We make sure it is perfect to send in, and then we call them. We track people. We help people who are just lost in the system.

Organizations like Edward's reduce the administrative burdens of racialized legal status that were built into the tedious process of applying for coverage. Obtaining the documents required to prove eligibility, however, still presented severe structural barriers for the undocumented. Although applicants for Health Safety Net did not need to submit any proof of documentation status, this information was mentioned only in a note at the end of the form. The request for documentation status on the first page could easily be perceived as excluding undocumented immigrants from eligibility. Furthermore, acceptable documents to prove state residency and income level are more difficult for undocumented immigrants to produce. In 2012 and 2013, Massachusetts did not issue driver's licenses to undocumented immigrants. Many of the undocumented share living expenses with documented immigrants whose names are on leases or mortgages and on bills with residential addresses. Immigrants without work authorization tend to be paid "under the table" in cash, which prevents them from documenting their income. All those who cannot produce these forms of proof are bureaucratically disqualified, making this obstacle difficult to overcome.

Documented immigrants I interviewed also expressed concern about applying for coverage. To determine whether they were eligible for Commonwealth Care, documented immigrants had to submit proof of their legal status. Distinctions between short- and long-term green card holders and naturalized citizens influenced the process. Although the statutory prohibition on admitting immigrants deemed likely to become a "public charge" gained national attention under the Trump administration, it already caused concern among providers, immigrant advocates, and documented immigrants in 2013. They wondered whether obtaining health coverage under the Massachusetts health reform would harm immigrants' prospects for obtaining green cards. Márcia, a Brazilian advocate, worried about the predicament created by the disconnect between state and federal health and immigration policy: "Here in Massachusetts, health insurance is mandatory, but some people can't pay for health insurance. I think the federal law is not compatible with the state law. . . . Some people end up not following the law. Because if you come with a green card, you sign a waiver that says you will not ask for [government benefits], but here, it's mandatory to have health coverage and if you ask for [or enroll in] a plan from the state [like MassHealth], you are violating federal law." MassHealth did not count against immigrants before the Trump administration proposed changing the public charge rule in 2018, so this concern was not founded in fact at the time of our interview. But Márcia's perception speaks to the level of ambiguity that existed in 2012 about what public benefits counted against applicants for lawful permanent residency.

Once immigrants completed the process and received or were denied coverage, cost still remained a barrier to care. This was especially the case for immigrants whose incomes were too high to qualify for Health Safety Net and MassHealth. Sebastião, a Brazilian advocate, emphasized the seriousness of this problem: "The price is really high for immigrants" who don't qualify for subsidized coverage.

> So, they try to avoid getting coverage, but then they would also have to pay a tax penalty. So, they get afraid about not having coverage. I see many immigrants who pay the tax penalty and cope with chronic illnesses. I see many painters with lead-related blood problems who don't go to clinics because they were denied by MassHealth. They wait until they are sicker to return to their home countries because they can no longer work.

Sebastião also alluded to the health consequences of the inability to afford coverage. Immigrants of various statuses felt they must have coverage to avoid the state penalty, but others remained uninsured. Bianca, the Latinx immigrant advocate who is quoted at the beginning of this chapter, described another catch-22: immigrants need to earn enough money to support their families, but if they earn too much to qualify for their current state-subsidized coverage, they may lose it without being able to afford private insurance.

While some applicants were denied access to subsidized coverage, those who were successful received letters in English indicating their coverage type: Health Safety Net, MassHealth, or Commonwealth Care. Depending on the coverage type, applicants were required to select a specific medical plan, and here again, some immigrants fell through the cracks. Daniel, a Spanish-speaking health advocate, explained that "sometimes they are eligible for Commonwealth Care, but they don't know what to do, . . . that they have to call to let them [MassHealth] know. . . . They [immigrants] are missing all the information, and also the letters. . . . A lot of them . . . don't speak English; plus I know some people, they don't know how to read."

In sum, while everyone in the state was eligible to apply, all applicants did not have the necessary language skills, documentation, or understanding of bureaucratic procedures to navigate the process effectively. Scholars refer to this as "bureaucratic disentitlement."[76] The combination of administrative burdens and bureaucratic disentitlement sent a shrewd message that potential beneficiaries should not apply. In his analysis of social welfare programs in Boston forty years ago, political scientist Michael Lipsky noted that similar processes constrained potential beneficiaries' ability to navigate the social welfare system. He argued that, in addition to governments eliminating or cutting back programs, "obligations to social welfare beneficiaries are reduced and circumscribed through largely obscure 'bureaucratic' actions and inactions of public authorities."[77] If application processes are made difficult and have onerous requirements, eligible beneficiaries are tacitly discouraged from applying, which in turn reduces the state government's responsibility and the costs of programs. Some immigrant advocates, such as Tiago, a Brazilian advocate, felt that this was especially the case for undocumented immigrants. Tiago thought Massachusetts intentionally raised the administrative burdens to apply for HSN after the 2006 reform. Before, coverage was easier to obtain "because FreeCare [HSN's predecessor] was a lot looser. I'm told that you can actually" use Health Safety Net "even without documents, but it's not as easy. . . . I believe they [Massachusetts legislators] tied in the regulations [regarding] documentation on purpose so people would not take a chance." Tiago thought that this reduced access to coverage for undocumented immigrants.

This observation aligns with other advocates' and providers' perceptions that the Massachusetts reform reduced access to health coverage for immigrants, especially the undocumented, by setting up overly complex application procedures, cutting benefits, and reducing funding for state navigators to assist disadvantaged residents with the enrollment process. Because Massachusetts has had the nation's highest healthcare costs, a large proportion of which is paid by the state, cost-saving or cost-cutting measures have been implemented over many years.[78] We know from other studies that increasing bureaucratic disentitlement and administrative burdens have enabled state and federal governments to limit total costs by decreasing the number of potential beneficiaries.[79] The disproportionate impact of these cost-cutting measures has negatively affected Black, Latinx, low-income, and immigrant residents' health coverage.[80] This pattern demonstrates that implicit racialized legal status discrimination is subtly inscribed in policy changes that result in exclusion for the most vulnerable.

"Now That I Have Coverage, What Am I Gonna Do with It?"

Some immigrants were persistent and resourceful enough to overcome the racialized legal status burdens that applying for and finally receiving health coverage entailed. But the next challenge was figuring out where and how to use their coverage. The United States has one of the world's most complicated and expensive healthcare and health insurance systems.[81] Most Americans lack health literacy and struggle to understand how their coverage works well enough to obtain care.[82] Differing levels of health literacy are associated with health disparities.[83] Latinx immigrants around the country generally have lower health literacy levels, particularly if they have limited English proficiency or are undocumented.[84]

Although most of the Boston-area Brazilians and Dominicans I interviewed had some type of health coverage, many spoke of their difficulty in finding out where, when, and how they could use it. Milton, a 45-year-old undocumented Brazilian with medium-brown skin who identified as Latino and switched from private to public coverage after leaving his job, did not know how to find help for his depression: "I had a really good job with really good health insurance, but I left it. I don't have that insurance anymore, I have FreeCare, but I don't know what my rights are. I don't understand very well what I can and cannot have. Right now, I need psychological help; I want to see a psychiatrist to treat my depression. But I haven't yet. I called a clinic, but I haven't heard back from them. I don't know how FreeCare works. That's the main problem I have." FreeCare, which became Health Safety Net after the 2006 reform, provided some psychiatric services if the HSN facility where a patient sought treatment had them available. At the time of these interviews in 2013, one BHC site had a psychiatric clinic specifically for Portuguese and Spanish speakers, and I spoke with some of its staff. Many said that the demand for psychiatrists was so high because only a few psychiatrists could provide services in these languages.[85]

These staff members spoke of being overworked, not having enough hours in the day to treat patients, and long waiting lists of patients to be seen at the clinic. Even if Milton had known that his coverage included treatment in Portuguese, the long waiting list might have still made it very difficult for him to get the mental health care he needed.

Advocates and providers shared the perception that lack of information about the health insurance system was a huge problem for their constituents and patients. Edward, a health advocate quoted earlier, said that for immigrants, "the whole concept of health insurance is difficult to understand." Those who come from countries "where health care is provided by the government" or patients pay for treatment when they receive it do not see "why they have to pay a premium" while they are healthy. The most common things that immigrants found confusing were the concept of a primary care physician or provider (PCP), the fact that coverage could not be used everywhere, and the distinctions between visits to the emergency department and appointments with regular physicians. Most health insurance plans require patients to see a primary care provider first, who must then make a referral to a specialist. Immigrants, especially those who had health coverage in their home countries, thought it was odd that you could not go directly to a cardiologist for a heart problem. In their home countries, Brazilians and a few Dominicans could go directly to see a specialist, and their insurance would cover the cost, no questions asked.

Finding a PCP, who serves as the gatekeeper to the US healthcare system, is never easy. The supply of PCPs has been declining nationally, as they are the least well compensated medical doctors, and many medical students choose to specialize in more lucrative fields, especially if they have education loans to repay.[86] Camila, a BHC medical interpreter, recounted that "in many countries, they don't know" what a primary care doctor is: "So, when people come here and you ask them, 'Do you have a primary care doctor, did you call your primary care doctor?,' you can tell, like there are nurses that kind of go like, 'Are you serious?' It's not their fault; it's just they don't have the knowledge, why you should have gone to your primary care doctor first or why you have to have one."

Moreover, PCPs in private practices can opt out of seeing patients with publicly provided coverage such as Medicaid because of its low reimbursement rates.[87]

The difficulty of figuring out how their coverage worked prevented many immigrants from getting optimal or even minimally appropriate care. Many did not understand the distinctions between appointments with physicians and visits to the emergency room. For some, ER visits remained the only way they could be sure of being seen without going through the hassle of making and then waiting for an appointment, which could be days, weeks, or months away, or even impossible to obtain. For others, the factor of out-of-pocket costs was decisive. Amelia, a BHC provider, discussed this problem at length: "We still have patients [who] struggle. They can't afford to pay a premium. Or they cannot afford to pay their co-pays for visits or medications. So, they avoid coming to the doctor unless they are extremely sick . . . and go to the ER instead. Even though they have insurance coverage. The reason is because if they go to the ER, they don't have that co-pay, but they can still be seen. . . . Now we are trying to work with that issue. It costs the state a lot of money for patients to go to the ER every time they are sick and then to come see a provider."

Remarking that the problem had snowballed recently, she pointed to an example that, although extreme, illustrated the trend and its cause: "We have one patient that has gone to the ER 28 times in the last 12 months. The provider is here and can see her anytime she would like. But she'd rather go to the ER to avoid the co-pay." This situation contributed to longer wait times in emergency departments and meant that patients did not receive follow-up care. Furthermore, such repeat ER visits increase healthcare costs for the state and private insurers.[88] Yet the expense of co-pays influences patients' healthcare decisions even when they have free or low-cost public coverage.

Some immigrants felt their coverage was sufficient and did not have expensive co-pays or premiums. Daiane, the Brazilian quoted earlier who identifies as Pardo and is a lawful permanent resident, recounted her experience in a hospital: "I used a government plan, and my surgery was entirely paid by the government. I think even the medication that I took home I didn't pay for." Other immigrants felt their coverage did not meet all their needs. The lack of dental insurance for most was particularly serious, given the high cost of dental treatment.[89] Jessica, the undocumented Black and Latina Brazilian quoted earlier, complained: "We don't have access to dental service, and we've suffered a lot, and I have to fix a tooth, and I don't have the funds." Among documented immigrant respondents, those with sufficient financial resources would return to their home countries for dental care and other medical treatments that were not covered by insurance in the United States and were more affordable elsewhere.

Twelve of the Brazilians and 8 of the Dominicans I interviewed had some sort of public coverage, placing them at a disadvantage in the stratified healthcare system. Miranda, a Dominican advocate, said she thought that lower-income immigrant patients of color with public coverage receive inferior health care than those with private coverage. "In the health centers, . . . the person who has private insurance gets taken care of more seriously. The clinics get those with public insurance." The same situation exists in hospitals: "The people with private insurance, they get [a] better experience. They get the best room, . . . the private room." Even in nursing homes, "I could see there is a big difference. Somebody with MassHealth [who] is Black or Latino or African or whatever, the room is like an old room, and they are put next to somebody that is the same as them, and they keep the nice room for White people that have private insurance."

Similar types of race and class-based discrimination have been documented in other studies of the healthcare system.[90] The enduring legacy of structural racism in the United States has contributed to a correlation between race and class so that Black and Latinx people, regardless of their actual socioeconomic and legal status, are perceived to be low-income and likely to be using public benefits. Bureaucrats and service providers treat them in a hostile or inferior manner because racialized legal status erases the particular characteristics and situations of individuals and associates them with an acutely marginalized group.[91] Conversely, this research highlights the perception Miranda voiced: that White Americans (and some White immigrants) receive better treatment than people of color, regardless of income level and insurance type.

The Challenge of Renewing Coverage

In 2012–2013, individuals receiving any type of public health coverage had to renew it annually. They were required to resubmit proof of state residence and income to determine their eligibility for coverage under the same plan, a different plan, or none at all. As the renewal deadline approached, the state sent letters in English explaining the process. Many immigrants told me that they either did not receive the correspondence or could not read and understand it. Those whose addresses had changed were supposed to notify the state, but if the letter went astray, they lost their coverage. Some of those who received the letter did not know where to go for assistance with the renewal process. Consequently, people might have coverage one year and lose it the next, a process referred to as "churning."[92] Paola, a health advocate, said that the state should make it easier for people to reenroll and retain their coverage. Many administrative burdens had to be overcome for immigrants to keep their coverage under the Massachusetts health reform. It is a wonder that most of the immigrants I interviewed had been covered long enough to be able to discuss their experiences in the healthcare system.

Yet the high cost of premiums and deductibles led some to cancel their coverage. Dania, a 50-year-old Dominican and naturalized US citizen with very light skin tone, dark-brown eyes, and short blonde hair, told me that she eventually let her coverage lapse because it was unaffordable: "I paid really high premiums for my insurance, about $1,000 monthly for Blue Cross Blue [Shield] with rent and food, that was a lot to pay. So, I got rid of my coverage and have not reenrolled. I know there is more affordable coverage available, but in this moment, I'm not at an economic level where I can afford to pay for it." In Dania's case, providing the basic necessities for her family outweighed her ability to keep coverage she could not afford. Despite being in Massachusetts, where coverage was required and supposed to be more accessible, the cost still remained a barrier. Her experience aligns with the perception of Sebastião, the Brazilian advocate, that the available coverage was not affordable for those without government subsidies. It also reflects the view of Amelia, a BHC provider, that patients were unable to afford the co-pays required for receiving care. These statements about the lack of affordable coverage and care in the commonwealth were confirmed by health insurance companies themselves. A 2013 report by Blue Cross Blue Shield of Massachusetts found that Massachusetts residents spent above the US average in every category of healthcare services.[93] So, even when immigrants managed to get coverage, whether or not their premiums were subsidized, some still could not afford the cost of care.

Finally Receiving Care, yet Encountering Discrimination

Racialized legal status burdens and high costs present barriers to care for immigrants, particularly those who are undocumented and who are not perceived as White. Moreover, those who did receive care found that they were sometimes subjected to discrimination, which diminished the quality of care. A substantial body of research has demonstrated that individuals' race, ethnicity, documentation status, and socioeconomic status affect their health and healthcare access for better or worse.[94] The intersections between these characteristics can magnify or mitigate the privileges or harms that people's experiences with the system entail. Racialized legal status discrimination has created and perpetuated disparities at every stage of the medical encounter for people of color, regardless of whether they are citizens, lawful permanent residents, or undocumented.[95] The facts are striking. Black Americans are less likely to be prescribed pain medication than White Americans with similar conditions because doctors think that Black people feel less pain than White people.[96] Latinx individuals of various legal statuses are more likely to be uninsured and less likely to have a regular healthcare provider than their counterparts who are ethnoracially categorized as White.[97] Generations of malign neglect and mistreatment have created a pervasive distrust of doctors and the US healthcare system in marginalized communities.[98] The explicitly racist and anti-immigrant rhetoric of the past decade has generated a climate of fear that has diminished Latinx and other immigrants' willingness to seek health care around the country and even in Boston.[99] These themes surfaced among the individuals I interviewed in 2012–2013. They encountered language-based difficulties in making and scheduling appointments and obtaining transportation, suffered from providers' implicit and explicit discriminatory treatment, and feared being profiled and detained on the way to appointments, which could lead to their arrest and deportation. Thus, racialized legal status discrimination was pervasive in Latinx immigrants' experiences with the Boston healthcare system.

How Language Hinders the Medical Encounter

Limited English proficiency (LEP) hindered immigrants' communication with healthcare providers, which intensified all the other forms of discrimination they might encounter. For the estimated 25 million individuals in the United States with LEP, language presents a huge structural barrier to obtaining health care, from scheduling appointments and seeing providers to filling and accurately taking prescriptions.[100] While the inability to obtain necessary information in one's primary language may seem an inadvertent consequence of migration, it represents a violation of anti-discrimination law. As I discussed in Chapter 1, Title VI of the 1964 Civil Rights Act protects the right of individuals to receive language-appropriate information and assistance in federally funded institutions. Consequently, the inability to receive such assistance is a form of racial discrimination, which compromises LEP individuals' engagement with meso-level institutions. Like many primary English speakers, I previously took for granted the privilege of making appointments and communicating with healthcare professionals in my primary language. As I interviewed stakeholders, I realized how many patients ran into these racialized legal status barriers when attempting to obtain health services.

I asked Brazilian and Dominican respondents about the quality of their interactions with medical providers. Francisca, the Brazilian who complained that the government made it difficult to apply for coverage, described the problem her family faced when getting care: "My husband speaks very little English, and today he went to the doctor and had an interpreter there. Where he goes, they have to have people who speak Portuguese there. . . . When neither my son or me can go with my husband to medical appointments, it takes him longer to be seen. If you need an interpreter, you could wait two or three months to get appointments."

At BHC sites, I noticed multilingual signs in elevators and hallways that included instructions on how to request a medical interpreter during check-in with the receptionist. These signs were primarily in Spanish and Portuguese, but also in Haitian Creole and Vietnamese, as well as other languages I did not recognize. Seeing these signs reminded me how important being able to read is for navigating the healthcare system. I heard from providers and advocates that illiteracy disproportionately affected Salvadoran patients, who had been unable to attend school regularly during their childhood.

Language barriers inhibit or prevent communication between patients and providers. A growing body of research has found that language minorities, who are typically also people of color, experience communication anxiety in healthcare settings, which can negatively affect their perceived quality of care and health outcomes.[101] For LEP patients, medical interpreters are a lifeline.

Immigrant respondents who were BHC patients (about half of those I interviewed) felt that they were able to receive language-appropriate care and that providers and staff cared about their health and overall well-being. This perception aligns with BHC's reputation as a place where patients are treated well regardless of their racialized legal status, ability to pay, or the type of coverage they have. BHC is also a federally qualified health center and a designated Health Safety Net facility. Many of the providers I interviewed, who trained at some of the nation's best medical schools, said that they chose to work at BHC to care for marginalized populations. BHC has medical interpreters available, and providers and staff work hard to make it a welcoming place for all its patients. Adriana, a BHC medical interpreter, said: "I think that working in this hospital, they [patients] feel really good about coming here. Many are surprised at how many services they can get here. Sometimes, I see people come here and they have no idea that all these resources are available, free or low-cost coverage for the undocumented. The finance department is well trained in explaining things and answering questions so as to not scare immigrants so that they will return."

Some providers with sufficient proficiency in other languages opt out of using medical interpreters and speak with patients directly. Usually, but not always, this works well. Jessica, the Black and Latina Brazilian who discussed her lack of access to dental care earlier and is fluent in English, explained that this practice could make patients uncomfortable: "In the doctor's office, for many years I no longer need an interpreter. But my primary care doctor is American and married to a Portuguese man [so] she insists on speaking Portuguese. Her Portuguese is horrible. I speak to her in English, but she speaks Portuguese, and when she speaks in English, she uses gestures. I don't know if it is a habit that the person creates to communicate or if it is intentional to show that you are not understanding." Later in the interview, she told me that she has no other criticisms about her BHC experience aside from this doctor: "I just have praise for them. For example, at the check-up I do annually, they have been trying to improve and streamline the service. Both in the hospital and in the clinic. But I can say that I don't like my doctor. I don't like her way of treating me, but as she is an expert that I always need, I stay with her. It took me years to remember her name because I don't like the way she treats me."

For providers and the patients who need them, medical interpreters play a vital role in communicating patients' health issues. The limited research that has been done on the quality and cost-effectiveness of medical interpreters finds that they improve the likelihood of patients receiving care, increase satisfaction, and reduce healthcare costs.[102] Very little research has explored how the presence of medical interpreters and the modality of interpretation (i.e., in person, by phone, or video) influence the medical encounter, however. Among BHC providers, those who used interpreters felt that doing so only minimally affected the patient-provider interaction. Yet, even with the most skilled interpreters, important information can be difficult to communicate or get lost in translation. Camila, the BHC medical interpreter quoted earlier, shared the heart-breaking story of struggling to tell a young patient that he had terminal cancer. Although he was from El Salvador, he did not speak Spanish, but an Indigenous language called Mam, for which there was no interpreter.

> Since he spoke mostly Mam, his cousin spoke a little bit of Mam, but mostly Spanish. So, I translated for the cousin, the cousin translated for him. We were trying to tell him that there was nothing we could do for him because he has terminal cancer, and he was only 18. So, the doctor was frustrated, I was frustrated, the family was frustrated. It got to a point that I could say, "You are going to heaven, you are going to meet God when the spirit leaves your body." . . . We were trying to find the words to say, "I am sorry you are going to die," and he couldn't understand it, and it took weeks. So finally, one day for him to finally say, "Oh, I am going to die"—I remember that moment as one of the hardest for me to communicate.

BHC staff were aware of how central interpreters are to meeting BHC's mission. In 2013, the primary mode of interpretation was in person: the interpreter would be in the same room as the patient and provider. Adriana, the BHC interpreter quoted earlier, explained the strengths and weaknesses of various modes of interpretation and her preference for in-person interpretation.

> In the past, you could, for example, go with the patient to schedule an appointment and walk with them through the hospital. This has ended and had an impact where patients say, "I feel alone." But BHC has a lot of capacity for phone interpretation and every place has a telephone. So, a person does not end up without an interpreter at any point. . . . Video interpretation connects the two types; you are not there, but you can see. For example, on the phone, if a patient speaks a little bit of English, I cannot see them to know if they responded.

Adriana also appreciated having time to walk and clear her mind between sessions. With phone and video interpretation, interpreters feel they are working nearly nonstop without any time to debrief, given the high demand for their services.[103]

Beyond language, cultural differences affect the healthcare experiences of immigrants who are fluent in English and have high socioeconomic status, as well as those who lack the resources that the US healthcare system demands. Marcos, the Brazilian law school professor, had observed differences between doctors in Brazil and those in the United States: "I think American doctors are not as warm and friendly as Brazilian doctors. They pay less attention to you and more attention to their computer screen. They have less holistic curiosity in terms of aspects of your life that could be relevant to your health." Sometimes these differences left patients feeling that US doctors were impersonal and lacked the *calor humana* that made for more positive healthcare experiences.

Discrimination in the Medical Encounter

Most immigrant respondents felt positive about their experiences with BHC interpreters and providers. Maria, a 37-year-old White Brazilian immigrant I interviewed in English the day after the Boston Marathon bombing, was ecstatic about the care she received at BHC despite the structural barriers she encountered getting coverage and navigating the system:

I do not know if I am lucky or have a great doctor and a great team, but it just works. They call you to remind you of your appointment, or when you get blood tests. They call you to go there and then the assistant nurse explains to you all the tests and makes [asks] like 50 different questions about how you are, how is everything, and she explains all this. My doctor is awesome. When my depression was [a] little like, kind of like bad, like I wasn't doing really well, like last year, her nurse called me to check on me.

Other Brazilian immigrants painted a less rosy picture. Gilma, a 34-year-old green card holder who classified as White, complained about mistreatment from a BHC provider: "Sometimes I think doctors see you as ignorant. . . . The last experience I had was with my digestion. The doctor said I had a problem with my placenta and I questioned him, and he ignored me, he just would say I am well. I said, 'Tell me the name of the conditions for me to research,' and he wouldn't say. I don't know if he is like that with all patients or thought I was ignorant." Gilma felt that her provider's behavior was discriminatory and based on her national origin.

The majority of immigrants I interviewed in 2012–2013 did not report having experienced any racial or immigration-based discrimination in their medical encounters. Other research, however, has found that limited English proficiency and lower levels of acculturation are associated with lower levels of perceived discrimination among Latinx people with various documentation statuses in the United States.[104] This surprising disparity might explain why only three immigrant patients, all Dominican, who received care at non-BHC healthcare facilities reported having experienced discrimination from providers. In those cases, the respondents felt that the discrimination was tied to their racialized legal status. Carlos, the undocumented Dominican immigrant with medium-brown skin quoted earlier, recounted what happened when he went to a hospital emergency room after he had been injured and needed his wounds cleaned. He told me that the Black American provider did not treat him because he was Hispanic. Eventually, a Puerto Rican staff member gave him the care he needed. He reflected: "I don't understand why this happened because many of the people who work here as doctors are Hispanics too. As soon as you go to the ER, . . . they should not look at you and think I am a Hispanic, I don't speak English, or am an immigrant. They should treat people in emergencies because a life is a human being, whether I am here in this country with papers or not." Outside of health care, too, Carlos said that his racialized legal status contributed to discrimination, and he felt it was affecting his mental health.

Documented immigrants such as Dania, the Dominican who let her health coverage lapse, said that having legal status does not remove or even decrease the likelihood of encountering anti-immigrant discrimination in everyday life and in healthcare facilities. Her statement about the discrimination she has encountered is at the beginning of Chapter 1;

she poignantly described how being Latina, being an immigrant, having darker skin color, and speaking Spanish resulted in routine mistreatment. For Dania, these factors undermined the legal privileges she received as a green card holder. Many Latinx Bostonians shared this view. Alma, a 42-year-old Black Dominican with US citizenship, shared that people like her are treated like "a rat, a thief, like you are nothing."

Dominicans were more likely than Brazilians to mention experiencing racialized legal status discrimination within and outside medical encounters. Despite being documented or naturalized, most were racialized by others as Black and stigmatized for speaking Spanish or Spanish-inflected English. Dominicans' darker skin tone made their non-Whiteness and presumed foreignness more visible. In contrast, many Brazilian immigrants were more often perceived as White due to their lighter skin tone and more European-looking features. Despite being more likely to be undocumented, which put them at a structural disadvantage compared with documented Dominicans, Brazilians' ability to blend in with White Americans made them less visible—at least until they spoke. Only then did their accents reveal their foreignness and otherness. In some ways, Brazilian and Dominican respondents' experiences exemplify those outlined in the racial profiling example I describe in Chapter 1 (see Figure 1-2). Brazilians were less likely to be racially profiled than Black Dominicans; but, once they were stopped or pulled over by police or immigration officials, their accent and the names on their license and proof of car insurance (if they had these documents) could reveal their undocumented and foreign background, which could subsequently lead to arrest, detention, and deportation.

These groups' differing experiences with racialized legal status discrimination shaped what each group thought was the basis of the discrimination they experienced in healthcare settings and US society generally. Dominicans thought race was a factor in discrimination, while Brazilians thought discrimination stemmed from their actual or perceived documentation status and foreignness because of their limited or accented English. For both groups, regardless of their physical appearance or documentation status, language differences led others to racialize them as immigrants. The significance of these findings is underlined by other studies showing that race and skin color differentially influence the lives and health of lighter- and darker-skinned Latinx people around the country.[105] Increasingly, being perceived as an immigrant—regardless of whether an individual was born in the United States or not—contributes to discriminatory treatment that has health implications.[106]

Latinx immigrants' negative experiences in encounters with health-care providers, coupled with their difficulties in securing coverage and navigating the healthcare system, highlight the importance of having a more ethnoracially and linguistically diverse workforce in health care and social services. In addition to providing medical interpreters, immigrants thought that governmental and nongovernmental agencies should address cultural differences that contribute to racialized legal status discrimination and reinforce the systemic exclusion associated with patients' and clients' language and ethnoracial backgrounds. This type of exclusion affects both US- and foreign-born individuals of color with limited English proficiency. Currently, most of the US healthcare work-force is White, while Black, Latinx, Asian, and Native Americans are underrepresented.[107] In the absence of a diverse workforce to meet the needs of diverse patients, it will be difficult to reduce the structural barriers and associated administrative burdens essential to providing equitable health care.

Racialized Enforcement Concerns in Seeking Care

At the same time that Brazilians and Dominicans struggled to navigate structural barriers within the healthcare system, they also had to cope with racialized immigration enforcement, which has increased dramatically in its scope and intensity over the past decade. Nationally, Latinx residents of all documentation statuses are targeted for arrest, detention, and deportation.[108] Although deportation rose under the Obama administration, President Trump's explicitly racist rhetoric describing Mexicans and, by implication, all other Latinx immigrants as criminals seeking to have "anchor babies" made Latinx people—whether US-born, docu-mented, or undocumented—feel that they were all being targeted.[109] This perception has not disappeared under the Biden administration, whose policies have been both pro- and anti-immigrant. Despite promising to have more compassion than the previous administration, the Biden administration has urged migrants not to come to the United States, deported migrants arriving at the US southern border, and built more walls along the border.[110] Thus, enforcement fears affect the decisions Latinx residents make about seeking health care. Those who are undocu-mented worry that they could be detained while in transit to or from medical appointments, while those who have legal status know that they may be perceived and treated as if they were undocumented because of their race, ethnicity, and language.

Alicia, a 39-year-old Black Brazilian with a green card, had been pulled over and screamed at by local police the day before our 2013 interview. Being a Black immigrant meant that she was met with suspicion: "The police see you and stop you, thinking you're an immigrant, driving with-out a license." These concerns were common, regardless of whether people got to their medical appointments by car or public transportation. Some, like Rosalicia, a 39-year-old White Brazilian with a work visa, worried that healthcare facilities might call the police or ICE: "Undocumented immi-grants live in the shadows, they can't be seen. You think twice before you go anywhere, driving, you live on the margins of society, you're not in-cluded. You can't go to school because you're afraid, or the hospital either." Despite her privileged racial and socioeconomic background and legal sta-tus, she still felt vulnerable.

The post-9/11 increase in immigration enforcement, particularly through the Secure Communities program, resulted in immigration raids in Boston and around the country.[111] In my interviews with immigrants, providers, and advocates, many mentioned that fear of being pulled over by police officers or ICE agents deterred immigrants from keeping ap-pointments. The new federal program favoring the cooperation of local and state police with federal immigration authorities meant that arrested immigrants could be turned over to ICE for detention and deportation. Gloria, a BHC social worker, recounted a particularly anxious moment in Boston: "There was a time, I think it was three years ago, that there were raids, especially in Maverick Station in East Boston and also Sullivan Station. That day we missed a lot of patients, and we did not know what was happening. I started to call my patients, 'Why didn't you come?' They were like, 'You know that there are raids happening in East Boston since 5 o'clock in the morning, we are not going to work, we are not doing anything.' So, when people learn that there are raids, they don't come to see the doctor." Other studies conducted around the country between 2010 and 2013 revealed that similar concerns affected immigrants' healthcare access and outcomes.[112]

Immigration enforcement is racialized in the same ways as other aspects of US society, including racially biased law enforcement and mass incarceration; racial disparities in employment, earnings, and wealth; and higher rates of morbidity and mortality among communities of color.[113] As the entire system is rooted in White supremacy, enforcement allows the punitive arm of the state to control and punish Black and Brown bodies. Consequently, racialized legal status put immigrants in my study at increased risk of being stopped and arrested by police or detained by ICE. Samantha, another Dominican advocate, contended: "When talking about immigration, you have to talk about racism because it is one of the ways that the system oppresses people. If you don't have documents, they can oppress you more. . . . So, when people are afraid, that affects their involvement in the neighborhood and how they seek out information that could help them." Furthermore, immigration has been racialized as involving Latinx people, so individuals who "look" Latinx are perceived to be immigrants and most likely undocumented and consequently are not viewed as legitimate members of society.[114] As discussed in Chapter 1, racial profiling in overlapping law and immigration enforcement disproportionately targets Latinx and Black men, who are more likely to be arrested and imprisoned or detained and deported.[115] The immigrants I interviewed over the course of this study were acutely aware of the pejorative stereotypes of Latinx people and undocumented immigrants, who are viewed as one and the same and regarded as deserving mistreatment.

Gloria, the BHC social worker who described immigrants' anxiety about being stopped en route to her clinic, concluded that "once they are here, I think they are safe." But that was not how all immigrant patients felt. Many worried that using publicly provided health services could lead to detention or deportation or undermine the prospect of obtaining green cards for themselves or their family members. Staff members recounted that being asked for identification, a Social Security number, or a date of birth at healthcare facilities caused some immigrants to panic. Requests for this type of information are common when people check in with receptionists and do initial intake interviews with medical assistants and as doctors try to ensure that they are reviewing the correct patient file. These requests make immigrant patients feel uncomfortable or excessively scrutinized. Camila, the BHC medical interpreter who discussed immigrants' lack of familiarity with PCPs, suggested an alternative way of proceeding: "I think that when somebody goes to the doctor or the emergency room and they get to the registration clerk or the greeters [who ask], 'Do you have a Social Security number?' and they respond, 'No, I don't,' then the staff should say something like 'Oh, it's okay, no worries, we treat everybody whether they have a legal status or not.'"

Another BHC provider, Kevin, heard similar concerns about public charge rules and federal patient privacy laws such as HIPAA that require asking for identification and birth dates during medical encounters.[116] "For the people who are trying to work towards citizenship, there's often—I don't know if it's an urban myth or accurate—the idea that if they use services without being documented, then that will count against them when they are applying" for legalization or naturalization. "Back when we had the FreeCare pool, basically state funds for undocumented people, they would say, 'Oh, I can't use that because I am trying to get my green card.'" Kevin worried that federal HIPAA policies designed to protect patient privacy and protocols intended to prevent medical errors resulting from confusion about patients' identities had created more problems than they solved. "I mean, the way that we ask for photo

IDs everywhere and we ask everyone their birthday a hundred times even before we talk, like I am supposed to do every single time I see my patient, it doesn't matter if I have had 165 visits with you, I don't have your date of birth memorized but I know who you are. It is absurd, but that kind of stuff breeds some suspicion." Quite reasonably, immigrants worry about how all this information will be used.

Immigrants feared that using healthcare services or incurring debt from medical bills could lead to deportation. I heard about this fear from Maria, the White Brazilian who earlier praised the care she received at BHC. Although Maria had a green card when I interviewed her, she was previously undocumented. "Every time I would go [to the doctor], I thought I would get like a $2,000 bill and if I did not pay, the police would go to my house and deport me. I don't know. Like when you are illegal you are afraid. You do not know that Homeland Security is not attached to" the healthcare system. "You just live . . . in fear. So . . . I was very afraid to have [medical] debt because, you know, immigration forces will find me and kick me out of the country."

Immigrant advocates like Glaucia, who assisted Brazilians, reported that some constituents without valid IDs or Social Security numbers waited for hours before anyone would treat them:

> Right now, in many places you have to provide a valid ID to get any kind of care. And right away, if you don't have that valid ID and you are not dying, they are not going to see you. That's one of the experiences that I had with someone. This person came in and didn't have a valid ID. They could not be seen. And then the second time around with someone else, this person had an accident, and the person wasn't treated adequately right from the get-go and the person didn't have a Social Security number and we actually waited around for three hours, and the person decided to leave because they didn't receive any care.

All too often, documentation status–based discrimination occurs in medical encounters either explicitly or covertly. When patients do not have or are uncomfortable with providing the identification and documents needed to verify their identity or process claims for coverage or payment purposes, the absence of this information may result in delayed treatment or none at all.

My interviews with stakeholders reveal the various ways racialized legal status indirectly shaped immigrants' healthcare experiences through the ever-present threat of enforcement from police and immigration authorities in 2012–2013. Even though Boston and some nearby towns had sanctuary policies minimizing information sharing between police and ICE, immigrants often perceived these uniformed officers as representing the same authority. Moreover, health providers' and facilities' frequent requests for personal information made immigrants feel that they were under government surveillance when using health services. For most US-born citizens, these requests seem benign, but in the current anti-immigrant climate, birth dates and Social Security numbers are constant reminders of noncitizens' precarious position and vulnerability to deportation. Noncitizen status shaped immigrants' experience in a healthcare system that has a long history of excluding and discriminating against citizens of color. Some immigrants even opt out of the healthcare system and other institutions providing services to remain under the radar from surveillance. According to sociologist Asad Asad, undocumented immigrants especially avoid what he calls "system embeddedness" as a protective strategy to reduce their deportation risk.[117]

More broadly, sociologists Cecilia Menjívar and Leisy Abrego define the increasing importance of documentation status in immigration law and the encroachment of the federal, state, and local government into immigrants' lives as "legal violence."[118] Menjívar and Abrego argue that the law can inflict violence through its harmful effects on immigrants, obstructing their prospects for work, at school, and in the family.[119] Sociologist Meredith Van Natta argues that a similar process, which she calls "medical legal violence," plays out in health care, where increased concerns regarding federal immigration policies lead immigrants to make risky calculations about seeking or avoiding care.[120] What I heard from Boston immigrants, providers, and advocates reveals that fears about immigration enforcement and the intrusion of federal authorities into healthcare facilities are damaging immigrants' healthcare access and health.

Conclusion

The intersection of race, ethnicity, and legal status had a significant impact on the ability of Boston Latinx immigrants to apply for health coverage and access health services after the historic Massachusetts health reform. Despite their legal inclusion as residents of the commonwealth, racialized legal status restricted immigrants' ability to use benefits for which they were eligible. Boston immigrants experienced structural barriers associated with RLS in the form of administrative burdens as well as explicit and implicit discrimination in trying to obtain health coverage and care. First, they encountered implicit discrimination in the application process as lack of language access increased their administrative burdens in an already complicated enrollment process. They experienced legally based discrimination as documentation status, along with income, stratified their public coverage options. For both low-income and undocumented immigrants, these coverage options were perceived as substandard because they could only be used at certain locations and did not cover all health services. For immigrants who earned too much to qualify for public coverage or subsidies, the high cost of private insurance meant that some purchased plans with high deductibles they could not afford to use or went without coverage and paid the state's tax penalty. For those who eventually received coverage, limited English proficiency and inadequate health literacy made it difficult for them to navigate the complex healthcare system. Finally, in some instances racialized discrimination led to problematic encounters with White and non-White providers who perceived immigrants as "difficult" patients or whose treatment decisions were affected by implicit racialized anti-immigrant bias.

Premigration demographic differences between Dominicans and Brazilians influenced their perceptions of discrimination in health care and the broader society. Dominicans with darker skin tones and lower socioeconomic status in their country of origin were more likely to mention negative racialized healthcare experiences even though most were longtime green card holders or naturalized US citizens and eligible for all public coverage options. Conversely, Brazilians with lighter skin tones and higher premigration socioeconomic status were more likely to perceive discrimination as anti-immigrant because more of them were undocumented. Ethnicity became more important as limited English proficiency and perceived cultural differences between Americans, on the one hand, and Brazilians and Dominicans, on the other, influenced health literacy and affected their ability to navigate the healthcare system and interact with providers.

Regardless of the differences in their healthcare encounters, Brazilians and Dominicans spoke equally often about the threat presented by racialized enforcement from police and immigration authorities to their movement to and from healthcare facilities. Many feared that police stops at subway stations or in their cars on the way to appointments could lead to their arrest, detention, and eventual deportation. Some perceived that using health services and being unable to pay medical bills could derail their future naturalization or lead to deportation. Racialized enforcement, which extended the heavy hand of the punitive state into health care, figured into the calculated decisions some Latinx immigrants made about their health. Living in a progressive state with immigrant-inclusive health reform and world-class medical care could not allay Latinx immigrants' concerns that racialized legal status negatively affected their lives. As we will explore in the next chapter, Massachusetts's decision to fully comply with ACA implementation alongside increased immigration enforcement intensified the impact that racialized legal status had on Latinx immigrants' healthcare experiences.

CHAPTER 3

The ACA Narrows, Rather than Widens, Healthcare Access (2015–2016)

[Immigrants] come to Massachusetts because Massachusetts law . . . says any person that declares the intention to live in the State of Massachusetts has the right to all benefits. It's not connected to the federal concept of legal or illegal; it's the basic right. So that's why in Massachusetts, to prove that you have the right [to health coverage], you just have to present an electricity bill or lease contract that shows that you live in Massachusetts. So [state officials] don't care that you live in Massachusetts legally or illegally. . . . In the other states you have to prove your immigration status.

—*Luisa, BHC provider interviewed in 2016*

Whoever provides [health care] or if it's an option, they probably don't want immigrants to hear about it, because they want them to get sick, they want them to be poor, they want them to go back. That's the ultimate goal, you know. I mean, it's better to be a dog than an immigrant, when it comes to going to the hospital, because if you find a dog that has been hurt, we will . . . accept it in any animal hospital, right away. But an immigrant will be rejected.

—*Manuel, Salvadoran pastor interviewed in 2016*

When I returned to Boston and began interviewing immigrants, providers, and advocates in the fall of 2015, it had been nearly 10 years since Massachusetts had passed and implemented its landmark Chapter 58 health reform, which included all state residents regardless of documentation status. The Affordable Care Act, often called Obamacare, had recently been implemented. When I concluded my interviews with stakeholders in the summer of 2013, some were thrilled that increased federal funding would allow more working and middle-income people to qualify for Medicaid as well as subsidies to purchase coverage in the state's health exchange. Others were concerned about how the commonwealth's health coverage information technology system would connect with the ACA and whether the shift would adversely affect immigrants with public coverage. Luisa and Manuel's statements provide insights into how immigrants, providers, and advocates I interviewed in 2015–2016 recalled what happened after the ACA was implemented in Massachusetts.

Luisa emphasized the inclusivity of the state's policy to grant benefits to all individuals residing within its borders regardless of documentation status. But Manuel spoke quite strongly about how immigrants remained excluded from care. He shockingly thought it was easier for dogs to get health care than immigrants in the commonwealth. I still shudder when I think about this remark from our interview. The juxtaposition of their views illustrates the contradictions that marked ACA implementation in Massachusetts. The ACA excluded federally ineligible immigrants, which meant that the commonwealth had to modify its rules to continue offering basic health coverage to all residents. Legal status increasingly stratified access to coverage for immigrants across the state, making it more difficult for some to retain their coverage and raising out-of-pocket costs for many.

This chapter analyzes the effects of the ACA on Latinx immigrants in 2015–2016. In addition to the federal-level restrictions based on legal status, more documents were required to determine income eligibility. The shift to an online enrollment process created more cumbersome burdens for state residents, particularly Latinx immigrants with limited English proficiency and little or no internet access. On the national and state level, the shifting sociopolitical climate was reshaping conversations about healthcare policy, and racialized legal status became more salient. Proposals for immigrant-inclusive legislation, such as issuing driver's licenses to the undocumented and making Massachusetts a sanctuary state, had not been passed.[1] Recently elected Republican governor Charlie Baker proposed drastic cuts to the state's Health Safety Net program, which remained the primary way that immigrants excluded by the ACA could get preventive health coverage. As the 2016 presidential campaign got underway, Donald Trump and other contenders for the Republican nomination promised to repeal Obamacare and implement more punitive immigration policies if they won the general election.

At the same time, the surge of unaccompanied minors from Central America seeking asylum at the southern border brought renewed attention to the Obama administration's immigration policies. Since the Boston area has a sizable Central American population, some of those minors were relocated there to be united with relatives. For that reason, in 2015–2016 I added Salvadoran immigrants to the study and interviewed 10 of them. I found new respondents among Brazilian and Dominican immigrants, interviewing 15 and 14 of them respectively, for a total of 39 immigrants. Among them, 6 Brazilians and 6 Salvadorans were undocumented; 3 Brazilians and 2 Salvadorans had green cards; and 1 Brazilian and 1 Salvadoran were naturalized US citizens (see Table I-3). Two Salvadorans had temporary protected status. In contrast, 11 Dominicans had green cards, and 3 were naturalized citizens. These documentation statuses aligned with the demographic characteristics of the Brazilians and Dominicans I interviewed in 2012–2013.

As in 2012–2013, I interviewed 19 healthcare providers from the Boston Health Coalition and 25 employees of immigrant and health advocacy organizations. Although the majority of these providers and advocates were new respondents, I was able to reinterview 7 providers and 10 advocates who had been interviewed in 2012–2013. Interviewing members of these different stakeholder groups was essential to understand the consequences of ACA implementation for immigrants' healthcare access in 2015–2016.[2] More important, the perspectives of Brazilian, Dominican, and Salvadoran immigrants were vital for comprehending the role that racialized legal status played in immigrants' lives as virulently anti-immigrant and racist rhetoric intensified. The ascendance of Donald Trump as the 2016 GOP presidential nominee made Latinx Bostonians fearful of his potential presidency, leading immigrants, advocates, and providers to discuss immigrants' disenrollment from health care and other public benefits. Respondents also described an uptick in RLS discrimination toward immigrants of various ethnoracial backgrounds in Boston.

From Chapter 58 to Obamacare in the Commonwealth

Because the Affordable Care Act was modeled after Massachusetts's Chapter 58 health reform, stakeholders anticipated that the commonwealth was well positioned to implement the national legislation. Most Massachusetts policymakers and health advocates viewed the ACA as a boon because it would extend Medicaid to those whose incomes had previously made them ineligible, provide more subsidies to middle-income people to purchase coverage through the state's health exchange, and increase funding for community health centers.[3] The federal reform would also guarantee that people could not be denied coverage for preexisting conditions and that young adults up to age 26 could remain on their parents' health insurance plans.[4] Although the US Supreme Court decided that states could opt out of the Medicaid expansion, Massachusetts never considered abandoning its existing commitment to coverage for low-income state residents without official federal documentation status.[5] Massachusetts and 26 other states expanded Medicaid, whereas 21 states had not done so by June 2014.[6] Consequently, individuals' state of residence determined their access to some crucial ACA provisions.

Nonetheless, inequality based on documentation status and income had been built into the Massachusetts reform (see Table 2-1, Figure 2-1). Under Obamacare, these forms of stratification became more powerful in determining access to health coverage. Those whose legal statuses rendered them ineligible for federally funded programs or whose incomes were too high to qualify for the available public options had fewer options in the private insurance market. Massachusetts state legislators and health and immigration advocates realized that, although most naturalized citizens and long-term lawful permanent residents would gain from Obamacare, some immigrants who were eligible for coverage under the Massachusetts reform would be deemed ineligible under the ACA.[7] Undocumented immigrants who previously used the state's health exchange to shop for private insurance coverage were now prohibited from doing so.[8] The application process as well as income eligibility cutoffs and some public coverage options changed.[9] Rather than applying to MassHealth, which previously sorted all applicants into the options they qualified for, ACA applicants completed online forms or submitted paper applications to the Commonwealth Connector for the state's new health exchange. That shift created massive confusion for many state residents, but it weighed especially heavily on immigrants who had not been naturalized and were not proficient in English. Many found the bureaucratic maze impossible to navigate by themselves, and some gave up after being summarily rejected even though they were eligible for coverage.

Figure 3-1 shows the most common types of public coverage options for adults ages 19–64, such as Health Safety Net, MassHealth Standard, and ConnectorCare, and includes the criteria for eligibility related to income and documentation status, what types of services each includes, and where they can be used.[10] Eligibility requirements for Health Safety Net and MassHealth Standard were similar to those under the original Massachusetts reform.[11] Moreover, because short-term LPRs and those with other special statuses were covered under the state's Commonwealth Care program before the ACA, state legislators revised the program to ensure that they would remain covered under Obamacare. Subsequently, Commonwealth Care was renamed ConnectorCare.[12]

Those with private ConnectorCare coverage still had wide access to medical facilities, but more income eligible long-term LPRs, refugees, asylees, and citizens were shifted to Medicaid under the ACA. Subsequently, Massachusetts further reduced state funding for the Health Safety Net program, which primarily covered undocumented immigrants and other low-income residents. Together, these income and documentation status requirements increased the stratification of coverage.

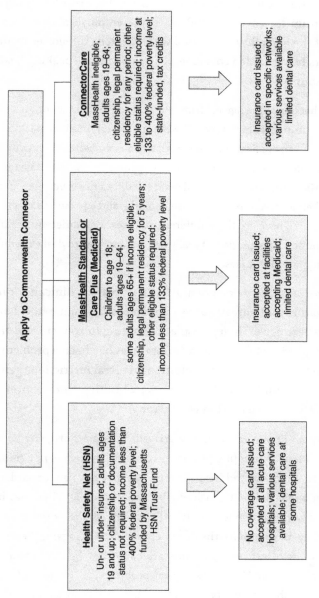

Apply to Commonwealth Connector

Health Safety Net (HSN)
Un- or under-insured; adults ages 19 and up; citizenship or documentation status not required; income less than 400% federal poverty level; funded by Massachusetts HSN Trust Fund

MassHealth Standard or Care Plus (Medicaid)
Children to age 18; adults ages 19–64; some adults ages 65+ if income eligible; citizenship, legal permanent residency for 5 years; other eligible status required; income less than 133% federal poverty level

ConnectorCare
MassHealth ineligible; adults ages 19–64; citizenship, legal permanent residency for any period; other eligible status required; income at 133 to 400% federal poverty level; state-funded, tax credits

No coverage card issued; accepted at all acute care hospitals; various services available; dental care at some hospitals

Insurance card issued; accepted at facilities accepting Medicaid; limited dental care

Insurance card issued; accepted in specific networks; various services available; limited dental care

Figure 3-1. Massachusetts Coverage Options for Adults (Ages 19–64) After ACA Implementation

In numerous interviews, respondents said that the range of documentation status categories created confusion for those helping immigrants sign up for coverage. Indeed, some employees' own incomprehension of the eligibility associated with different categories resulted in immigrants being denied coverage. Kelly, a Spanish-speaking health advocate, recounted:

> I think that one of the biggest frustrations that I've dealt with . . . is when I get calls from clients that say, "I went to the community health center to complete an application and I was turned away because I am undocumented." Some people are hired to help people apply, but they are not necessarily trained to understand what the difference is between an asylum seeker, a person that has a case pending, and a person that actually is an asylee. Those are three different statuses with different qualifications, and some people do not really understand how to deal with different immigration statuses.

If the range of existing documentation statuses was difficult for health-care navigators and bureaucrats to understand, imagine how hard this must have been for ordinary people attempting to apply for coverage.[13]

The complexity of documentation statuses had been a problem under the Massachusetts reform, but additional federal restrictions generated more confusion under the ACA. Maggie, a health advocate interviewed in 2015, described what often went wrong:

> Let's say an immigrant is newly arrived, they are not going to ever pass the identity proofing process because the system is not going to be able to verify their address. That means they can't go forward, they can't get a real-time automatic eligibility decision. . . . Then they have to fill out a paper application [that] they are who they say they are, which they may not have the documents to do. And again, the worker inputs an incorrect immigration status and they [get an] erroneous eligibility decision. That's the biggest problem: lots of cases of immigrants who should qualify for greater benefits than they're getting because of these errors.

Undocumented and other immigrants lost or did not obtain coverage, even when they might have been eligible for some state-funded programs.

The lack of language-appropriate assistance, another marker of racialized legal status, continued to pose a structural barrier when applying for coverage. Most application materials online and on paper were in English, and educational materials explaining what health insurance was and how it could be used were rarely provided. According to Penelope, a health advocate, LEP immigrants often remained "eligible but unenrolled." Julia, a Dominican health advocate, saw the same lack of communication between providers and patients she had observed before and told me frankly that "we're still working on this question I'm sure you've heard millions of times: Is it a duty . . . is it *our* duty, to make sure everything is available" in the languages that patients understand?

The ACA required health facilities receiving federal funds to have qualified interpreters available for LEP patients when doing so was necessary to provide them with "meaningful access" to health care. It also restricted the common practice of having adults or minors who accompanied LEP patients serve as interpreters, since it can lead to dangerous misunderstandings. But as I learned in my 2016 interview with Angelica, the language access attorney who explained the connection between language access and Title VI of the Civil Rights Act in Chapter 1, the ACA had no provision for enforcing this rule. When coupled with the inability to obtain coverage due to documentation status, the result can be deadly for the most vulnerable.

Romina, a 31-year-old undocumented Salvadoran immigrant, eloquently explained how these conditions led to deteriorating health:

> The truth is many people, . . . I have seen this in families . . . where people who don't have documents or don't have health coverage, I have seen people who are really sick and don't go to the hospital and nearly die. Many of us have come to this country with dreams, but without documents or health coverage return home in a coffin. There are opportunities, but there are also limitations without health coverage or speaking the language. People work, don't take care of themselves, don't eat well. And

because they know they'll try to apply for coverage and won't get it, sadly, they give up on their dreams.

Romina described the intersectional barriers of language, documentation status, and lack of health coverage that she and others faced. She was one of the two immigrants interviewed in 2015–2016 who said they had personally experienced racial discrimination in the healthcare system. With medium-brown skin and long, straight black hair, she was perceived as a Latina as well as undocumented. Despite living in Massachusetts, where undocumented immigrants theoretically had more access to coverage than in other parts of the country, Romina and many like her lived under perilous health conditions without proper access to care.

In fall 2013, the rollouts of both the federal Healthcare.gov website and the state's Commonwealth Connector website were disasters.[14] I heard countless stories from health advocates about the resulting chaos. State residents with a wide range of documentation statuses were inadvertently kicked off their coverage.

The shift from paper to online enrollment created significant barriers. Levels of English proficiency, computer literacy, and access to high-speed internet were lower among immigrants, communities of color, and those with fewer financial resources.[15] But most Massachusetts residents found the jargon in the ACA application confusing. Jenny, a health advocate, emphasized that "you may read English, or you may read Spanish, but if . . . you don't understand what's a deductible, what's a co-pay, what's a premium, what are tax penalties and advance premium tax credits, well, are you really able to make informed decisions about health care and health insurance?"

The website's new, instantaneous process for verifying applicants' identity and eligibility was a major source of problems. Everyone was told to include information on their residency in the state, income, and documentation status. If applicants or their navigators made any mistakes, however trivial, applicants were deemed ineligible for coverage. Even experienced navigators such as Kelly, the Spanish-speaking health advocate quoted earlier, had great difficulty enrolling people: "It took so much time to complete the application process with each person who called that it was impossible to help more than a few of them each day." Lucia, a Brazilian who worked as a healthcare navigator, described what she and the applicants experienced: "There were steps in the electronic application process where you had to stop filling it out and submit your proof of identity in the mail. You could not move forward in the process until you did so." After the application finally got processed, "applicants would receive a letter stating 'because of your documentation status, you don't have the right'" to coverage. "It was just one line" in the letter. "So, for people who don't speak English well, what do they do? They receive the letter and [think] 'Oh my God, my immigration status!' So they bring the letter to me. It causes so much confusion!"

Up to 310,000 Massachusetts residents of various legal statuses had to be enrolled in temporary and free MassHealth coverage for 2014 due to these bureaucratic problems.[16] I could hear the exasperation in her voice when Maggie, a health advocate, described the fall 2013 enrollment process:

> We were bombarded by . . . sick people that really counted on their health insurance to get them access to healthcare services. . . . People calling us saying "I reapplied, I did everything they said, but my coverage is ending, . . . and I don't have a new plan and they can't tell me . . . what's going on." And we didn't really have an answer for them because the state didn't initially say they were going to start this temporary MassHealth coverage program . . . to extend Commonwealth Care. So many people were calling us, and we couldn't give them answers, which is extremely frustrating and stressful for advocates across the state trying to help these people.

After listing many causes for interruptions of coverage, Maggie said that health advocates spent a lot of time "helping people that had already been on the program and needed help getting back on" after "falling off for mostly administrative reasons." Many stakeholders made similar remarks about the initial enrollment period. At the time I interviewed health advocates in 2015–2016, they said that the process had improved. Later in our interview, Maggie acknowledged those improvements, but emphasized that for "the most vulnerable immigrants, as well as the disabled population in the state, the system still can't determine eligibility appropriately."

Immigrants themselves attested to the lack of information about the shift to Obamacare. Just half of the 39 immigrants I interviewed in 2015–2016 recalled hearing anything about the ACA. I usually asked, "What, if anything, have you heard about health reform in Massachusetts or the United States?" Most of the 20 who responded that they had heard something mentioned hearing about the Massachusetts reform or Obamacare but were vague on the details. This was true regardless of their nationality, educational level, and English proficiency.[17] Like those interviewed in 2012–2013, more Brazilians had at a least college degree than did those from the Dominican Republic or El Salvador.[18] In terms of English language skills, 6 of 15 Brazilians, 3 of 14 Dominicans, and 2 of 10 Salvadorans reported excellent or good proficiency.[19] These factors most likely shaped individuals' knowledge of health reforms.

Jazmin, a 40-year-old Salvadoran with temporary protected status, said, "I have heard that . . . everyone is supposed to have insurance and they will check your income. Depending on your income, you may qualify for free insurance coverage or have to pay a certain amount. . . . But I don't understand it much or what [health conditions] it treats." Adelia, a 50-year-old Brazilian with a student visa, was more skeptical about the ACA: "It's very confusing with rules that change at a speed that I cannot understand. . . . The only thing I understand . . . is that people are not satisfied with it because if you no longer have insurance through your job, . . . you have to enroll in Obamacare and pay for coverage that some people say is not cheap."

This criticism of Obamacare was common among some US-born and naturalized citizens. Amalia, a 53-year-old Dominican who is a naturalized citizen, complained that people who did not buy insurance had to pay a penalty even if they did not use any healthcare services. She spent much of our interview criticizing the high cost of coverage and her family's inability to maintain it and concluded that "Massachusetts is the worst" and its "healthcare system is a piece of garbage." State residents such as Amalia who objected to the individual mandate, which was in both the Massachusetts reform and Obamacare, did not understand its rationale. Rather than being an infringement on individual choice, the tax penalty spread the risks and costs of care across the whole population. If young and healthy people decided not to buy health insurance while only those who needed to use healthcare services did, this imbalance would undermine the principle that makes health insurance work. Other immigrants I interviewed felt that the exclusion of the undocumented from Medicaid was discriminatory, even though Massachusetts retained the Health Safety Net program for those who could not afford to buy private insurance.

The shift to Obamacare created enormous barriers for those enrolling in coverage for the first time or renewing their existing coverage. Black, Latinx, immigrant, and low-income Massachusetts residents were all disadvantaged, as individuals in these groups were disproportionately unable to surmount these obstacles and unlikely to know people who could assist them with the enrollment process.[20] Racialized legal status discrimination compounded these barriers for Latinx Bostonians, however. As federal policy transformed the contours of eligibility, disparities in health coverage, care, and outcomes became more severe, demonstrating medical legal violence in action.

Latinx Immigrants' Difficulties in Accessing Care Under the ACA

Providers and advocates agreed that the available resources were insufficient to accommodate the growing numbers of people seeking health care under the ACA. It became increasingly difficult to find doctors who accepted Medicaid for patients who benefited from the program's expansion. According to Thomas, a BHC provider, "for MassHealth, less than 50% of physicians in Massachusetts take it, and far less than that take Health Safety Net." The number of primary care providers did not rise, despite the ACA's requirement that everyone have a PCP to coordinate their care. The results of increased demand for services included longer waiting times for authorization and gaps in coverage that disrupted both preventive and critical care.

Most of the immigrants interviewed in 2015–2016 had health coverage (32 of 39), and a majority had a regular healthcare provider (26 of 39).[21] Salvadorans had difficulty identifying what type of coverage they had, although some told me they had coverage. I am not sure whether this was due to their fear of disclosing that they had public coverage or their inability to comprehend the question despite my posing it in different ways. Nevertheless, as in 2012–2013, most of these Boston-area immigrants were able to access coverage and see a provider regularly despite tedious (re)enrollment processes, major policy shifts, and language barriers. According to census data from 2015–2016, 91% of the US population was insured.[22] Unfortunately, Latinx people accounted for 40 percent of the uninsured in 2016.[23] The immigrant respondents I interviewed in 2015–2016 were more likely to have coverage compared with their counterparts elsewhere in the country.

Lorena, a 55-year-old undocumented Brazilian who was ineligible for Obamacare, had little sympathy for her insured friends when they complained about the high cost of coverage. "I try to tell them, 'It is better this way, at least you know there is assistance.' And they continue complaining, 'No, it is not, because I have to keep paying and I'm required to have coverage,' blah blah blah. . . . I turned around and told them, 'Do you want to trade places? I would pay $1,000 because I found work and would pay.' It's easy to complain . . . when you already have something that others don't."

Respondents with coverage thought that their healthcare costs had risen, mainly because of higher premiums, co-pays, or deductibles for publicly subsidized or private nonsubsidized care. Patients who paid these costs out of pocket either did not make appointments with specialists or had high no-show rates. Aware of these challenges, providers spent extra time helping patients navigate the system and expressed frustration that coverage did not meet patients' needs. Greg, a BHC provider with mostly Brazilian patients, recounted: "Those who are insured, they've been complaining actively to me about paying more both for medications and for visits. . . . Some of them will say, 'Oh, I have Health Safety Net but I got a bill for a thousand dollars from the hospital, why?' Because they have to pay down a deductible. Health Safety Net and MassHealth say, 'We cover you once you paid this much money.' It's not [something] you pay to MassHealth, it's a deductible you pay" when you first receive services. Deductibles can be high "because some immigrants make a reasonable amount of money. I'm not saying they're doing great, but enough so they're above the [eligibility] cap, but not enough that they could get private insurance or through the ACA. So [Health Safety Net] will say, 'Well, you have to spend this much money before you get covered for everything.'"

A significant number of patients and providers expressed concerns about the reduction in services that accompanied the shift to Obamacare. Although some individuals with Health Safety Net and MassHealth had previously received dental and vision care, these services were not included in most insurance plans after ACA implementation. Renata, a 47-year-old Dominican and naturalized US citizen, said that her insurance used to include some vision and dental services but now it does not, so her coverage "is worse than it was before." Agustina, a 34-year-old Salvadoran with temporary protected status, said "When I have to go to the dentist and pay, it is too expensive. . . . In my country, I could afford to go to the dentist. But here, no. So, we don't have the same benefits that a person born here has, [or a person] that has their documents." Agustina, like many other immigrants, did not realize that dental care is typically not included under most health insurance plans in the United States.

Thus, despite the ACA's efforts to reduce the cost of health coverage and care, some immigrants shared the view expressed by Silvana, a 33-year-old Brazilian with a green card: "Here, I can't afford to get sick. Even if you are middle class here, . . . you can't get sick as it will wreck your budget."[24] This perception was also common among US-born residents of Massachusetts, as healthcare premiums and other costs rose after the Massachusetts and ACA reforms.[25] Nationally, studies indicated similar increases that kept the cost of coverage out of reach, estimating that the ACA raised premiums by about 60%.[26] So individuals and families ineligible for public coverage or subsidies purchased cheaper plans with higher deductibles and co-pays to avoid the tax penalty; but they might not be able to use their coverage at all because of the cost.[27] Zoe, a health advocate, described the situation facing immigrants and other state residents: "Affordability is [a] big challenge. . . . A lot of the plans that are being offered on exchanges have limited networks and you might not be able to see the providers that you want to see or that you need to see." In Zoe's view, the focus on cost containment jeopardized the quality of care: "So, our costs are high, but the outcomes are also bad."

These systemic problems posed such immense difficulties for the state's immigrants that some opted out of the US healthcare system. Adelia, the Brazilian on a student visa, said, "If it is not a critical health problem, an emergency, I try to resolve [it] on my own. I'll take medicine brought from Brazil. Here is too bureaucratic." Alexis, a BHC provider, described how the denial of a test led one of her patients to seek care in her home country: "I had a lovely Columbian patient who has a very strong family history of colon cancer in her family. . . . I thought it was perfectly reasonable to get a screening colonoscopy on her because she has actually a risk factor. Insurance denied it, so she went back to Columbia and got a colonoscopy for $100 and handed me the records, and I was thrilled." Rather than dealing with the bureaucracy and exorbitant costs of the US healthcare system, some immigrants received medication and remedies from abroad and consulted with medical providers online or in person while visiting their home country.

Racialized Legal Status Makes Latinx Immigrants' Lives Harder than Before

When I conducted these interviews in 2015–2016, the local sociopolitical climate for immigrants had been altered by the influx of unaccompanied minors at the southern border in the summer of 2014. I vividly remember the heart-wrenching media images of Central American children crossing the US–Mexico border to seek refuge from the violence in their home countries.[28] When I returned to the Boston area, I heard how directly and deeply the local Salvadoran community had been affected by this humanitarian crisis. Gabriel, the director of a Central American advocacy organization, described the process of reuniting some of these children with Boston-area relatives and the difficulties they faced applying for asylum in the two years since their arrival. "If the parents of the kids . . . are under temporary protected status here in the United States, and the children there are under 20–21 years old, the parents here can petition to help the kids who come here to United States through their refugee status." With "around a thousand Salvadorans" who have applied or reapplied for TPS, "we have been guiding many of them . . . through the process [so] they can bring their kids here."

The racialized legal status burdens in the bureaucratic process for the relocation and legalization of these children were extremely onerous. In addition to meeting the requirements for asylum applications, the federal government demanded extensive documentation and DNA tests to prove the legal and biological kinship between parents and children. Applications in English posed a challenge for those with limited English proficiency. Gabriel also expressed concern that undocumented relatives in the US who were or sought to become legal guardians for these children could be detained and deported in the process of picking up the children from US government custody. Some had already been appointed legal guardians by the children's parents, but those documents were not regarded as valid without further proof, and the guardians themselves had to be vetted, which was very risky if these adults were undocumented.

Given the size of the local Central American enclave, immigrant and health advocates immediately addressed the crisis. Raquel, a state government employee, commented that state funds for refugees had to be reallocated to assist with the "influx of unaccompanied teens and their difficulties" in adapting to life in Boston. These events drew attention to the precarity of temporary protected status, under which at least 400,000 people, many of them from Central America and the Caribbean, live in the United States.[29] As discussed in Chapter 1, TPS is a documented status that grants work authorization, Social Security numbers, and some public benefits to recipients for 6–18 months after arrival. It is not a path to citizenship, however, and must be extended by the US government and renewed by recipients to maintain their legal status.[30] For this reason, sociologist Cecilia Menjívar has described TPS as a "liminally legal" status that does not provide full security from deportation.[31]

Salvadoran advocates and immigrants I interviewed discussed the stresses of living in limbo. Only 2 of the 10 Salvadorans I spoke with had TPS. Gabriel, the director of the Central American organization quoted earlier, emphasized the difficulties this status causes in their daily lives and the grave uncertainties it creates about their future. "While renewing [TPS], paying $465, waiting for the work permit, sometimes we lose our jobs. Because the [employers] said, 'Well, you need to bring your work permit authorization, if you don't bring it . . . you are out [of] work.' People who have been here for more than fifteen years . . . feel that they need their legal status regular[ized]." Hondurans have been in the country with TPS since 1990, and Salvadorans have had TPS eligibility since 2001. "Many people are doing well but want to become permanent residents as soon as possible." Until the United States allows them to gain a more secure status, Gabriel concluded, "they go to bed wondering what is going to happen tomorrow, and they wake up again" with the same uncertainty.

The shifting sociopolitical and economic climate in Brazil contributed to a rise in immigration to Massachusetts after 2015. While some upwardly mobile Brazilians left amid an economic freefall, other Brazilians fled in response to criminal or political violence. Despite coming from differing socioeconomic backgrounds in Brazil and arriving in the United States either through the southern border or with visas, these migrants experienced tremendous hardships after they arrived. Micaela, a Brazilian advocate I also interviewed in 2012–2013, described their desperate situation: "Once people get here, it's very difficult. Some arrive with their families and have nothing [except] the clothes on their backs. Immigration takes everything from them at the border, even their Brazilian passports. They have no documents."

The Racialization of Latinx Immigrants

Much of my discussion in this chapter so far has focused on legal status; I now turn more attention to the "racialized" aspect of racialized legal status. The analysis begins with how migrants ethnoracially classified themselves. Using US categories, most Brazilians (9 of 15) and Dominicans (8 of 14) self-classified as Latino, whereas most Salvadorans (8 of 10) self-classified as Hispanic.[32] Interestingly, only 1 Salvadoran self-classified as Latino, and only 2 Dominicans self-classified as Hispanic. Three Brazilians and 2 Dominicans self-classified as Black; no Salvadorans did. One Brazilian, Dominican, and Salvadoran each self-classified as White. Thus, most of these immigrants viewed themselves as non-White in the United States, regardless of their appearance.

Most Dominicans and Salvadorans felt that the categories of Hispanic and Latinx were synonymous and interchangeable. But a few, such as Cristobal, a 32-year-old Dominican with medium-brown skin tone, dark-brown eyes, and short, curly black hair who had a green card, refused to call himself Hispanic. When asked whether he identified as Hispanic, Latino, or both, he replied: "Hispanic, I don't like it much. I like Latino better." When I asked why, he said: "Hispanic is . . . a lot more cliché. Like a very popular term, but Latino unites us more." He added, "I think that Latino is more American. Hispanic feels like we were colonized by Spain."

Brazilians, along with most Dominicans and Salvadorans, agreed that Brazilians are Latino but not Hispanic.[33] Some Dominicans and Salvadorans also perceived Brazilians as different from other Latinos but found it difficult to describe the difference. Other studies indicate that individuals of Latin American descent in the United States do not share a consistent interpretation of the Latino and Hispanic categories, which were created by the US Census Bureau.[34] Unfortunately, because Brazilians are not Hispanic, they are often excluded from research on Latin Americans, and their ethnoracial classification and identity in the United States are more complicated. The ambiguity around Brazilians' relationship to these categories and their place in the US ethnoracial hierarchy has rarely been investigated.[35]

An important way to highlight the significance of racialized legal status to immigrants living in the United States is by exploring how they believed other people in this country racially classified them and comparing it to their own sense of identity. How others perceive immigrants shapes their experiences of ethnoracial discrimination in everyday interactions. I found that immigrants' self-classifications mostly aligned with how they perceived that *other people* classified them in ethnoracial terms. This was particularly true for Salvadorans: 7 of 10 believed others classified them as Hispanic.[36] While 7 of 15 Brazilians believed others classified them as Latino, 4 believed others classified them as Hispanic. And 8 of 14 Dominicans believed others classified them as either Hispanic or Latino. Although no Brazilians or Salvadorans believed other people classified them as Black, four Dominicans felt this was the case. Strikingly, when asked how other people classified them, two Brazilians and one Dominican rejected the categories provided. They replied "Other" and said they were seen as "immigrant." These respondents directly connected being perceived by strangers as an immigrant with a racial classification, demonstrating the salience of the intersection between race and legal status in the United States.[37] Comments from other immigrants implied their racialization. They thought they were perceived as outsiders and foreigners because they were not White relative to those who were considered "real White" Americans. Notably, only one Brazilian and one Salvadoran believed that others classified them as White.

The Financial and Housing Insecurity of Immigrant Families and Communities

The racialized legal status of immigrants shaped their economic situation in Boston, as it did across the United States. Although the economy had recovered to some extent from the Great Recession, levels of employment and earnings remained highly skewed by class and race. Social mobility was still limited for poor and working-class people, whether citizens or noncitizens.[38] Nationally, income and wealth inequality had increased by about 20 percent from 1980 to 2016, with middle- and lower-income individuals and families benefiting significantly less from these decades of economic growth than those in the top 5%.[39] Boston was deemed the country's most unequal major city in 2016, mainly because of the disproportionate gains made by high-income earners and the lack of affordable housing for lower-income residents.[40] According to 2020 census data, Massachusetts ranked 4th of 50 states in housing values, and housing was most expensive in the Boston metropolitan area.[41] Rising rents and property values have been attributed to gentrification, particularly as city and state officials encouraged economic development by attracting pharmaceutical and biotech companies.[42]

Black and Latinx residents did not benefit equally from this economic boom but were disproportionately affected by the housing crisis.[43] In 2015, a landmark report found that nonimmigrant Black Bostonians' household median net worth was $8, compared with $0 for Dominicans and $247,500 for Whites.[44] Most working families' main asset is the home they own. Unable to purchase and get mortgages for houses and condominiums, many Black and Latinx residents struggle to find affordable rental housing and accumulate wealth. Persistent structural racism has limited the housing prospects of African Americans and, by extension, immigrants who are racialized as Black, including some of the Dominicans and Brazilians I interviewed.

While taking public transportation or driving throughout the metropolitan area to conduct interviews, I listened to local news stations (usually GBH, one of two National Public Radio affiliates in the Boston area) report on the severe shortage of affordable housing. Respondents brought up the effects of economic inequality and gentrification on formerly inexpensive neighborhoods and areas that were once ethnic enclaves for Brazilians, Dominicans, Salvadorans, and other immigrant communities. Jeff, a community advocate in Somerville, an exceptionally diverse small city where immigrants and their children once formed most residents, described the consequences of this transformation: "The whole area . . . [is] gentrifying very quickly. Somerville is no longer a 'gateway city' [for immigrants]. It still functions that way in the sense that it has established Brazilian, Salvadoran, and other communities where people come in initially. They are doubled up for a while, and there are a few slumlord situations where you get three families [living] in two bedrooms. As soon as they have the economic capacity they move out. But those cities are beginning to gentrify in the same way." As immigrants moved to neighboring cities, some of which were predominantly White, their presence revitalized local economies. But it also led to debates about the lack of racial and ethnic representation in local governments and the need for English for Speakers of Other Languages (ESOL) programs in schools and language interpretation to access social services.[45]

As economic and political crises in other countries led to an influx of new immigrants and economic and racial inequality in the Boston area increased, immigrants were increasingly unable to find affordable housing and were thus forced to move to less expensive neighborhoods. These circumstances were exacerbated by the more noticeably racist and nativist national sociopolitical climate as the 2016 presidential contest got underway. Boston immigrants, and especially people of color, began to feel the heat, which heightened the impact of racialized legal status on their healthcare access and health.

The Intensifying Racialized Anti-immigrant Climate amid the Rise of Trump

When I was halfway through the 2015–2016 interviews, the campaigns for the presidential nomination began. Hillary Clinton was regarded as the front-runner for the Democratic Party nomination. The Republican Party, which was anxious to regain the White House, had a much wider pool of candidates. Among them was Donald Trump, a real estate tycoon, reality TV celebrity, and political newcomer who had gained notoriety for challenging Barack Obama's eligibility for the presidency by alleging that he was not born in the United States. Trump also falsely claimed that Obama was Muslim, which made him unfit to be president of a Christian nation. The racist, xenophobic, and anti-Muslim biases Trump exhibited in office were visible even before he declared his candidacy.[46] In seeking the Republican nomination, Trump vilified "illegal" immigrants as criminals and promised to build a wall on the US–Mexico border to keep them out.[47] Although he was initially considered a long shot, Trump tapped into the resentment that many White Americans, especially those who were in regions experiencing economic decline and identified as evangelical Christians, felt about the country's changing ethnoracial demographics and declining economic power.[48] He explicitly stated that he would repeal Obamacare and undo other policies Obama initiated, including the DACA program that allowed many undocumented immigrants whose parents had brought them to the United States as children to remain and work in the country.

Because of Trump's lack of political experience, the numerous scandals that tarnished his reputation, and his explicitly racist, sexist, anti-immigrant, and other offensive social media posts and campaign statements, I, like many political spectators, did not think he would be a viable candidate, let alone become the nominee. I was stunned to see his unprecedented campaign take off and push out more politically savvy and better-established contenders. My shock was shared by respondents and those at events I attended around Boston. Unprompted, Trump's name came up in interviews when I asked stakeholders about changes in health and immigration policy, how they thought immigrants were affected by them, and what life was like for immigrants in Boston. A Brazilian health advocate, Alcione, worried that "Trump's rhetoric triggered, woke up the wolf that was dormant in a lot of people." She and others recognized that if Trump won the presidency, the well-being of many marginalized groups living in the United States would be at risk.

Many immigrants I interviewed were acutely aware of the shift in the national sociopolitical climate and felt it was affecting them locally. Of the 39 immigrants interviewed in 2015–2016, 21 reported experiencing perceived discrimination during their time in the country. Those individuals were nearly equally distributed across nationalities. Of those 21, 18 (half of all those interviewed) felt that the discrimination they encountered was specifically tied to their being immigrants.[49] Among Brazilians, Dominicans, and Salvadorans who thought they had experienced anti-immigrant discrimination, six members of each group connected it to their appearance and to having limited English proficiency or speaking English with an accent. This opinion was noticeably more common than it had been in 2012–2013, when 12 of the 31 (less than 2 out of 5) Brazilian and Dominican immigrants interviewed reported what they perceived to be anti-immigrant discrimination. In 2015–2016, those in all three nationality groups who reported perceived anti-immigrant discrimination tended to self-classify as Black, Hispanic, and Latino. Interestingly, only two Brazilians who experienced discrimination attributed it to their race.

After Trump appeared on the national stage, many respondents felt that their lives had become more difficult and thought it had become socially acceptable to discriminate against immigrants both implicitly and explicitly. While these respondents themselves did not use the phrase "racialized legal status" to describe this discrimination, their statements clearly indicate their recognition that being perceived by others as foreigners who were likely to be undocumented because they were non-White shaped how others treated them.

Some directly attributed this shift to Trump's influence. Micaela, the Brazilian advocate quoted earlier, said that the "very strong anti-immigrant climate" was clear at a Housecleaners' Cooperative that she coordinated: "Recently, a client from the cooperative called and said she wanted to see her cleaner's documents. I said, 'Ma'am, you can call another cleaning company because here we don't ask about the immigrant's migration status. We work with human beings and human beings don't need documents.' [The client] said, 'But you have to have a work permit.' I asked, 'Did you ask your plumber if he has a work permit?' [The client replied,] 'It is different.' [I asked,] 'How is that different?'" Expressing her own opinion to me, Micaela concluded: "It's because if a person doesn't speak English, they are considered different. And this Trump, for me, he's a terrorist. He provokes violence, division, and hate."

Manuel, the Salvadoran pastor quoted at the beginning of the chapter, observed that the shifting political situation and heightened immigration enforcement meant that the undocumented who were hired as day laborers faced greater problems than before. "We have a lot of people that gather to go to work in the morning. Some of them have been picked up by contractors and when they are done with the job, they [contractors] say, 'I can't pay you and if you say something, I will call ICE.' So, it's crazy."

Jenny, the health advocate quoted earlier, said that her immigrant friends who were Muslim were reluctant to apply for citizenship because of the extra scrutiny it might bring. "In this political climate . . . people are really afraid, and understandably so. We work with a lot of undocumented people, and even folks who are immigrants here legally, they are also worried. . . . I think these are legitimate concerns." Some told her that they were targeted for discrimination from law and immigrant enforcement since they were perceived as foreigners because of their appearance alone.

Charles, a 53-year-old Black Brazilian and naturalized US citizen who arrived without papers and felt that his origins would prevent him from being fully accepted as an American, stated: "It is hard for immigrants here to rent an apartment, it is so expensive, and we are not seen in a positive light. An American is treated differently if they want to rent an apartment. If the rent is $2,000, the rent will be increased for an immigrant. They [rental agents] think immigrants don't have the money to pay and they keep adding requirements, it never ends. That is discrimination." Like Micaela, Charles connected this discriminatory treatment and the presumption that immigrants do not belong in the United States to Trump's campaign rhetoric.

Respondents often made the connection between racism and anti-immigrant sentiment, which together indicated the salience of racialized legal status in their lives. Federico, a 33-year-old Salvadoran who regarded himself as Hispanic and did not report his legal status, recalled being racially profiled: "Once, I made a mistake when I was driving with a permit and not with a [Massachusetts] license. I had the license from my country and the police stopped me. He got mad and said that we Hispanics are coming and ruining everything. I knew I'd made a mistake, but he was upset with all Hispanics. I acknowledged my mistake, was respectful, and apologized and he said nothing. . . . It's like we provoke them [Americans] just based on our appearance and because we are Hispanic, we are not on their level."

Federico and Charles were acutely aware of how they are racialized by others, which contributes to their experiences of discrimination regardless of documentation status.[50] They said that Latinos and Hispanics are perceived as non-White and, correspondingly, as noncitizens who are subjected to substandard treatment before the law and in other settings.

Racialized legal status is associated with presumed foreignness and denial of belonging for Latinx immigrants, particularly in encounters with police and others who identify with the dominant White society. This assumption by others lends additional weight to immigrants' sense that in the United States, they are classified as non-White.

Racialized Legal Status Discrimination Among Latinx Bostonians

Although immigrants agreed that the worst discrimination they encountered came from White people who were born in the US, some thought that they also experienced discrimination from other immigrants based on documentation status, nationality, or both. Undocumented immigrants often felt that documented co-ethnics mistreated or looked down on them. Respondents in all the stakeholder groups perceived that Brazilians were not Latinx like Dominicans and Salvadorans and were sometimes regarded as socioeconomically and culturally superior. Brazilians' racialization as comparatively lighter and their higher premigration socioeconomic status likely contributed to this perception.

Mariana, a 42-year-old undocumented Brazilian with light-brown skin, dark-brown eyes, and long, straight, dark-brown hair who identified herself as Latina, used "we" and "them" to refer to Brazilians and Hispanics, respectively: "We are often mistaken for them. I think Americans and Hispanics know that we speak Portuguese and that our culture is different. I believe most Brazilians come to study and make a life here. They [Hispanics] need to make money to support their families at home. They don't have time to study, read, or understand what is happening here. They want to work, earn money, and not declare taxes." Agustina, the 34-year-old Salvadoran with TPS quoted earlier, reflected on her experiences with discrimination from documented Latinx people: "Sometimes, it's really curious that the same Hispanics or Latinos who get their green cards or citizenship are more discriminatory than Americans. It's like they get their papers and forget where they came from and think they are so much more [than us]." Samuel, a 48-year-old Dominican with a green card who identifies as Latino, expressed puzzlement and criticism: "I have experienced more discrimination from Latinos than North Americans, which is really odd. For example, a Puerto Rican told me, 'You are Dominican and here you don't matter.' I told him, 'You don't matter because I have more education than you.' And it's the same with the Colombians who discriminate against other [Latinos]."

In recent years, Latinos' "linked fate"—the extent to which Latinos feel that their experience is connected with that of other Latinos—has attracted attention from scholars. Together, that research indicates that experiences of discrimination from non-Latinos, documentation status, national origin, skin color, and income level shape this sense of commonality.[51] These studies, however, focus on Mexicans, Puerto Ricans, Cubans, and "Others." The Brazilians, Dominicans, and Salvadorans at the center of this book are lumped together with immigrants with different national origins in the "Other" category. Furthermore, the scholarship that examines discrimination from others in the same ethnic group or among Latinx people finds that discrimination from other Latinos reduces group identity.[52] But most of that research centers on Latinxs of Mexican descent.

Immigrants' Responses to Fear

The most common word used by respondents across the different stakeholder groups to describe the sociopolitical climate for immigrants in 2015–2016 was "fear." Joshua, an attorney who worked with a health advocacy organization, discussed immigrants' new hesitations about seeking healthcare and other social services: "People are afraid, particularly with . . . anti-immigrant sentiment which is way too prevalent these days, Donald Trump, and the flames of hate, and such misguided ideas about policy. . . . It really does create a culture of fear in some immigrant communities. What I hear from my clients and from my partner organizations is that people really are afraid and that this kind of rhetoric that we hear really does drive people away. . . . They stay in the shadows. They don't want to apply for coverage, [even] if they have legal status." Joshua's perceptions align with the research of sociologist Asad Asad, who argues that documented immigrants are more visible to the bureaucracy than undocumented immigrants, who regard invisibility as a protective measure.[53] The climate of fear sparked by Trump made documented immigrants want to be less visible in engaging with social service bureaucracies, too.

Fear of negative repercussions if Trump were elected became a major driver in decisions immigrants made on a daily basis. Some Latinx immigrants in Boston disenrolled from health plans and became reluctant to share personal information with advocates and providers. Some reconsidered their decisions to naturalize or adjust their status. In contrast, others who were eligible for naturalization responded by applying for citizenship, which they felt would bring more security. David, an immigrant advocate, observed that both applications for naturalization and participation in his organization's citizenship clinics had spiked: "Through sheer coincidence Channel 5 news called and said we're interested in a story on the Trump Effect. And we were having a clinic right downstairs. . . . So, I think [Trump] definitely had an effect. Of course, you know there's fear. But at least for those people who are eligible, it's something they can do." Yet those who are undocumented have no path to citizenship. And "Muslims . . . who are citizens" and should "have no reason to fear" were being targeted.

Trump's anti-immigrant rhetoric was directed specifically, though not exclusively, at Mexicans and other Latinx ethnic groups. Those who were naturalized or US-born citizens did not feel that their status would protect them from detention or unfair treatment under the law. As I discussed in Chapter 1, scholars' distinction between legal and sociocultural citizenship highlights the powerful roles that race, ethnicity, and religion play in determining individuals' full inclusion in the United States.[54] Sociologists Nilda Flores-Gonzalez and Ariana Valle have found that Latinx people of various ethnicities are criminalized, stigmatized, and regarded as not belonging to the body politic, a position they share with Black Americans.[55] Respondents I interviewed for this study felt similarly: being racialized as Latinx led to their being profiled as undocumented and targeted by law and immigration enforcement even if they were citizens.

While Trump's campaign was inciting fear in Latinx communities, David, the immigrant advocate previously quoted, pointed out that the Obama administration's policy of conducting raids inside the US rather than concentrating enforcement efforts on the border had led to increased racialized enforcement in Boston.[56] He explained that ICE raids were part of "a very deliberate effort to try to stem the tide" of unaccompanied minors from Central America by detaining and deporting undocumented immigrants whenever and wherever they could be found. Tony, a BHC provider, said that the combination of ICE raids in nearby Massachusetts towns and police checks in Boston's mass transit stations created enough fear that immigrants altered their daily lives. Immigrants "send alerts to each other when they see police in the T stations, like when they do the checks of bags, . . . they'll turn around and . . . choose not to go through security, because they are so afraid of the officers at the turnstile."

Despite the perception that Massachusetts and Boston were more welcoming to immigrants than other places, respondents recognized that immigrants were not protected from either Homeland Security or the national sociopolitical climate, a finding echoed in other studies of sanctuary cities.[57] Jenny, a health advocate, put herself in the shoes of the undocumented immigrants that her city health agency served:

> The political climate in Massachusetts is just so different than the rest of the country. That being said, East Boston has a huge number of immigrants and I have gone over there for outreach. And I see Donald Trump signs, which everyone has the right to their political views, . . . and I know that there are immigrants who support Donald Trump. But I would feel really uncomfortable like, if I was surrounded by—if it were me, and I saw those signs. . . . And then you see that and you are like, who can I trust, where can I go, does that mean that person is saying, if they know I am undocumented, they don't want me here.

The consensus among stakeholders was that the racist, anti-immigrant climate was making life much harder for immigrants. This problematic situation affected their overall health and encounters with the healthcare system.

The Health and Healthcare Implications of Amplified Law and Immigration Enforcement

In interviews, I heard countless stories about the harmful effects of this hostility on immigrants' physical and mental health. Like the immigrants interviewed in 2012–2013, most immigrants interviewed in 2015–2016 reported having good or excellent physical and mental health before coming to the United States. At the time I interviewed them, the majority also reported being in good or excellent physical and mental health. Compared with Brazilians and Salvadorans, a higher number of Dominicans reported having average physical health (8 of 14) and mental health (3 of 14). Interestingly, about a third of all immigrants reported having been diagnosed with diabetes, high blood pressure, cardiac conditions, stress, anxiety, or depression.[58] As an interviewer, I found it odd that so many immigrants had such positive health assessments despite having serious health conditions. Maybe this was the case because the immigrant respondents had regular providers and felt their conditions were being sufficiently managed without impeding on their daily lives. Or perhaps they did not want to disclose their issues with the stranger interviewing them.

Nevertheless, immigrants' chronic health diagnoses reflected what I heard from advocates and providers such as health advocate Carolina, who assisted immigrants who spoke Portuguese. For "anxiety, depression, they have to take the medication. High blood pressure has to do with their physical health, but it's also most of the time related to their mental health because they [have] been at work too much. They are tired. They go through all those stresses." In a pernicious cycle, not having health coverage or being unable to obtain the health care they need intensifies their stress. Some providers and advocates directly attributed immigrants' health problems to structural and social conditions such as neighborhood segregation, restricted housing and employment options, and increased immigration enforcement. Brazilian advocates emphasized the high levels of depression and rising number of suicides among immigrants. Lucia, who served as a healthcare navigator for Brazilians, told me: "There have been many cases of suicide in our community. And many people sit in that chair where you're sitting now and tell me that they are depressed and that they can't find work, both documented and undocumented. People feel really isolated, they can't do anything. They feel like they're in prison. So, that feeling of not having freedom to do what you want is difficult: 'I want to go to Brazil, but I can't. If I leave, I can't return.'"

Gabriel, the Salvadoran advocate who described the plight of Salvadorans with temporary protected status, spoke poignantly about the additional stresses the presidential campaign rhetoric was creating for undocumented immigrants in his community. "With the Republicans saying 'we are going to deport every single undocumented over here,' that doesn't bring you peace of mind. . . . You get sick because you are thinking, 'Am I going to be deported, what about my kids, what about this, what about [that], what I have been working [for] here?'"

In this distressing political situation, increased racialized surveillance and enforcement from law and immigration officials had a chilling effect on immigrants' decisions about health coverage and care. While my findings reflect what was happening in the Boston area, other studies conducted around the country demonstrated similar health and healthcare impacts on immigrants in 2015–2016.[59] Sociologist Meredith Van Natta's research in a "red" state during this time finds that this more exclusionary setting made immigrants view healthcare institutions as punitive sites of surveillance; the result was that they delayed getting health care.[60] Sociologist Asad Asad's research with mostly undocumented immigrants in Texas finds that their awareness of government surveillance through engagement with social service institutions such as healthcare facilities led them not to utilize such services.[61]

Racialized Legal Status as a Deterrent to Coverage and Care

Racialized legal status became even more important in limiting Latinx Bostonians' healthcare access under Obamacare. Omarina, a 49-year-old

Dominican green card holder with fair skin, dark-brown eyes, and short blonde hair, observed that "my daughter and I, we go to doctors' offices and where we want; those with green cards can move around more openly. But others" without green cards, "no, they are afraid. They don't want to go to doctors, they don't want to go anywhere because they don't feel free. It's really sad. . . . It's not good to be here without papers, in any situation." She and other immigrants commented that the situation for them, especially the undocumented, had worsened since they arrived in the United States decades ago.

Healthcare providers and advocates reported an uptick in the encounters their immigrant patients or their relatives had with immigration enforcement that jeopardized their household's stability and well-being. Grace, a BHC provider, recounted that when "the family member of one of my patients has been picked up for documentation status, and is going to be incarcerated or is in the process of being deported, . . . patients will come in and ask me to write . . . letters of support, that the breadwinner of the family with small children" has been detained and is being sent out of the country. Those incidents were becoming more frequent, but her letters on their behalf did little to change these decisions.

Advocates knew that some Boston immigrants responded to the enforcement risks they faced by disenrolling from health coverage or removing themselves from the entire health and welfare system. In some cases, immigration attorneys advised clients who were applying to adjust their status to preemptively decline all public benefits they might receive. Carolina, a Brazilian health advocate, disagreed with this advice: "I think sometimes because of the language barrier, even immigrant lawyers . . . try to simplify and they are afraid that the immigrant [will] make some mistake." So, they advise immigrants to stop accepting any services—but Carolina thinks "it's worse if you don't have the insurance. . . . If you get sick and you're waiting on your immigration status and you don't go to see a doctor because you can't afford [it] and you don't have coverage," your life is at risk. "I think it's better if you . . . get your treatment, [and] then get your immigration status." When she counsels immigrants, she does not contradict their lawyers but explains her clients' options. She concluded: "It's so painful, these people go through a lot and then you still have to pay a penalty for not having insurance. So, immigration, tax law, and health care all come together."

Providers, too, were aware that immigrants might delay or discontinue getting care if they were applying for a green card or citizenship and expressed concern about the negative consequences for their health. Aurelia, a BHC provider, said, "I've had many patients with diabetes or other chronic diseases not seek care for up to a year while their papers were in what they felt to be [a] precarious position. And, in spite of our reassuring [them] and trying to make sure that they understood how separate these systems are, some patients just didn't believe it." Despite the harms of deferring treatment for diabetes, some immigrants consider the benefits of remaining under the radar and less embedded in the healthcare system worth the risk.[62]

The problems that arise at the intersection of health and immigration policy must be addressed for everyone to receive vital healthcare services. Sociologist Meredith Van Natta also writes about the complicated dance that immigration attorneys and social workers must perform when advising immigrants about whether to remain enrolled in social services. While such individuals may want immigrants to keep services for their well-being, often attorneys and social workers err on the side of caution to make immigrant clients less vulnerable to penalties that could occur from keeping such services when they apply to adjust their legal status. It really is a catch-22.

The combination of the barriers immigrants faced in getting health care with overt hostility to immigrants and intensified enforcement convinced Manuel, the Salvadoran pastor whose powerful quote is at the beginning of this chapter, that the powers that be do not want immigrants to access health care. As troubling as it might seem, he feels that dogs have an easier time getting health care than immigrants. Although it is illegal for emergency departments to turn away patients due to their documentation status, Manuel was aware of the implicit and explicit signals that our society sends about who is deemed worthy of medical treatment. As an immigrant and a pastor who serves immigrants, Manuel recalled the deteriorating treatment of immigrants over time and felt that most presidential administrations, including those of Clinton and Obama, had not done much to ease their plight. Instead, he felt they had used immigrants as political pawns and made their situation worse.

Increased law and immigration enforcement deterred immigrants from obtaining health care because they were concerned about being apprehended while en route to medical facilities. Although most immigrants and other respondents felt safe getting care at the hospitals and clinical offices where they were usually treated, I heard more about heightened surveillance and its effects on immigrants' healthcare decisions in 2015–2016 than in 2012–2013. Alcione, the advocate who helped Brazilian immigrants obtain health coverage, said that information about enforcement is often shared on social media to warn community members: "Today on Facebook, I saw a post that said, 'Please don't drive at night on Highway 495 if you don't have a license. The State Police are stopping everyone.' This is creating a new terror in our community."

The stress of fearing and evading enforcement affects immigrants' health, as well as their mobility. Recent research has found that biased and excessive enforcement can increase cortisol levels, which have been associated with more negative health outcomes.[63] Research has also indicated that persistent systemic racism generates "weathering" in Black Americans, which reduces their bodies' ability to fight disease and can result in higher maternal and infant mortality rates. Similarly, increased enforcement tied to racialized legal status is producing a "weathering" effect on Latinx immigrants' health, affecting citizens and noncitizens alike.[64]

The cumulative impact of racialized legal status on healthcare access combined with working long hours in physically taxing jobs can be lethal, particularly for Latinx immigrants and other immigrants of color. Fabiana, a BHC provider, underlined the long-term damage that resulted for her patients:

They express fears . . . about not being able to perform in jobs that make them survive here and help the family in Brazil or in Portugal or anywhere. So, because of the exhaustion of the physical body and some accident, especially in the construction field where my folks come from and cleaning houses, . . . it just kills them every day in the end. If you think about the boom of immigration starting in 1995, it's been 20 years of daily cleaning . . . and daily putting up [with] stuff. So, it's taken a toll on their bodies.

Taken together, these testimonies and observations illuminate the immense and contradictory pressures that immigrants feel when they are trying to make decisions about their health and well-being. These stories delineate how medical legal violence operates through the enforcement apparatus of the state: immigrants fear interacting with the healthcare system because of the possibility that information might be shared with government authorities and lead to detention or deportation for themselves or family members.[65] The health implications of racialized legal status enforcement demonstrate how closely connected people perceive US social institutions to be, their ability to conduct surveillance, and the significant overlap between immigration and health policies that shapes immigrants' health and health care.

Patient–Provider Interactions Along and Across Cultural Lines

Immigrants I interviewed in 2015–2016, like their counterparts in 2012–2013, had mixed experiences with healthcare providers. Jimena, a 63-year-old Latina Dominican and naturalized US citizen with a Latinx provider, enthused, "For me, my doctor is my friend, my adviser, my psychiatrist, she's everything to me." Another Dominican respondent, Yleana, a 58-year-old naturalized US citizen who identifies as Hispanic and Latina, praised the staff at her doctor's office: "The secretary, the nurses, all of them know my name when I arrive." Interestingly, I found that Dominican respondents reported more positive healthcare experiences than Brazilians and Salvadorans. This difference was somewhat surprising, since Dominicans' typical racialization by others as Black would make them more likely to have negative experiences. Perhaps because fewer of them had health coverage and regular contacts with physicians in the Dominican Republic, they had lower expectations of the US healthcare system than Brazilians did.

Conversely, Brazilians, who were more likely to be racialized by others as White and least likely to report experiencing any type of discrimination, felt that providers did not always listen to them, lacked patience and cultural sensitivity, or refused to write prescriptions for them. These perceptions were likely based on Brazilians' comparisons to providers in Brazil, whom they regarded as more attentive to patients' needs. Brazilians' relatively privileged premigration socioeconomic positions gave them a different frame of reference for assessing their experiences with "cold" and "distant" American providers. Mariana, an undocumented Brazilian immigrant who discussed the difference between Brazilians and Hispanics, struggled to get a health issue diagnosed for several years. She expressed frustration with a very rude provider who lacked "the sensibility to listen to the patient and the ability to diagnose or treat" her condition. Another undocumented Brazilian, Clara, who had medium dark-brown skin, dark-brown eyes, and straight black hair and identified as Black, said: "Once I had kidney stones and told my doctor about this issue. The doctor told me, 'Well, you can live with that.' But I didn't think it was normal to have to live with kidney stones. It became difficult to stand and got worse" because the doctor did nothing.

Salvadoran immigrants shared the perception that their race reduced the quality of their care. Federico, the Salvadoran who was racially profiled by police, also felt that immigrants encountered discrimination in healthcare facilities: "When you go to a hospital and need medical attention, you can see how the doctors treat an immigrant; usually they treat them last. If it's anyone else, like an American, the doctor will treat them first." Federico, like other immigrants, did not know that patients with life-threatening conditions, such as heart attacks and strokes, are treated before those with less severe medical problems, rather than everyone being treated in order of arrival. The absence of signs in Spanish and other languages and the staff's inability to communicate how patients are prioritized to those who are not fluent in English contributes to immigrants feeling disregarded when seeking care. Thomas, a BHC provider, underscored the importance of providers' cultural competence and acknowledged that patient–provider interactions are "influenced by perceptions of discrimination . . . I think there is plenty of nonobvious discrimination, or at least that's felt and that influences care."

Amid the climate of harsher enforcement and extremely negative racialized anti-immigrant rhetoric, Latinx Bostonians' healthcare access declined, even though most immigrant respondents had health coverage. This grim reality indicates yet again that having access to health coverage does not guarantee adequate care if the appropriate linguistic and cultural resources are not available for people to communicate with their providers and navigate the healthcare system. Furthermore, structural discrimination rooted in racialized legal status within the system enables providers and bureaucrats whose practices and decisions are shaped by implicit and explicit bias to continue without being educated in how to provide appropriate and culturally competent care and extending effective services to all who are eligible for them.

State-Level Policies Further Diminish Immigrants' Healthcare Access

Immigrants' awareness of the increasingly hostile sociopolitical climate nationally was reinforced by the more subtle but nonetheless consequential changes in Massachusetts's policies toward its immigrant residents. The shift from Democratic governor Deval Patrick to Republican governor Charlie Baker set a new tone toward immigrants and placed greater emphasis on saving the state money than on providing health care and other social services to those who needed them most. Immigrant advocates saw Baker as less willing to protect and advance immigrants' rights. As the Republican governor of an overwhelmingly Democratic state, Baker had to work in a bipartisan manner. The high approval ratings that led to his being dubbed "America's most popular governor" in 2020 suggest that he succeeded in doing so, and Massachusetts has been considered a model for effective state government.[66]

But immigration and health advocates thought that his administration left much to be desired.[67]

David, an immigrant advocate quoted earlier, expressed this shared sentiment:

> I think the . . . interesting challenge for us . . . has been the change in administration. A lot of us were worried. We knew, I mean, Charlie Baker is obviously not . . . [like] the governor of Arizona [Jan Brewer]. But at the same time, he came into office saying he'd basically veto all of our priority legislation with a focus on the undocumented. So . . . he's been a very mixed bag. In some ways, he's been very supportive and interested in high-skilled [immigration]. But it's also been very hard to get him on the record around any sort of immigrant agenda.

Raquel, the state government employee quoted earlier who worked with newly arrived Central Americans, was particularly troubled that Baker supported local police cooperation with federal immigration enforcement, despite objections from many communities and their police departments. His position was that "if you pull over a person who's not lawfully living here, who doesn't have papers, you can basically turn them over to ICE. That wasn't something that we were working with over the last few years and that's kind of a big deal."

Governor Baker's proposed changes to Health Safety Net, the state's program for immigrants ineligible for other public options, in early 2016, were the most consequential. Those changes included lowering the maximum income level that allowed applicants to qualify for the program; reducing the retroactive payment of services under the program from six months to 10 days after applying; and imposing new charges on seniors and the working poor.[68] Most important, the proposal aimed to eliminate the state's annual contribution of $30 million to the program's budget.[69] For the estimated 285,000 HSN recipients, many of whom were already lower-income, these changes would have serious consequences.[70] HSN-designated healthcare facilities, which were struggling financially, worried that the state was shifting the cost of care for these patients onto them. Immigrant and health advocates whom

I interviewed in 2016 told me about a public hearing in February 2016 where concerned Massachusetts residents could comment on the proposal. The changes the governor proposed were not announced until about a month before the meeting, and the local media provided little coverage. According to Stella, who worked in a human services advocacy organization, the public hearing was a mere formality: "The administration is able to make regulatory changes without the permission of the legislature. This is why it's actually key and very hard to stop."

When I attended the public hearing, I was reminded of my privileges as an English-proficient citizen with a car and a flexible schedule. The hearing took place in Quincy, a city south of Boston, at the Executive Office of Health and Human Services (EOHHS), which was difficult to access via public transportation. Concerned residents who wanted to comment had to preregister. The proceedings were held in English, and no translators were available. Of the 20 members of the public who attended, I was one of three visible people of color. The majority of those in attendance appeared to be White, female, and middle-aged. I was struck by the irony that very few of the people in a position to decide or comment on the proposal were HSN recipients. The lower-income residents, immigrants, and citizens of color who would be most affected by the proposed changes were not able to advocate on their own behalf.

The state's assistant general counsel and an EOHHS employee presided over the meeting, which began with the director of HSN giving an overview of the proposed changes. These reductions were framed as though they would be beneficial for the state and its residents. The information in the handout stated that there would be no fiscal impact on cities and towns. Nothing acknowledged the effects of these changes on HSN facilities where patients go for treatment and the communities where they are located. The reduction in resources to HSN would likely result in layoffs to compensate for the loss of revenue and state support. Essentially, the state wanted to bring HSN more in line with the MassHealth and Health Connector insurance programs to reduce costs. The state estimated that these changes would "reduce HSN demand" by $60 million each year.

When public comments began, some healthcare providers and health and immigrant advocates I had previously interviewed came forward to outline the detrimental impact of these changes. Nearly everyone who spoke in opposition to the proposal agreed that this was not a cost-saving measure. Rather, it was a cost-shifting measure, moving healthcare costs that were being paid by the state onto its most vulnerable low-income and immigrant residents and the healthcare facilities that served them. They argued that the state should not treat HSN as an insurance program because it was really a safety net that allowed people to get basic health care even though they were ineligible for health insurance or unable to afford the available supplemental insurance. I was most struck by the comments from a representative of the Massachusetts Legal Association of Community Health Centers, who stated that although Massachusetts had been "the envy of other states when it comes to health care," these changes would take away that status by damaging HSN.

I saw these changes as another step in chipping away at the uncompensated care pool, an incremental process that, as one speaker pointed out, had been ongoing in Massachusetts since the 1980s. The representatives of healthcare organizations and advocates who mentioned these changes in our interviews were frustrated. Jenny, the health advocate quoted earlier, said at the meeting: "Everyone is in it together." Those who served immigrants and low-income residents were "really upset about" the changes in Health Safety Net.

These changes in HSN were implemented in July 2016, just as I completed my interviews. I could not help thinking about the thousands of HSN recipients who would lose coverage and the remaining uninsured who would become ineligible for the program. With a presidential election looming, I realized that the future of Obamacare was also at risk. Like the people I interviewed, I feared the prospect of even greater changes in the sociopolitical climate and in public policy. I was also concerned about the racialized legal status implications such shifts could have for immigrants and citizens' healthcare access in Boston and around the country.

Conclusion

The shift from the original Massachusetts reform to Obamacare in late 2013 significantly affected immigrants' healthcare access after ACA implementation. Racialized legal status became a more salient factor shaping Latinx immigrants' experiences amid changes in eligibility based on documentation status, insufficient language-appropriate enrollment materials and navigators, and the increase in racist and anti-immigrant rhetoric in the lead-up to the 2016 presidential election. Although the ACA was supposed to provide Americans with greater access to affordable health coverage, the restrictions based on documentation status under federal law, the more stringent requirements for income, and the heavier burden of proof for both decreased the health coverage options of immigrants in the commonwealth. Immigrant-restrictive policies at the federal level undermined immigrant-inclusive policies at the state level. In addition, the shift from a paper application to an online enrollment process created chaos for immigrants and other state residents during the first two years of Obamacare. Many felt uninformed about the changes that were coming and lacked the language and computer literacy to navigate the Commonwealth Connector website. These technical difficulties compounded the racialized legal status burdens that many Latinx immigrants had encountered in 2012–2013 under the Massachusetts reform, which resulted in some losing coverage.

At the same time, opposition to immigration increased as Donald Trump's campaign brought racialized anti-immigrant sentiment to the forefront of national political debate. It became socially acceptable to express racism and xenophobia. Latinx immigrants in and beyond Boston felt targeted by this rhetoric. Furthermore, rising deportations and increased cooperation between law and immigration enforcement under the Obama administration, coupled with the surge of unaccompanied minors at the southern border, sent a powerful message to immigrants and citizens of color that they were not wanted or welcome. Their racialized legal status made Boston's Latinx immigrants feel more vulnerable to being racially profiled, arrested, detained, and deported by anyone in uniform or who appeared to exercise government authority.

Growing racialized legal status enforcement had severe consequences for health and health care. The stresses of being hyper-surveilled and fearful of potential arrest or deportation had negative physical and mental health effects on a vulnerable population that was already predisposed to health problems from working in physically taxing jobs for meager wages. Among Brazilian immigrants, this pressure was regarded as the cause of increased suicide rates. Among Salvadoran immigrants, this pressure made them wary of using health services. And Dominicans, most of whom were green card holders or naturalized citizens, were not immune; being racialized as Black and Latino made them subject to profiling. In all three ethnic groups, immigrants responded to this hostile sociopolitical climate by disenrolling from health and other public social services, becoming hyperaware of their surroundings, and sharing information with community members on social media to warn of potential police traps or ICE raids. These responses signify attempts to become less visible and less socially embedded in the system to minimize detection and avoid potential removal.[71] Some Latinx immigrants postponed or stopped seeking health care despite having chronic conditions. As Fabiana, a BHC provider emphasized in an earlier quote, "it just takes a toll on their bodies."

All of this unfolded in Boston, a city in a state that should have been better prepared for Obamacare than other places and might have done more to mitigate the impact of punitive immigration policies at the federal level. But the election of Charlie Baker, who did not support immigrant-inclusive state policies, meant that Massachusetts did not become a sanctuary state. State lawmakers, including some Democrats, were unable to pass reforms that could have made immigrants' lives marginally easier in the commonwealth. Despite advocates' best efforts, lack of legislative action took a toll on immigrants' access to health care. Most seriously, the Baker administration's decision to eliminate state funding and reduce eligibility for the Health Safety Net program in 2016 was a severe blow to this program of last resort for those who were poor or undocumented.

Racialized legal status was having a more significant impact on the lives of Boston's Latinx immigrants in June 2016 than it did in 2013. When Trump won the presidency in November 2016, it was clear that the salience of racialized legal status would increase and have grave implications for immigrants' health and healthcare access.

CHAPTER 4

Deterring Immigrants from Using Services Under Trump (2019)

I think the challenge is dealing with this administration every single day. There's something new and it's like a bomb. And then, they [immigrants] don't know how to react, they don't know how or what to do about it because it instills fear in them.

—Daniel, health advocate interviewed in 2019

The truth is that health [care] in the United States exploits people. They exploit people too much, it's absurd. You have a [medical] emergency, do two or three exams and leave with a debt of $9,000, $10,000. . . . When it comes to health [care] here, they are thieves.

—Sabino, Brazilian immigrant interviewed in 2019

After the election and inauguration of President Trump in 2017, members of many marginalized groups and their advocates voiced their collective opposition to his anti-immigrant and racist rhetoric and policy proposals. In Boston, advocates, service providers, and concerned community members mobilized to reassure everyone, especially immigrants of color, that they remained eligible for health and other social services and could seek them safely despite the hostile national sociopolitical climate. Advocates such as Daniel discussed how the Trump administration's constant barrage of draconian immigration policy proposals made it difficult to connect local immigrants effectively with the services they needed. Concerns that Trump and the Republicans would make good on their threats to repeal Obamacare also prompted Massachusetts lawmakers to bolster existing health coverage and policy protections, while advocates pushed for stronger state-level measures to protect immigrants from increasingly punitive federal immigration policies. Joshua, a healthcare advocate I also interviewed in 2015, said that the "chaos" was aimed "to create confusion and sell fear." He emphasized that racism was at the root of the Trump administration's stance on immigration in 2019: "If we don't recognize the systemic White supremacy aspect of it, we're ignoring a really key piece of what is really going on in the underbelly of these policies." Many of the 56 immigrants, providers, and advocates I interviewed in metropolitan Boston in 2019 were conscious of the increasingly significant role that the intersection between perceptions of their race and assumptions about their citizenship status played not only in rhetoric and policymaking but also in local communities of color. The effects of what I call racialized legal status on Latinx people's daily lives, mobility, and access to services became more acute, affecting citizens and legal residents as well as those who were undocumented.

While Latinx immigrants continued to experience confusion about their eligibility for coverage under the complex array of legal statuses, they expressed more serious anxiety about increased racialized enforcement in 2019. They had to decide what information they felt comfortable sharing with bureaucrats and providers when (re)enrolling in coverage and obtaining services, given the heightened risks that doing so might jeopardize their ability to avoid summary deportation and to regularize their legal status in the future. In addition to worrying about making, keeping, and paying for medical appointments, they reported more experiences of discrimination in their encounters with healthcare professionals.

State- and national-level changes in immigration and health policy alongside explicitly racist and anti-immigrant rhetoric meant that Latinx

Bostonians' access to health care and their use of health services deteriorated in 2019. Combined with the heavy administrative burdens that Latinx immigrants had previously experienced, the intensified consequences of racialized legal status created more substantial barriers to accessing coverage and care. Markers such as race, ethnicity, skin color, limited English proficiency, or speaking English with an accent made immigrants stand out from "Americans" and heightened the discrimination they faced. The Trump administration's haphazard announcement of executive orders and policy proposals designed to curtail immigration and persecute the undocumented generated pervasive fear of leaving home, going to work, taking children to school, and seeking preventive and specialty health care. Therefore, although Massachusetts remained one of the few states with robust coverage options for state residents, immigrants' anxiety about surveillance and enforcement deterred them from seeking medical care except in dire emergencies.

The intense fear created by the Trump administration made many immigrants unwilling to participate in this study in 2019. Aiming to replicate the design I had used in previous years, I hoped to interview 30 immigrants, 10 each from the Brazilian, Dominican, and Salvadoran communities. Despite my volunteer work with local organizations, my visible identity as a Black woman, my proficiency in Brazilian Portuguese and Spanish, and the offer of $25 gift cards to participants, I was able to interview only 12 immigrants: 8 Brazilians, 2 Dominicans, and 2 Salvadorans.[1] Two of these immigrants were reluctant to allow me to record our interviews despite my assurances that none of the information we discussed could be traced back to them. Given their hesitation, I also felt uncomfortable taking notes. Before 2019, no immigrant had ever declined my request to record our interviews. I understood the difficulty of recruiting immigrants in 2019, because I myself might be fearful and reluctant to participate in a study if I thought that my documentation status could threaten my or my family's ability to remain in the country.

Most of the dozen immigrants I interviewed rated their physical and mental health between excellent and average, regardless of their country of origin.[2] As in previous years of the study, most respondents had public or private health coverage and a regular provider.[3] In terms of education, the majority had at least completed some college. As before, immigrants' English proficiency varied widely.[4]

In contrast to immigrants, healthcare providers and immigrant and health advocates were eager to talk with me about their concerns (see Table I-1). I interviewed 14 BHC providers; half of them were new respondents, and the other half had been interviewed in 2012–2013 or 2015–2016. I interviewed 30 immigrant and health advocates, 10 of whom had spoken with me in 2012–2013 or 2015–2016.[5] The difficulty of finding immigrants who were willing to take what many perceived as the risk of talking with a researcher means that this chapter has more quotations from the other stakeholder groups. Yet providers' and advocates' in-depth engagement with immigrant communities at the Boston Health Coalition and local immigrant and health advocacy organizations provides valuable insights into immigrants' experiences during this turbulent period.

After discussing the sociopolitical climate from President Trump's election to when I began interviews in 2019, this chapter explores the implications of heightened hostility to immigrants and people of color for Boston's Latinx immigrants, with statuses ranging from undocumented to naturalized citizen. Next, the chapter outlines the policy choices Massachusetts legislators made regarding state health and immigration policy in response to federal policy changes and proposals. In the 2019 interviews, respondents emphasized that the Trump administration's rhetoric, threats, and actions targeted a vulnerable population and sent them into hiding. The withdrawal of many Latinx immigrants from the health and social services for which they were eligible had serious consequences for their well-being, despite the best efforts of providers and advocates to reassure them. To reveal the impact of racialized legal status beyond immigrant respondents, I rely on advocates and providers of color who told me about personal attacks they experienced and insecurities they felt in their work and personal lives because of discrimination aimed at the groups others thought they belonged to. Weary and wary from the constant policy changes that made their jobs more difficult, those who served immigrants shared how they coped with the chaotic environment the Trump administration created.

In sum, this chapter reveals the cascading effects of policy and rhetoric that spread far beyond those who were directly targeted. All the quotations in this chapter come from interviews I conducted in 2019, when Democrat Marty Walsh was the mayor of Boston, Republican Charlie Baker was the governor of Massachusetts, and Republican Donald Trump was president of the United States.

Immediate Responses to Trump's Presidency

Many providers and advocates I interviewed began our conversation by emphasizing the alarming decline in the number of immigrants seeking the services they offered in January 2017, when Trump's presidency began. Latinx immigrants suddenly became much less likely to utilize healthcare facilities and organizations providing social services. Javier, an immigration attorney at a legal advocacy organization, recalled:

> Before the Trump administration, you know, you would go into the health center and the health centers would be full. Full of people seeking services, whether it's related to a medical need, or otherwise just coming to the health center to be connected and referred out to different services. . . . Early in [Trump's] presidency, the health center was empty. Nobody was coming. So much so that the hospitals across the city and across the country started posting signs saying this is a safe space, so that people who would arrive would feel more comfortable, and so that . . . people would then be able to speak about it with their friends, family, neighbors, to spread the word that they should be coming and accessing services.

Physicians and agency staffers described a confusing array of politicized proposals for policy changes that made it difficult for them to serve their patients and clients. The steps taken by the Trump administration to dismantle protections for *documented* immigrants were terrifying indicators of what the government could do to those who were undocumented.

Immigrants told providers and advocates about their worries that using services to which they were entitled would make it easier for ICE to track their movements and impair their future ability to adjust their status. A chilling effect had definitely set in even before major policy changes were enacted. Providers and advocates recognized that they would have to stay on top of policy proposals and proactively educate immigrants about keeping their public benefits and obtaining needed services.

Aria, a Brazilian health advocate, worked tirelessly to convince Brazilian immigrants that they could safely retain their coverage and obtain preventive health services for themselves and their families such as WIC, a federal program that provides nutrition for pregnant or breastfeeding women, infants, and young children. "So, right in the beginning, there was this 'Oh my God, what's gonna happen' among our constituents" after January 2017. "There were a number of clients who were afraid." She said, "Many . . . would ask us, 'What's going to happen, how will we be affected? When I apply for my citizenship, will they see that I used MassHealth or WIC?'" Aria went on: "Our job was to tell them: 'Even though you are afraid, you must continue to take care of yourself and look after your health, you have to take care of your family, and we will keep fighting regardless of what [Trump] says or does.'"

Daniel—the Spanish-speaking healthcare advocate who, at the beginning of the chapter, described the Trump administration's haphazard but dangerous policies as a bomb—recounted the concerns expressed by anxious immigrants: "They were calling me and saying, 'All right, so are we going to lose everything because of the new president? So, are we going to have to pay more? How is this going to work? Is this economy privatized?' All these kinds of questions were up in the air for them, because the new president came attacking the immigrants." Daniel, whom I interviewed each year of the study, had recounted the numerous challenges he faced connecting immigrant constituents with essential healthcare information and coverage. In 2019, the constantly changing policies and threatening atmosphere made his task even more difficult.

Among the vast assortment of proposals and policies restricting legal immigration and deterring and punishing the undocumented, immigrants were most fearful of the proposed "public charge" rule change, which was based on a century-old federal law that was rarely invoked but loomed large amid stepped-up immigration enforcement.[6] Even before the Department of Homeland Security announced that a new interpretation of the rule refusing admission to anyone who was "likely to become a public charge" would be implemented in October 2019, confusion about who was subject to the rule and what public benefits it applied to generated disenrollment in services by documented immigrants already in the country.[7] Essentially, immigration officials could deny green cards to lower-income applicants whom officials suspected might use certain public benefits in the future.[8] The change was not officially implemented until February 24, 2020, as concern about the global coronavirus pandemic superseded more generalized anxiety about immigration.

Once information about the proposed public charge rule reached the public, however, many advocates and providers whom I interviewed in 2019 thought that it prompted Boston-area Latinx immigrants to disenroll from public benefits, cancel medical appointments, and delay or terminate health services. Javier, the immigration attorney quoted previously about empty health centers after Trump's election, discussed the detrimental impact he observed: "People have not just stopped showing up in the same numbers at places like the health center. But we also see people actually taking themselves off of public assistance, housing lists, removing themselves from public benefits like food stamps, right? 'I am going to take myself out of this to avoid any problems, because I don't know if this is going to be or if I'm going to be penalized for participating in this program that I may be completely lawfully entitled to.'" The proposal to disqualify any applicants for permanent residency (green cards) who had used publicly funded services during the previous five years "generated so much fear . . . that people [would] rather not place themselves in harm's way," Javier concluded.

Other advocates shared stories of immigrants wanting to pay out of pocket for services they had previously received through public benefits. Joshua, the healthcare advocate who earlier emphasized the racism embedded in immigration policy, discussed the situation of an immigrant applying for asylum. Asylum seekers "shouldn't have to be afraid," he declared. But this person "wanted to pay back all these benefits and drop benefits." Because the proposed policy was not yet official, Joshua responded by saying, "At this point, you know, there's nothing to be afraid of, right at this very moment. The future, potentially." Joshua explained, however, that "people make their own calculation about their risk. . . . It's a really tough decision to make in this environment." The proposed public charge rule, coupled with all the confusion it (perhaps deliberately) aroused, led to a decline in immigrants' use of benefits, including health care, in Boston and around the country.[9]

The constant barrage of Trump administration announcements about possible and actual changes in immigration policies made it difficult for advocates and providers to effectively communicate with immigrant communities.[10] They struggled with the tension between remaining informed and combating confusion among their constituents and patients. At the same time, immigrants unintentionally shared information that was not always accurate among themselves on Facebook and WhatsApp. These social media platforms enabled Latinx immigrants to warn other community members about real or rumored ICE raids and checkpoints. Immigrants adapted their behavior to reduce their risk of being detained and deported.

In response, advocates and providers mobilized and collaborated with immigrant communities to allay unfounded fears whenever it was realistically possible. They agreed that the most beneficial approach was to organize educational campaigns to help immigrants get accurate information and learn their rights so they could make more informed decisions. Paola, a healthcare advocate, explained that they created "flyers with the seven healthcare rights that immigrants have access to. We thought they were common knowledge, but they're not." Advocates and providers encouraged immigrants to deal with the anti-immigrant climate proactively. They urged eligible immigrants to apply for citizenship. For undocumented parents, who faced more imminent threats, advocates offered assistance in developing family preparedness plans that designated legal guardians to take care of their children in case they were detained and deported. Damian, a lawyer who works with the same organization as Javier, planned a workshop for the Student Immigrant Movement (SIM), which represents and serves those with DACA and other statuses. SIM members told him that "we need lawyers to set up a transfer of property and custody documents for us. So, when our parents or . . . family members are deported, the houses that they've bought can be transferred to us. [So] our uncle can get custody of us, so we [can] continue to go to school and continue to have rights." Damian added that "naming citizen relatives who would take legal responsibility for those who remained in the country . . . doesn't just apply to folks that are undocumented." Those with the whole range of legal statuses short of birthright citizenship also faced threats. The Trump administration made documented noncitizens and naturalized citizens feel that their presence in this country was less secure than that of US-born citizens.

Massachusetts Combats Federal Health and Immigration Policy Changes

State lawmakers and agencies made a serious effort to modify Massachusetts's health programs to insulate immigrants and other residents from the harmful consequences of new federal policies under the Trump administration. These measures were more successful in relation to health coverage and care than they were in relation to immigration law and enforcement. In both domains, however, advocates, providers, and immigrants were frustrated by the limitations of these state-level actions, which cannot be entirely explained by the US Constitution's granting of authority over immigration and citizenship to the federal government. The intersectional character of racialized legal status, coupled with long-standing reservations about immigrants and people of color among Massachusetts's predominantly White voters, meant that harsh immigration policies and practices had substantial negative effects on the health coverage and care available to the commonwealth's immigrant residents and to members of other racialized groups.

Keeping the Commonwealth Insured While the ACA
was Being Diminished

Following the implementation of Obamacare, Massachusetts continued to provide access to coverage for nearly all its residents. Just 2.8% of the population was uninsured in 2019.[11] Yet some groups—particularly male, Hispanic, and low-income noncitizens—remained disproportionately uninsured.[12] Some state residents were ineligible for Medicaid and subsidies because of their federal documentation status. Many of them could not afford coverage without a subsidy, and others purchased lower-cost plans with high deductibles even though their coverage was nearly useless.[13] People continued to struggle with reenrollment processes and had difficulty understanding where and how to use their coverage.[14] These challenges were magnified for people of color, lower-income residents, and those with limited English proficiency.[15]

Magna, a 35-year-old "un-DACA-mented" Brazilian with dark-brown skin, long curly black hair, and Indigenous facial features who identified herself as Latina, discovered that she had lost MassHealth coverage after "I just started receiving bills. And I was really confused."[16] When she found out that her coverage had lapsed, she canceled her upcoming medical appointments. But by then she had accumulated "close to $2,000 in bills from hospitals from when I wasn't aware I didn't have insurance and I was going to the doctors." Medical debt is crippling for low-income residents, and it is a needless burden when it results from a lack of communication with the healthcare bureaucracy.

The changes that were made in 2016 in the state's Health Safety Net program, the primary public coverage option available to lower-income Massachusetts residents of any documentation status, negatively affected immigrants in 2019. Some were no longer eligible and lost coverage. Carolina, a Portuguese-speaking healthcare advocate I had interviewed in previous years of the study, said that some immigrant patients did not discover that they had lost their HSN coverage until they went to medical appointments. "When they contact [us] here, it is sometimes too late. That's when I tell [them], it seems like their income is too high" under the new rules. Sebastião, another Brazilian healthcare advocate, emphasized the consequences that undocumented immigrants experienced because of their exclusion from HSN. "One day, I saw an older person who has been living here undocumented for some time, and he said that he needed insulin and they [the state] are not renewing his coverage. He needs to treat his diabetes and they are cutting his coverage." Sebastião said he thought the state was doing that "intentionally for people to die or return to their home country."

Advocates and providers reported that changes in MassHealth, the state's Medicaid program, also led to confusion and serious lapses in coverage and care. In 2018, MassHealth moved its 800,000 patients into networks of hospitals, doctors, and organizations, called Accountable Care Organizations (ACOs), to coordinate their care.[17] By shifting financial risks from insurance companies to providers, ACOs were supposed to improve the quality of patient care and lower healthcare costs—two goals that are not always compatible.[18] In Massachusetts, this transition was so complicated that the counselors who staffed healthcare helplines found that many patients lost access to their previous primary care physicians. Quinn, who works at the Health Connector for the state's health exchange, said that even the documentation the state sent to inform MassHealth recipients about these changes and assure them that their rights were still protected was more "overwhelming" than useful. Cumulatively, these state-level changes amplified the significance of immigrants' racialized legal status as they applied for and renewed their coverage. These increased burdens also complicated figuring out where that coverage could be used. Some BHC providers also shared a perception that their patients had a more difficult time getting and keeping coverage. Kevin, a BHC physician I had interviewed before, said that "since 2012, I feel like there's a lot more problems with people maintaining their health insurance."

Nationally, despite Supreme Court challenges and some states opting out of the Medicaid expansion, the ACA was successful in reducing the country's uninsured population.[19] Toward the end of President Obama's second term, Republican lawmakers repeatedly but unsuccessfully attempted to repeal the ACA.[20] The ACA's individual mandate requiring people to have health insurance was ended by the 2017 Tax Cuts and Jobs Act, which removed the federal tax penalty.[21] President Trump and the Republican-dominated Congress were also unable to repeal Obamacare, but their efforts were nonetheless consequential. Thomas, a BHC primary care physician, said that Trump had "been doing things all along to try and undermine coverage, like cutting funding for navigators and limit[ing] the number of days that the health insurance exchanges are open, getting rid of the individual mandate, and offering these short-term insurance plans that, basically, don't give you anything, but undermine people getting real insurance."

Although Massachusetts maintained the state's individual mandate along with its coverage for undocumented residents, the disparities between state and federal policies were confusing for everyone. They also posed special difficulties for immigrants who worried that the state mandate could jeopardize their own or their family members' ability to obtain green cards or naturalization under the proposed change in the public charge rule. Isla, a healthcare advocate, described a case in which these inconsistencies created a conundrum she was unable to resolve. A recent caller who was a US citizen and had a US-born daughter, but whose husband had a temporary green card, asked what would happen if she enrolled him in ConnectorCare.

> [After] we talked about the eligibility criteria . . . she said, "Wait a minute. So, it's mandatory to have health insurance. But at the same time, if public charge becomes effective, then I am jeopardizing my husband's immigration status. But at the same time, when I file taxes for next year, because we didn't sign up for tax credits because I'm afraid that this [public charge rule] will come in place, then I'm going to be penalized for each month that he did not have insurance. . . . But at the same time, . . . what if my husband cannot renew his green card?"

Isla reflected on this problem: "That's a tough one. I know that their [hands are] tied." The conflicting federal- and state-level policies regarding health and immigration and the wide range of complex legal status categories posed difficult and even impossible choices for immigrants in mixed-status families.

Nationally, the Trump administration reduced funding for outreach programs and federal healthcare navigators and terminated reimbursement to insurers for low-income enrollees.[22] By 2018, the cumulative impact of those changes led to an increase in the proportion of people who were uninsured.[23] Though the national healthcare debate shifted quite substantially, Massachusetts lawmakers, advocates, and community members at the state, city, and county levels attempted to bolster and buffer the state's health policy and healthcare system. Although these efforts were not entirely successful, state residents were more severely affected by the Trump administration's immigration proposals and policies, which directly influenced the healthcare decisions of immigrants in the Boston area.

Taking Action Against Trump Immigration Policies

Massachusetts lawmakers were more proactive in protecting the state's healthcare system from the Trump administration's efforts to dismantle Obamacare than they were in directly addressing the other problems that immigrants in the state faced. Given the rapid and sweeping changes in federal immigration policy, advocates, immigrants, and concerned citizens urged Massachusetts lawmakers to provide some relief through more inclusive state policies. There were renewed pushes for driver's licenses to be available to undocumented residents and for sanctuary legislation to limit cooperation between state law enforcement and federal immigration enforcement. Advocates recognized that federal actions would always supersede state-level policies as far as immigration was concerned. Michele, an immigration attorney at a legal advocacy organization, said that all states can really do to assist immigrants "is financial. The state can create programs, separate from the federal programs, with its own dollars."

The inability to drive legally, combined with the absence of a statewide sanctuary policy, prevented many undocumented immigrants from using the health coverage for which they were eligible because they could be penalized and turned over to ICE if they were pulled over while driving to a medical appointment. By 2017 and in response to Trump administration immigration policies, only 49 of 351 Massachusetts municipalities passed sanctuary ordinances, and their practical rather than symbolic meaning was not always clear.[24] Nationally, an estimated 400 locales had sanctuary policies by 2018.[25] While such policies may limit cooperation with federal immigration enforcement, they do not adequately address the sociopolitical exclusion that curtails immigrants' access to social services, health care, and financial assistance.[26] They do not make immigrants feel completely safe, as was the case for the father of Magna, the Brazilian immigrant who was burdened by medical debt. She told me her undocumented father was so fearful that he and his family could be deported that he was uncomfortable "everywhere," including in local stores. Ethan, who worked on immigrants' issues at Boston City Hall, commented that the legal definition of a sanctuary policy was so blurry and subject to dispute from the federal government that advocates focused on creating trust in local government among immigrants and encouraging all city residents "to welcome immigrants." This statement suggests the limitations of municipal actions, no matter how positive their intentions, in the wake of punitive federal policies.

Boston's 2014 sanctuary policy, known as the Boston Trust Act, came under scrutiny in 2017 when Jose Martin Paz Flores, an undocumented worker who had been injured on the job, filed a lawsuit against his employer, Tara Construction, for not paying the workers' compensation claim to which he was entitled.[27] Tara Construction retaliated by asking a high-ranking Boston police detective on a joint ICE / Boston Police Department (BPD) Task Force to investigate Flores's identity, which led to his arrest by ICE. The incident called attention to the BPD's continued practice of sharing information with ICE, even though the Trust Act was intended to limit it.

Widespread publicity about the BPD's ongoing cooperation with ICE, along with earlier high-profile incidents of immigrant Boston Public School students being arrested by ICE, led to passage of a revised Trust Act in December 2019.[28] This measure explicitly banned police from getting involved in deportation matters or providing information about a person's immigration status to federal authorities for immigration enforcement purposes. These examples of information sharing between the BPD, Boston Public Schools, and ICE effectively demonstrate the limits of sanctuary policy in restricting federal-level enforcement. Despite the state's inclusive health policy, Boston immigrants' concerns about racialized immigration enforcement constrained their healthcare access.

Elsewhere around the country, the Trump administration significantly increased immigration enforcement, deliberately targeting localities with sanctuary policies.[29] It extended enforcement to places that had been previously designated as "sensitive locations," such as places of worship, healthcare facilities, and courthouses, where ICE had not been allowed to detain immigrants.[30] ICE officials argued that in jurisdictions where sanctuary policies limited the agency's ability to detain immigrants, they had no choice but to surveil and pick up immigrants with warrants everywhere they found them.

Cyrus, an immigrant advocate, explained that in a 2017 decision, *Lunn v. Commonwealth of Massachusetts*, the state's Supreme Judicial Court invalidated detainers issued under ICE's Secure Communities Program.[31] "ICE's argument has always been, 'Hey, look, if local police aren't going to hold folks for us, well, now we have to go to the courthouses to pick them up.' Basically, they're just blaming our local policies" for their "uptick in courthouse enforcement." Advocates were especially concerned because the new policy applied to the undocumented whenever they were in a courtroom, whether they were accused of a crime, seeking redress for a crime committed against them, or testifying as witnesses. A federal judge issued a temporary stay on ICE's courthouse detentions in June 2019, but it was overturned in September 2020 amid a continuing standoff between the commonwealth and the federal government. Then, Cyrus explained, because the Obama administration order banning ICE from detaining immigrants in sensitive locations referred specifically to actions *inside* those places, the Trump administration directed ICE agents to detain undocumented immigrants *outside* them—for example, at schools when parents were dropping off their children.

Jeff, a local immigrant advocate I also interviewed in 2012 and 2015, reported that the practice of detaining undocumented immigrants any time they came to the attention of law enforcement had harmful consequences for a child. After the child's parents separated, the father had visitation rights even though he "had some kind of domestic violence record." Then the parents "got into a fight" when he came to the mother's house. "So, the police were called, and she was taken away because she had an immigration warrant just because she missed" an appointment with US Citizenship and Immigration Services (USCIS). "It was . . . a mad scramble because the child needed the Department of Social Services, and then the father took the child [and] disappeared." Stories like this circulated widely in immigrant communities, underlining the vulnerability of undocumented women to domestic violence and the risk that a mother could be separated from her children if she needed protection from an abusive father.

Advocates were directly involved in lawsuits to overturn the Trump administration's racialized anti-immigrant policies. Advocacy groups collaborated with Massachusetts attorney general Maura Healey on the nearly 70 lawsuits she and other state attorneys general filed against the administration.[32] I especially observed this type of activism among advocates and providers with immigrant backgrounds or who identified as people of color. Other Boston-area residents, especially citizens of color, mobilized to support immigrants' rights as well. Ethan, the City Hall employee previously quoted, told me that Puerto Rican and African American community leaders "are increasingly trying to educate themselves and be more sensitive and aware and trying to be allies" of immigrants. Recognition of shared struggles against racial oppression amid Trump's attacks on immigrants and communities of color facilitated the formation of coalitions to combat federal policies that inflicted harm on immigrants of color.

In the absence of federal immigration reform and in the presence of severe federal restrictions on residents' rights based on documentation status, subnational contexts have become increasingly important sites for shaping immigrants' experiences.[33] Sociologist Angela García argues that differing approaches to inclusion or exclusion generate an uneven burden of illegality, so where immigrants are physically situated affects their incorporation into the larger society.[34] Other cities, including New York and San Francisco, have become more inclusive by granting their immigrant residents access to municipal identification cards, driver's licenses, and voter registration for local elections, as well as health care.[35] Boston and Massachusetts have not done as much as they could to ensure immigrants' security, but local and state governments have limited power to prevent federal agencies from enforcing policies that threaten immigrants' presence and undermine their well-being. In light of such limits, we now turn to the experiences and perspectives of immigrants, providers, and advocates as discrimination based on racialized legal status intensified in Greater Boston.

Rising Racialized Legal Status Discrimination and Hate Crimes

The increasingly more racist and xenophobic sociopolitical climate under the Trump administration coincided with a rise in overt discriminatory rhetoric and behavior as well as hate crimes associated with people's racialized legal status.[36] This was especially the case for individuals racialized as people of color and immigrants around the country. In Greater Boston, respondents across the three stakeholder groups noted that the national climate shaped local immigrants' experiences. Immigrants, providers, and advocates perceived that racialized legal status discrimination manifested in two ways, attributing both to the Trump administration. The first way was through interpersonal interactions with laypersons in immigrants' daily lives. Specifically, immigrants were more likely to themselves experience or report experiences of discrimination to advocates and providers. Some immigrants even feared going places and encountering discrimination in those spaces. The second way RLS discrimination was more salient was through interactions with law and immigration enforcement, which immigrants feared could lead to arrest, detention, or deportation. Both forms of RLS discrimination jeopardized Latinx immigrants' comfort, safety, and well-being.

Interpersonal Interactions

The majority of the 12 immigrants I interviewed in 2019 described the sociopolitical climate as more difficult for immigrants, regardless of documentation status, than it had previously been. Some described specific incidents of discrimination they witnessed or personally experienced. In terms of racial classification, these respondents were less diverse than those interviewed in previous years. Eight of the Brazilians classified as White or Latino. One of the Dominicans classified as Hispanic and the other as Latino. One Salvadoran classified as White and the other as Hispanic and Latino.

The fact that most of the immigrants I interviewed classified as White makes it particularly striking that 7 of the 12 (4 Brazilians, 2 Dominicans, and 1 Salvadoran) reported that they had experienced discrimination. Of those who did, 4 (3 Brazilians and 1 Salvadoran) felt that this discrimination was due to their being an immigrant. The other 3 (1 Brazilian and 2 Dominicans) thought that they were discriminated against because others perceived them as different from and inferior to White Americans, a sentiment that confounded their racial and immigrant identities. Thus, despite the smaller numbers of immigrant respondents, racialized legal status definitely registered in their experiences with discrimination in 2019.

Leticia, a 34-year-old undocumented Brazilian who described herself as "Morena," said she felt "apprehensive but not completely frightened," which I found surprising. She explained her reasoning: "Trump is only doing this because of his base, making immigrants his target to get more votes. There are Americans who are fanatics about not liking, hating immigrants. But they should consider that without us, where would they be? [American] women don't clean their own bathrooms or houses. Who will do the laundry? . . . They should realize that immigrants are here to help themselves, not to hurt anyone. But it seems they want to hurt us. If all the Brazilians, all the immigrants who are here were deported, what would happen to the US?"

Magna, the Brazilian woman who was burdened by medical debt and whose undocumented father was afraid to venture outside the house, told me that the heightened racism Trump promoted had "definitely taken a toll [on] my mental health." She lived and worked in Somerville, a diverse, densely populated small city adjacent to Boston. Her parents brought her to the United States as a child, and her lack of legal status had prevented her from fulfilling her dream to graduate from college and become a parole officer. Because of her skin tone and hair texture, she was racialized by others as Black. She had been called a "monkey," experienced racism from her classmates, and had numerous negative encounters with local police who racially profiled her. Magna and a friend recorded one incident in which other civilians called the police when she was hanging out with four friends at a shopping center. The first officer who approached them asked one of her friends for ID.

> And she's like, "Why?" And he goes, "Because I want to know how old you are." And she's like, "No." And we just continue to walk. He immediately pushed her, like, "You need to give me your ID"; he did that twice. And right away, I started recording. So, I have an 18-minute clip from this night. My other friend records, too. . . . First, we're like, "You are so rude. So, we're not going to cooperate with you." . . . He wants to just ID [her] and she's just saying no. And we're asking him like, "We're doing what you said. Are we detained?" And he's like, "No." I'm like, "Then we can go," and he's like, "No." That's actually against the law. I'm pretty sure that's kidnapping when you don't let people leave. . . . He just wasn't having it. He called for backup. There's five of us. It ended up being eight officers at the scene.

Madelyn, another BHC provider, reported that her patients mentioned discrimination mostly when they "are complaining about how the police treat them. So many, many patients of color in particular, will say, 'Well, they treat me this way because I'm Black or because I'm Hispanic.' That's real. Then people come in with agitation. . . . Very commonly, in those encounters people are like, 'All the police officers don't like me or have something against me.'"

Being perceived as Latinx or Black was usually associated with experiences of racial discrimination. Despite most immigrants self-classifying as White, 8 thought that they were racialized by others as non-White. Of those 8, 5 thought they were racialized as Hispanic or Latino, and 3 said they were regarded as "Other: immigrant." Respondents were perceived as immigrants because of their lack of English language proficiency or because they spoke English with an accent, which affected Brazilians, Dominicans, and Salvadorans regardless of their physical appearance. Looking non-White or sounding like an outsider might result in discrimination. Magdalena, a 26-year-old Salvadoran who self-classified as White and had a green card, recounted: "When I was trying to resolve an issue by telephone, I called a call center, customer service, and tried to get help in Spanish. But I was told I couldn't. So, I decided to call the customer service center in English. When I did, they didn't give me any problems." Magdalena's contrasting treatment depending on which language she spoke underlines the fact that not speaking fluent, unaccented English can be a source of mistreatment in public and private settings.

Josefina, a Dominican advocate, encountered a particularly absurd response from a stranger: "Once I was having a nice conversation with a woman. And when she asked where I was from and if I spoke Spanish, she said, 'Look, I don't speak with anyone who speaks Spanish.' But we weren't speaking Spanish. Racism has always existed. It's just that now, with Trump supporting all these people, the president has woken them up more and they are showing their racism in their really disrespectful comments about the Latino community."

Public places became increasingly dangerous. A local incident that shocked Bostonians took place in February 2020, when a Salvadoran immigrant and her 15-year-old daughter were verbally and physically attacked for speaking Spanish while walking in their East Boston neighborhood.[37] Two White women yelled at them, "This is America," told them "to go back to their country," and punched and bit them. The perpetrators were charged with violating the victims' civil rights and with assault and battery. At an emotional press conference, the Salvadoran mother stated, "We were attacked based on our race, our language, and our identity."[38] Nearly two years later, the two perpetuators struck a plea deal and received 15 months' probation, which some considered too lenient for a hate crime.[39] This incident was unusual mainly because it involved a crime of violence and became publicly known. In our interviews, stakeholders recounted numerous occasions when Latinx immigrants' presumed race and the language they spoke resulted in discrimination.

Oliver, a BHC provider, spoke at length about how he saw discrimination play out among his patients. He heard more complaints about discrimination from those who were "from the Caribbean, from the Dominican Republic [or] Puerto Rico" than from those who were from Central America. He thought that members of the former groups were aware of "the African American experience of discrimination," while those from Central America were "afraid to say, 'I've been discriminated against.'" Describing this as "my intuition," he continued: "They don't feel that they have the right to say that, because they're undocumented or that they should be thankful to their bosses because they need that job. But that does not give [employers] the right to not treat them well . . . or to make excessive demands." The occasional complaints about discrimination Oliver heard from Brazilian patients, in contrast, mainly involved "discrimination . . . from other Brazilians" who "have been living here a long time or have documented status" and "treat them differently." Some people who are undocumented complained about encountering hostility "from people from El Salvador with [legal] status." Puerto Ricans expressed antagonism toward Dominicans, and Dominicans did the same toward Central Americans.

In Oliver's analysis, having legal status, especially US citizenship, makes a difference. Puerto Ricans have the "full" rights and privileges associated with their legal citizenship when they are in the mainland United States, though those privileges are diminished in Puerto Rico.[40] Dominicans are also usually documented, while Central Americans and Brazilians are more likely to be undocumented. Immigrants with legal status may exploit those who lack it. Although, in previous years of the study, I noticed similar experiences of discrimination by immigrants with legal status against those who were undocumented, these instances came up more often in the 2019 interviews. This difference may be due to the more explicitly racialized anti-immigrant climate that enhanced the advantage of documented co-ethnics over their undocumented counterparts. In times of social strife, marginalized group members who have some structural power, such as citizenship, may use it against co-ethnics with less power.[41]

The 2019 data evinced another pattern that was less prevalent in previous years of the study: more advocates and providers who identified as citizens and immigrants of color reported experiences of discrimination in their work and personal lives. I have not included the ethnoracial classification of advocates and providers in previous chapters to protect the anonymity of those who could be easily identified in their predominantly White work settings. I mention those classifications here, however, to show how the overtly racist rhetoric and policies of the Trump administration led these advocates and providers to contemplate the meaning of their own US citizenship. Nicholas, a healthcare administrator who is Black, said: "You know . . . it's too bad that . . . we have a central government that is very divisive. I remember when Trump . . . commented about Africans and Central Americans coming from 'shithole countries.' . . . He forgot that we too are Americans, and that we have a vested interest in what's happening." Cecilia, a medical interpreter from Central America and naturalized US citizen, attributed an encounter with a xenophobic White woman on the street to the atmosphere created by Trump. "She throws coffee [at me] and then she's like, 'You should be out of here. Go back to your country.' . . . I was speechless. I didn't know what to say. . . . Because I had my jacket [on] and it was cold, I didn't feel like it burned or anything, but it was just a shock."

Many of the advocates and providers of color who shared experiences like these were US citizens. Sebastião, the Brazilian healthcare advocate who previously described immigrants' reduced health coverage access, explained that he carried his passport card and REAL ID driver's license with him everywhere he went as proof of his US citizenship. As a Brazilian with medium-brown skin tone and short black hair, he felt insecure about the protections his citizenship provided:

Even though I am a citizen, in this climate, I don't always feel like one. When I renewed my passport, I got my passport card to carry in my wallet next to my driver's license, to feel more, at times, I don't know—I still don't feel secure. I feel like I have to stay alert in case I am in a situation, even when I go somewhere. To be honest, we are on the defensive all the time. So everywhere I go, in public spaces, if I feel that people are treating me differently, I get defensive. Without realizing it, we get a little apprehensive because we don't know why people are treating us in certain ways: Are they being indifferent, or aggressive towards us?

Such accounts from providers and advocates who were immigrants and were racialized as Latinx or Black demonstrate that racialized legal status affected them in their personal and professional lives. Despite being citizens, they felt targeted and constantly on the defensive because of their race and ethnicity. Like the immigrant respondents I interviewed throughout the study, these providers and advocates' experiences reflect renowned scholar W. E. B. Du Bois's concept of "double consciousness," a sense of twoness people feel from belonging legally but not socially in the United States.[42] Their experiences also reveal the important distinction between legal and sociocultural citizenship, because their legal citizenship did not confer recognition as equally deserving members of the American family. My conversations with Black and Latinx advocates resonated with me because of my own personal experiences as an African American woman. Like Sebastião, I carry my passport card and driver's license everywhere I go. Because I have research and personal connections with immigrant communities, I figured these documents would prove my citizenship if there were an ICE raid at a community meeting or social gathering I attended or if I were stopped by police. I am Black in a time when "driving while Black" can be treated as an offense and police shootings of Black Americans are all too common. Having my passport card would at least prevent police from reporting me to ICE.

Law and Immigration Enforcement

The people I interviewed in 2019 were more likely to report that immigrant, Black, and Latinx residents of metropolitan Boston had frequent and hostile encounters with police than those I interviewed in previous years of this study. That increase is not surprising, given the rising number and heightened visibility of instances in which Black and Latinx men and women, regardless of documentation status, have been killed by police in recent years. Public protests have drawn attention to long-standing but previously less widely known patterns of police violence toward members of marginalized racial-ethnic and immigrant groups. Racialized legal status dramatically affected the encounters of all immigrants and people of color with law and immigration enforcement as federal policies and practices focused on and criminalized them. The increased presence of police and ICE agents in neighborhoods as well as near public schools, healthcare facilities, and courthouses eroded community residents' trust. Advocates explained that mistrust puts everyone's public safety at risk. Immigrants feel they cannot report crimes with confidence that they will not be treated as criminals by the very officers whose assistance they seek.

This problem extends to institutions where people go to access social services. Rachel, an immigrant advocate I also interviewed in 2016, said that the discovery that Boston police were communicating with ICE became part of "the social memory of the community." Her organization met with the staff at a community health center to plan how they would respond if ICE showed up in a waiting room. "For them, that could sink their entire health center. . . . If ICE came by one of the WIC offices . . . 500 families" would immediately disenroll from the nutrition program.

Advocates and providers heard immigrant constituents and patients express anxiety about information sharing between government and healthcare institutions. Quinn, the Health Connector employee quoted previously, reflected on the predicament she faced in her work:

> I'm thinking about . . . how difficult it is to provide people with accurate information that we and they can feel safe about. . . . For example, immigrant eligibility information has to be verified by the federal government. And there are legal protections around that right, so you can look at the law and say, this information ought only be used for health coverage-related, not for any immigration-related, purposes. But being

able to say that in a clear way, that we feel comfortable enough to put on paper, that you will be safe, you can trust us—this has been challenging.

The connection between policing and immigration enforcement aroused criticism when some Massachusetts jails and prisons were used to detain immigrants, most of whom were Latinx and Black, who had been refused entry to the United States or were awaiting deportation. At community meetings, advocates and grassroots activists pressured state and county officials to end contracts with ICE and Homeland Security. For example, Bristol County sheriff Thomas Hodgson, a fervently anti-immigrant Trump supporter, rented space in the county jail to ICE to hold detainees, including those from outside the state. This policy was met with protests as soon as it began, and opposition deepened with revelations that guards used excessive force against detainees who were protesting the inhumane conditions of their imprisonment.[43] This situation shed a bright light on the shared racism and xenophobia embedded in the criminal legal system and the immigration enforcement regime in Massachusetts, despite the commonwealth's reputation for liberalism.

In recent years, scholars have pointed to troubling connections between mass incarceration and immigration detention, as private prisons are now profiting from housing large numbers of immigrants held by the federal government.[44] Felicia, who formerly worked for the Mexican Consulate in Boston, was aware of this practice because she was responsible for trying to ensure that detained Mexican nationals were treated in accordance with international standards. While acknowledging that "people in immigration detention here . . . have some access to health care and [a] nurse," Felicia explained that the conditions of their detention were inadequate to meet their needs. The authorities "can call it a detention [center], but . . . it's just a different cell block. It has exactly the same problems that you would see in a prison. I saw people who had . . . terrible physical injuries. They wouldn't have [adequate] access to health care, [or for] dealing with the mental shock and trauma of what they've gone through."

Trump administration policies jeopardized the security of documented as well as undocumented immigrants. Noncitizens with a range of documented statuses worried that their legal status was under threat and that they could be targeted for deportation. In recent decades, these statuses have applied to immigrants of color from Central America, the Caribbean, and Africa who are almost uniformly racialized as Latinx and Black—indicating yet again that racialized legal status doubly disadvantaged immigrants. Moreover, the reverse was also true: US-born citizens of color could be profiled as "illegal" immigrants and subjected to violence and arrest.

The increasing presence of federal immigration enforcement agents in Massachusetts was evident in several well-publicized incidents. In October 2020, ICE officials stopped and questioned a Black man jogging in West Roxbury about his immigration status.[45] The jogger, a lifelong state resident, videotaped some of the interaction, which was posted on Facebook and led to a public outcry. Mayor Marty Walsh and three members of Massachusetts's congressional delegation—Representative Ayanna Pressley, Senator Elizabeth Warren, and Senator Ed Markey—questioned ICE about why officials stopped the jogger, who was mistakenly identified as being under ICE investigation. This incident illustrates another dimension of the racialized legal status discrimination that heightened insecurity and fear among Boston's Black and Latinx residents regardless of their legal status. Their encounters with police and ICE could lead to arrest, detention, incarceration, and deportation or death.

Immigrants' Health and Healthcare in Trump's America

As I conducted interviews in 2016 and 2019, BHC providers noticed that many Latinx patients dropped MassHealth while seeking to legalize their presence in the United States. Aubrey, a BHC physician, described a case in which a child had "likely had a congenital heart attack," but "the parents were getting deported," so the family urgently needed a lawyer. In cases where "it's an imminent health problem that either cannot be addressed in their own country or needs to be addressed here [first], . . . their immigration status is just getting in the way. So, we as health providers" feel that "a legal need is actually a health need."

Immigrants witnessed the fear other immigrants felt about seeking health care. Alexandre, a 56-year-old Brazilian and naturalized US citizen, said, "Now, many Brazilian immigrants and those of other nationalities are afraid to go to hospitals. Because Trump, I don't know if it's Trump or Congress, [but] if you want to get your green card or become a citizen and they discover that you received medical help or anything, that will be an impediment." Similarly, Josefina, the Dominican advocate who shared her own experiences of discrimination, said that immigrants "suffer from many medical problems." Sometimes they "take natural medicines . . . using old remedies that our Indigenous ancestors used" rather than risk going to a health clinic.

Making immigrants too fearful to seek medical attention was among the most damaging effects of the toxic sociopolitical climate. Those with minor health problems might forgo treatment or rely on home remedies without serious risk, although no one can be sure that a condition is actually minor without a proper diagnosis. For those with more serious health conditions, not seeking medical attention could have fatal consequences. Rachel, the immigrant advocate who discussed how ICE's presence could tank immigrants' health service use, shared a tragic case: "There was an incident right after the election, where we know that a young Brazilian family in Somerville, their toddler son was in [an] acute condition, and they were afraid to call in the EMT. And so, they try to drive their son to the hospital, and he died in route."

The anxiety that led immigrants to defer or avoid needed medical treatment had a significant impact on their physical and mental health. For immigrants of color, the consequences of being unable to obtain health care were exacerbated by their frequent encounters with racism. It has long been known that experiences of racial discrimination negatively affect Black Americans' health.[46] Recent research has established that discrimination against immigrants can pose similar health threats, especially to those who are Black or Latinx.[47] During the Trump administration, numerous scholars documented the negative effects of racialized legal status on the health of Latinx citizens and noncitizens around the country.[48]

The advocates, providers, and immigrants I interviewed in Boston made similar observations. Because I was conducting interviews while Trump administration policies were being announced, I heard about the real-time responses interviewees witnessed and their implications for health. Respondents repeatedly used the words "stress" and "trauma" to describe the impact of the daily assault on immigrants. Kiara, a Brazilian advocate, stated that "there's no way to not lose sleep at night or to not have a high level of stress or anxiety. Even if you tell yourself, 'Nothing will happen to me,' it could happen to someone I know. I think that immigrants are living in a situation with extreme instability, a situation of terror. I think that's the appropriate word, 'terror.' I think it's bullying and a politics of terrorizing people."

The descriptions and media images of families being separated and children being locked in cages at the southern border were especially distressing. Although Massachusetts is geographically thousands of miles away, these events were felt locally, as some of these family members were relocated to the commonwealth. Local providers and advocates tried to help them find physical and mental health services. Citizens and noncitizens in mixed-status families and communities also felt the pain caused by family separation policies. Manuel, the Salvadoran pastor who perceived that dogs could get better health care than immigrants in 2016, explained:

> Kids who know that their parents are illegal, they are afraid. Because if a kid is watching Telemundo, and it's said that Immigration is going to come and it's time to be careful and if they knock at the door, don't let him in. And that kid, a seven-year-old watching the news, is going to get afraid that mom could be taken, or that dad be taken. Imagine that kid going to school the following day, thinking that when I get back home, mom is not going to be home. The father is going to work, and he doesn't know if he's going to get arrested at work and is never going to see the kids again. So, it is affecting [them] psychologically, kids and adults.

As in previous years of the study, BHC providers thought that the most common physical health problems among immigrants were obesity, high blood pressure, high cholesterol, diabetes, cancer, lack of access to dental care, and workplace injuries. The mental health issues they mentioned most often were anxiety, depression, and substance abuse. Providers and advocates felt that stress brought on by the worsening sociopolitical climate exacerbated those physical and mental health conditions. Some, like Cecilia, the medical interpreter who had coffee thrown at her, thought that documented and undocumented immigrants alike were feeling the health effects. In her view, somatic complaints and substance use were clearly linked, so providers were trying to treat pain without medications such as opioids. Anxiety and stress tended to lead to weight gain, high cholesterol, and hypertension. "All those factors affect their physical health as well as their mental health."

Similarly, Noah, a Dominican advocate, stated, "I believe that the political climate creates the conditions to develop and make mental health issues worse." He noticed this pattern "through conversations, . . . going to community events, seeing families and friends." In the past, he said, "I used to joke about it: We [Latinx people] don't have time to get depressed. We need to go about . . . trying to make our lives better. We do not have [time] to stop going. It wasn't an option." Now, in contrast, you "try to hang in there. You fight your fight." But "your system tells you, your own [body] tells you, your brain tells you" you need to stop. "Then you collapse. That's what I see happen, and I think . . . there's not much we can do."

The accumulated stresses arising from racialized legal status discrimination and the blatant devaluation of immigrants' lives, particularly of Latinx people who were disproportionately targeted by toxic rhetoric, could produce illness and despair. At the same time, their concerns about aggressive and punitive enforcement, language difficulties, and costs they could not pay contributed to delayed or canceled medical appointments and the inability to fill prescriptions. Too many found themselves caught in this vicious circle.[49]

The vitriolic rhetoric and harsh proposals and policies of the Trump administration affected providers and advocates, along with the immigrant patients and constituents they served. Paola, the health advocate who discussed the difficulty of combating misinformation, appeared exasperated as she described the struggle.

> You can get tired because every week you have something to fight, . . . whether they are attacking the ACA, proposing [new] Medicaid requirements [or] Medicaid block grants, . . . reducing funding for your health center, or CHIP [the subsidized insurance policy for children] was on the line. . . . Every single week, you have something. And then you have the immigration stuff: the travel ban, the detention centers, the census citizenship question. Then public charge, DACA, TPS, immigration detention, now the fact that they cannot even apply for asylum at the port of entry. . . . You can get frustrated because you might win a battle, but then the next day, there's something else, if not three things at the same time.

I often wondered how advocates were managing on the front lines, working with immigrants who were living in fear and trying to convince them to keep their benefits and take care of their health. Sometimes patients took out their frustrations on advocates and providers, as Penelope, a healthcare advocate, recounted: "We deal with really complicated cases sometimes. We hear from people who've . . . been trying to fix their health coverage for many months or even years. They're really upset. And it can be hard . . . it feels personal when people are yelling at you. So, being able to step back, and remember, they're not actually yelling at you, they're yelling at the whole system" was vital.

Michele, a previously quoted immigration attorney, described the stresses of dealing with a constant barrage of "arbitrary" policy changes. It was even harder for "core community groups that work exclusively with downtrodden immigrant populations," she acknowledged. "I feel that collectively our communities, grassroots, nonprofit sector, lawyers, anybody in this immigration space has been mentally attacked. I mean, our mental health has been under siege."

BHC providers like Christopher, who did psychological evaluations of asylum applicants, carried an especially heavy burden:

The stories that I hear from asylum seekers . . . can be dramatically painful and hard to hear and hard to sit with. . . . You're meeting with someone one time and you have to hear everything that happened to them. That is quite different than if you're seeing someone for therapy: that can evolve over time, or if they say, "Hey, I don't want to talk about it in therapy often" or "Let's not talk about it," [you can] let them move on. But in these evaluations, I have generally one meeting . . . to hear stuff with my own ears so that I can put it in a report. That means I'm hearing a lot of horrible, often tragic things. It means the client has to say things that they would almost always prefer never to think about again. That's just emotionally fraught.

Christopher coped with this overload of secondary trauma mainly by exercising every day, talking with his wife, and drinking more often than he thought he should.

Those who did such difficult work at this particularly distressing time found inspiration and support from other advocates, providers, immigrant communities, and concerned citizens. They felt they were doing their part to create a more equitable society where immigrants and other marginalized people could live without overwhelming fear and access the social services they needed. As I interviewed them and heard their stories as well as those of immigrants, I sometimes felt overwhelmed by the magnitude of what immigrants and those who assist them were facing on a daily basis. I dealt with the situation in some of the same ways they did, by talking with my partner and exercising. As I attended community meetings, policy advocacy planning sessions, and public hearings at Boston City Hall and the State House alongside these various stakeholders, we found solace and solidarity in what we perceived to be a valiant and necessary struggle for social justice.

Conclusion

Shifts in health and immigration policy at the national and subnational levels under the Trump administration made racialized legal status more salient for Boston's Latinx immigrants when obtaining coverage and care in 2019. Consequently, access to health coverage and healthcare services deteriorated for Latinx immigrants in Boston and beyond. The explicitly racist and anti-immigrant rhetoric and proposed and actual policy changes, particularly in the public charge rule, made Latinx Bostonians more wary of using their coverage and any other public benefits.

Massachusetts lawmakers bolstered protections to strengthen the state's health coverage system amid GOP threats to repeal and undermine Obamacare. But the 2016 changes in the state's Health Safety Net program contributed to many immigrants losing eligibility for coverage in 2019. Furthermore, even in Massachusetts there was still little political appetite to pass and implement more immigrant-inclusive policies. The voters' and legislators' decisions not to offer driver's licenses to undocumented immigrants and not to adopt a statewide sanctuary policy made the commonwealth less hospitable for its immigrant residents. These choices had health consequences, as paralyzing fear of law and immigration enforcement made Boston's Latinx residents less likely to seek needed medical services or to report hate crimes and discrimination against them.

While immigrants struggled to navigate the increasingly difficult terrain created by their racialized legal status, advocates and providers of color, many of whom were also immigrants, felt targeted in their personal and professional lives. They sought to support their constituents and patients amid what some described as a situation punctuated by bombs and others compared to a war. Like the immigrants they worked with, advocates' and providers' health suffered from the stress of dealing with the Trump administration's chaotic campaign against all those it regarded as enemies.

Yet those who were committed to providing the health coverage and care all state residents needed were as resilient as immigrant families and communities in the face of this onslaught. Supporting one another and working together, immigrants, advocates, and providers resisted the federal government's punitive measures whenever possible. Collectively, they sued the Trump administration, advocated for stronger immigrant-inclusive policies at the Massachusetts State House, and kept showing up to provide services and care for those who needed them. Although 2019 proved to be the most challenging year of the study, when racialized legal status exclusion seemed to be at its worst, that time also provided more clarity about possible solutions to the challenges Boston's Latinx immigrants had contended with in the local healthcare system since I began the study in 2012.

Conclusion

I have been here [in the United States] for 21 years, and unfortunately, I haven't seen things improve [for immigrants]. It's only gotten worse. It's really sad to say, but I was in a meeting last week and said the same thing and everyone agreed with me. Because we started this struggle for immigrant rights [and] immigration reform. [Now,] 21 years later, we're still fighting for the same things.

—*Micaela, Brazilian advocate interviewed in 2016*

It's frustrating . . . to try to help patients. But you can't help patients because [of] the way the system is. . . . We're talking about equity care for all patients, and the patients . . . you just can't do much . . . because [a] patient says "I don't have insurance, I don't have transportation, . . . I need housing." . . . Even for us, providers, to try to navigate the system for [our] patients . . . it's frustrating for me to spend so many hours on the phone to try to get them covered. I can imagine how that is for a patient to try to navigate the system. So, they give up.

—*Olivia, BHC provider interviewed in 2019*

After spending nearly a decade interviewing people to understand how policy shifts reconfigured Latinx immigrants' access to health care in

Boston from 2012 to 2019, I must conclude that healthcare access and the sociopolitical climate worsened over time. Micaela, the executive director of a Brazilian advocacy organization whom I interviewed each year of the study, emphasized the lack of progress for immigrants since she arrived in this country more than two decades ago. Olivia, a BHC provider I also interviewed in 2012, highlighted the challenges she and her colleagues encountered while helping patients who belonged to marginalized groups in 2019. Their predicaments reflect larger social determinants, such as transportation and housing, that affect health but are external to the healthcare system. Ironically, these are the same challenges that Greg—a BHC physician interviewed in 2013, whose quote opens the book's introduction—articulated in the aftermath of major changes in health policy that were intended to extend coverage. Many of the structural problems in and outside of the healthcare system that made it difficult to provide patients with quality care still remain, even for people *with* coverage. And this is despite the passage and implementation of the Massachusetts and federal ACA healthcare reforms. Public policies that extend *beyond* the healthcare system are needed to address societal structural problems that exacerbate healthcare and health disparities.

Consequently, this book underscores a sobering truth about the US healthcare system: having health coverage and insurance does not guarantee access to care, especially given the pervasive power of racialized legal status for the most marginalized communities. The intersection of race, ethnicity, and documentation status is important both at the individual or micro level, in shaping encounters with providers, and at the meso level, as immigrants interact with bureaucracies and social service institutions. Being racialized as a person of color and treated as if one lacked legal citizenship regardless of documentation status magnifies the likelihood of exclusion and discrimination. At the macro level, the federalist structure of US governance and the ongoing dance between the state and national governments in health and immigration policy create unanticipated complications. These incoherent and sometimes contradictory policies compounded the heavy administrative burdens and procedural barriers that Boston's Latinx immigrants experienced in (re)enrolling for health coverage. In daily life, their racialized legal status generated concerns about encounters with police and immigration enforcement officials en route to hospitals and clinics. This intersectional form of discrimination was so severe that it created medical legal violence within the healthcare system, placing those in need of health care at risk of arrest, detention, and deportation. Thus, racialized legal status represents a consequential form of social inequality in the 21st-century United States, as citizens and noncitizens of color are not guaranteed full access to health coverage and minimally adequate care.

This situation is the opposite of the Massachusetts and ACA health policy reforms' goal: to increase access to care and coverage for un- and underinsured populations. Micaela and Olivia described the difficulties immigrants faced in obtaining health coverage and services in an increasingly hostile sociopolitical climate, even in places with immigrant-inclusive policies. The root of the problem is that healthcare policies do not fully address the actual problems that immigrants face in the healthcare system and broader society. Although those who are undocumented encounter more categorical exclusion, those who are legal residents and naturalized citizens also encounter difficulties because of the dynamics of racialized legal status.

The limits of healthcare policy to redress socioeconomic and racial-ethnic inequality had life-threatening consequences during the COVID-19 pandemic. I completed the interviews for this book before the COVID public health emergency led to global quarantines. I realized, however, that the social and healthcare challenges I observed in Boston's Latinx communities would leave them especially vulnerable to COVID. Unfortunately, I was right. As COVID case counts increased exponentially in Massachusetts, the immigrant neighborhoods where I interviewed people were some of the hardest hit, demonstrating a painfully clear connection between immigrants' healthcare access and collective public health. The sociopolitical climate in Trump's America was exacerbating a public health crisis. Just a few months before the pandemic, Javier, a civil rights attorney I interviewed in fall 2019, explained that it was vital for immigrants to feel safe obtaining health care "because if we have any type of dip in" immigrants obtaining medical services such as vaccinations, "it can have a ripple effect on broader public health. . . . We need to talk about these issues as public health threats . . . that affect not just immigrant communities but broader populations as a whole. And we need to talk about the public health consequences of immigration enforcement." Thus, in this concluding chapter, I summarize the major findings of the book, highlight their implications in light of the COVID pandemic and for other regions of the country, and close with some policy recommendations that would make health coverage and care more equitably available to all.

Racialized Legal Status in the US Healthcare System

Racialized legal status pervades the US healthcare system. First, policies operating at multiple levels of government include and exclude immigrants based on their documentation status and negatively affect immigrants and citizens of color through structural and systemic racism. Second, racialized legal status exacerbates the administrative burdens involved in applying for coverage and navigating the healthcare system. Third, the rise of "crimmigration"—the criminalization of immigrants and close collaboration between law and immigration enforcement agencies—is a major deterrent to seeking health services for immigrants and citizens of color, particularly those in mixed-status families. People's racialized legal status (see Figure 1-2) can heighten their experience of legal violence and medical legal violence.

The Tensions of Federalism

One resounding theme throughout this book has been the conflict between policies of the state and federal governments, which is a basic feature of federalism and can exacerbate political polarization. The immigrants I interviewed were at the mercy of macro-level policies that neither they nor most others understood. Often, they were caught between federal-level exclusion and state-level inclusion that required detailed evidence of their residence, income, and documentation status to prove eligibility. Significant confusion and effective exclusion ensue when federal and state policies contradict each other. The impact of Massachusetts's implementation of Obamacare illustrates this point. Immigrants, providers, and advocates commented that this policy mismatch often led to immigrants being told that they were ineligible for coverage under Obamacare even though they were still eligible under the state's policy.

The Trump administration's proposed change to the public charge rule sent shock waves through immigrant communities in 2019. In Boston, noncitizen immigrants responded by disenrolling from all types of public benefits, including state-funded health coverage. They believed that remaining enrolled would place them or their family members at risk of deportation or jeopardize their prospects for naturalization. Although that interpretation was inaccurate, it had its intended chilling effect of pushing immigrants outside the social safety net. These perceptions persisted beyond Trump's presidency. At a local immigrant health advocacy coalition meeting I attended virtually in fall 2021, advocates and providers said that many immigrants believed that the Trump-era public charge rule was still in effect even though the Biden administration had abandoned it in March 2021.[1] In the midst of the COVID pandemic, despite concerted efforts to convince immigrants that they could safely obtain coverage and care in Massachusetts, they remained worried that getting tested and vaccinated for COVID would endanger their status in the country. These accounts reveal the limits of state-level inclusive policies in the face of restrictive federal policies.

At the same time, the increasing devolution of responsibility for administering federal funds for health programs such as Medicaid and Medicare to states underscores just how important state legislatures are for extending or denying access to federal programs to their residents, particularly immigrants.[2] Access has remained exceedingly difficult and treatment much more expensive for immigrant and lower-income people in states that did not expand Medicaid under the Affordable Care Act.[3] Conversely, some states included immigrants in health and social services. California expanded access to its Medicaid program for low-income undocumented people in specific age groups who are unlikely to be fully independent: children and young adults up to age 26 and adults over age

50. Adults ages 26 to 49 became eligible in January 2024.[4] Illinois became the first state to extend health coverage to undocumented seniors.[5] Recent studies have revealed, however, that increased cooperation between federal immigration enforcement and state and local law enforcement agencies had a chilling effect on immigrants' willingness to seek health services even in states with immigrant-inclusive health coverage.[6] Thus, factors that extend well beyond health coverage prevent immigrants from obtaining appropriate care.

Massachusetts is among the few states whose health policy provides access to health care for most lower- and some middle-income immigrants with a range of legal statuses. That access has been restricted over time, however. Some providers I was able to reinterview throughout the project felt it was more difficult for immigrants to get and keep coverage in 2019 than it was before the Massachusetts and ACA reforms. Kevin, a BHC provider I interviewed in 2012 and 2019, recalled: "There's no question how different it is [now], but since my career [started] 16 years [ago, it] is a dramatic difference. . . . People have less coverage. So prior to 2006 . . . was the heyday of getting proper care for undocumented persons. . . . Then it [gradually] got worse."

Beyond health care, the commonwealth excluded immigrants in other policy domains while I conducted research for this book.[7] In these instances, federal and state policies aligned to exclude the undocumented. For example, undocumented immigrants' inability to obtain driver's licenses in many states, including Massachusetts, perpetuated racialized legal status exclusion in health care. A sizable proportion of the undocumented population consists of people of color, who are likely to be racially profiled and stopped by police. The ability to drive without the risk of being detained is essential to obtaining health care in the absence of adequate public transportation. During the COVID pandemic, the risk of taking public transportation to a healthcare facility outweighed the possible benefits of care.[8] Massachusetts's refusal to extend driver's licenses to all residents had been debated under both Democratic and Republican governors and in the Democratic-controlled state legislature, but the unfounded fear that noncitizens with driver's licenses would fraudulently be registered to vote blocked any change for more than a decade. As of July 1, 2023, under Democratic governor Maura Healey, Massachusetts became the 15th state to issue driver's licenses to undocumented immigrants.[9]

Finally, while many federal and state policies explicitly exclude people based on their documentation status, those policies have the appearance of being race neutral, but this does not mean they are devoid of racial implications. This country's democracy is based on structural and systemic racism, so policies that make no explicit reference to race are applied unequally. Racial and ethnic groups differentially experience the consequences, as people of color are unable to enjoy equal benefits and even endure particular harms. The impact is even greater for immigrants of color, who are often excluded because of their legal status or because White Americans presume they are undocumented due to their non-White appearance or the way they speak. In both policy and practice, racialized legal status has restricted Boston immigrants' healthcare access even under an inclusive health policy. Studies conducted by scholars elsewhere reveal a similarly stark reality in health care for immigrants of color in rural and urban locales as far west as California, as far south as Texas, and in midwestern states such as Illinois and Kansas—unfortunately, from sea to shining sea.[10]

Racialized Legal Status and Administrative Burdens

Beyond the contradictions produced by federalism in shaping eligibility for health coverage, racialized legal status influenced Boston immigrants' ability to use health services through time-taxing administrative burdens.[11] These burdens operated in an intersectional manner, so that both race/ethnicity and actual or presumed legal status limited access to coverage and care for Brazilian, Dominican, and Salvadoran immigrants. A myriad of structural barriers confronted them at every step, from trying to sign up for coverage under the Massachusetts and Obamacare reforms to using that coverage to obtain services. In light of these obstacles, spending huge amounts of time seeking coverage and care seemed futile. Amalia, a 53-year-old Dominican I interviewed in 2016, lamented,

"Everything is hard, it costs you a lot to do anything. You have to be very resilient for you [to] get something as an immigrant." When they had to choose between a prolonged search for health care and their primary commitments to family and paid work, they prioritized the most immediate needs they felt confident they could help to meet. Cumulatively, these obstacles interfered with immigrants' ability to take care of their health by seeing providers for preventive and specialty care.

Perhaps the most formidable structural barrier was the bureaucratic maze that constitutes the US healthcare system. This "kludgeocracy" imposes administrative burdens such as deciphering the byzantine rules determining eligibility; completing paper or online forms to sign up for coverage; understanding the differing requirements for obtaining primary care, referrals to specialists, and prescription medications; and navigating huge medical facilities to find appointments.[12] Essential tasks proliferate: producing required documents to prove eligibility, scheduling initial and follow-up appointments, organizing transportation to and from appointments, and finding the money for required co-pays and medical bills. Although some of these barriers could be overcome with assistance from knowledgeable family members, acquaintances, or advocates, others—especially those posed by documentation status—are impossible to evade and dangerous even to confront directly. Individuals navigated the system as best they could or gave up after wearisome and fruitless efforts. My 209 interviews with immigrants, advocates, and providers over the past decade substantiate this harsh reality. Simply put, these multiple structural barriers pose enough difficulties for most people. Those in marginalized groups, however—especially noncitizens, people of color, those with low incomes, and those with limited English proficiency—face cultural and financial barriers that translate into discrimination and exclusion.

Among the many barriers noted by participants in the study, those regarding language accessibility and racialized immigration enforcement were the most troubling. These problems shaped every aspect of navigating the healthcare system. The inability to find assistance in their primary language constrained many immigrants' ability not only to obtain and use coverage but also to communicate effectively with providers. Having a diverse medical staff and robust medical interpretation services is essential to providing quality health care.

Another consequence of limited language accessibility was immigrant communities' reliance on information from those who speak their language, whether directly through their social networks or indirectly through social media. This information, which was sometimes inaccurate, shaped their healthcare decisions. For example, rumors were spread on WhatsApp and Facebook about ICE agents near medical facilities and the public charge rule that deterred people from seeking health care even if there were trusted providers in these communities.

Nevertheless, immigrant and healthcare advocates and agencies play crucial roles in helping immigrants navigate the system. The dedication of these individuals in Boston and elsewhere is reducing the impact of racialized legal status discrimination on marginalized populations around the country.[13] Advocates' policy expertise and experience with the bureaucracy reduce the barriers built into the system, provided that people know where to find help. Social networks are vital sources of useful information. In interviews with immigrants and advocates, I heard story after story about people who were at the end of their rope trying to meet Massachusetts's health insurance requirements but were unsure of how to do so given the confusing English language enrollment process. Being able to call a health consumer helpline and get assistance in Portuguese or Spanish made all the difference.

Unfortunately, the barriers posed by racialized legal status seemed to worsen each year of the study, becoming so formidable that only the most persistent were able to find a way over or around them. I consider it a miracle that most of the immigrants I interviewed had some type of health coverage and could provide the name of their regular provider and facility—but what about the many others who could not? These burdens can be impossibly heavy, the barriers insurmountable. For hourly workers, taking time off for appointments may be impossible. Yet many respondents invested significant amounts of time seeking care for themselves and others. As scholars such as Victor Ray, Pamela Herd, Donald

Moynihan, Bruce Link, and Jo Phelan have pointed out, the weight of those burdens falls most heavily on the least privileged among us.[14] Racialized legal status not only steals time but also makes daily life and obtaining health care more taxing for immigrants and communities of color in Boston and beyond.

Latinx Heterogeneity, Crimmigration, and Intensifying Legal Violence

The different ethnoracial and socioeconomic backgrounds of the Brazilians, Dominicans, and Salvadorans I interviewed shaped their experiences with health care. Despite being grouped together under the "Latino" label, they were remarkably heterogeneous in their premigration backgrounds and current social situations. Cultural differences between the US healthcare system and the systems in Brazil, the Dominican Republic, and El Salvador also affected these immigrants' interactions with bureaucrats, advocates, and providers. All these differences mattered for shaping how racialized legal status operated among these groups, who are typically unrepresented or underrepresented in health-related or broader research on Latinos.

Given the power of legal status to shape eligibility for access to health care and other public benefits under most federal and state policies, we might think that Dominicans would benefit significantly because the majority were green card holders or naturalized citizens. Their legal status offered them more formal access to services and, for most citizens, freedom from deportation. But many were racialized as Black and had darker skin tone, came from lower socioeconomic positions, lacked health insurance before migration, and had limited English proficiency. The confluence of these factors limited the scope of their legal inclusion. While aware of their Blackness, Dominicans often identified as Latino or Hispanic. Their encounters with racism in structural and interpersonal forms played out in negative interactions with providers and, more broadly, in their concentration in residentially segregated communities such as Jamaica Plain, where they were being pushed out by gentrification. My data indicates that Dominicans tended to have serious health problems and public coverage. Given what we know about the impact of racism on health for Black Americans and immigrants racialized as Black in this country, Dominicans' experiences are not surprising.[15]

Like Dominicans, most Salvadoran immigrants came from low socioeconomic classes without health insurance in El Salvador and had limited English proficiency. Having undocumented or temporary protected status further constrained their access to public benefits and services. Furthermore, their medium-brown skin tone and black hair quintessentially marked them as Latinx. These physical features stigmatized them as "illegal," "criminal," and "not American."[16] Salvadorans tended to identify as Latino or Hispanic and felt that others classified them in the same way. Many were clearly aware of how others' racialization of them sometimes resulted in discrimination in health care and other settings. Some directly connected this problem to their exploitation at work and their resulting physical and mental health problems.[17] Both Salvadorans and Dominicans attributed the discrimination they experienced to their racial and immigrant backgrounds. They felt they were viewed and treated as outsiders regardless of how long they had been in the country and that looking "Black" (among Dominicans) or "Latino" (among Salvadorans) generated significant harms in their daily lives.

Brazilians had a range of documentation statuses, but a sizable proportion had been or were still undocumented. We might think that their legal status would have put them at a significant disadvantage, explicitly excluding them from public benefits. But the fact that most had lighter skin tones and came from working- or middle-class backgrounds in Brazil benefited them in their daily lives and healthcare encounters. Having had access to health coverage and regular healthcare providers, along with higher levels of formal education, before migrating enhanced Brazilians' ability to navigate the US healthcare system. At the same time, they faced challenges finding appropriate help in Portuguese, which is relatively unfamiliar to Americans compared with Spanish. So, Brazilians' social networks were crucial conduits for information. Because racial stratification in Brazil shapes who migrates, many Brazilian immigrants self-identify and are classified by others as White. While they may not be considered

White in the United States, their appearance privileges them relative to Dominicans and Salvadorans. No Brazilian respondents identified as Hispanic, and only a few called themselves Latino. Most preferred being identified as Brazilian. Many of the Brazilians I interviewed attributed any discrimination they experienced to being an immigrant or speaking English with an accent, rather than regarding it as racially motivated.

Advocates' and providers' perceptions of these groups were closely aligned with the immigrants' self-perceptions. In the eyes of advocates and respondents, Brazilians were more adept at navigating the healthcare system than Salvadorans and Dominicans were. Indeed, some advocates and providers discussed Brazilians and Latinos separately, just as some Brazilian respondents refused to be lumped together with Latinos. Recognizing the heterogeneity hidden under this umbrella term is vital, as Dominicans and Salvadorans, as well as Brazilians, differ significantly from Mexicans, who are the largest group of Latin American origin and descent in the United States and are the focus of most studies on "Latinos." The differences I found in premigration background, racialization, and healthcare experiences affect the ways in which various members of this large pan-ethnic group navigated their daily lives, the healthcare system, and other social service bureaucracies. Collectively, these differences may contribute to diverging health outcomes among Latinx ethnicities, which should be examined in future studies.

The main problem that Brazilians, Dominicans, and Salvadorans shared was fear of immigration and law enforcement officials. Their experiences in the Boston area, a sanctuary city located in a nonsanctuary state, reveal the extent of crimmigration in the commonwealth. Across these groups, respondents mentioned their fear of police and ICE, which intensified over the duration of the study. Stakeholders mentioned actual raids and threats of raids in subway stations or on highways, and immigrant respondents thought they could easily be profiled, detained, arrested, and deported. While Dominicans and Salvadorans more often thought they were targeted because they looked Black or Latino, Brazilians thought it was due to their perceived immigrant status and the inference made by these authorities that they were undocumented. Numerous members of all these groups recounted instances when they or others in their communities were pulled over for questioning by police or ICE. Their experiences were like those of other Latinx individuals—citizen and noncitizen—around the country.[18]

Intensified enforcement, coupled with racialized anti-immigrant rhetoric, created so much fear in some communities that it deterred people from seeking health care. Many opted not to attend scheduled appointments when raids occurred or were rumored to be planned in their neighborhoods. People used social media to warn others of police or ICE stopping people on the highway and in the subways. Crimmigration inflicted significant legal violence on these communities, not only by inhibiting them from getting the care they needed but also by exacerbating their physical and mental trauma. This trauma was heightened by experiences of racialized legal status discrimination and intense frustration with the administrative barriers that blocked them from getting much-needed health care. Research has shown that such cumulative trauma can create a pernicious cycle of deteriorating physical and mental health.[19] Other studies have found similar connections between threats of deportation and worsened health outcomes around the country.[20]

In response to these challenges, some immigrants sought health care in their home countries. Those whose financial resources and legal status in the United States allowed them to visit their home countries took this course because the costs were lower, language was not a barrier, and they felt more comfortable with co-ethnic providers. Those who were undocumented consulted with physicians online or received advice, medications, and medical advice from trusted relatives in Brazil, the Dominican Republic, or El Salvador. These practices demonstrate immigrants' resourcefulness and resilience in getting around the various barriers that impose excessive burdens on finding care in the United States.[21]

Implications Beyond Boston

The most important takeaway from this book is that access to health coverage does not guarantee equal access to care for immigrants and other marginalized groups. The legacy and ongoing patterns of exclusion associated with racialized legal status show the inadequacy of health policy alone to rectify disparities in coverage and care. Exclusion on the basis of documentation status is still legally entrenched in policy, and seemingly race-neutral policies produce differential outcomes among racial groups. Consequently, existing policies in a country with embedded structural and systemic racism exacerbate RLS discrimination in health care and society. Although this study focused on a particular time period, its findings reflect ongoing problems with the US healthcare system and healthcare access that have long existed and will continue to exist because of how the system is set up. As long as there is discrimination in law, practice, institutions, and interpersonal interactions, there will be health and healthcare-related inequities based on race, ethnicity, legal status, and socioeconomic position. Until policies effectively address structural and systemic discrimination in the broader society, discrimination will continue to manifest itself in the healthcare system, leaving the most marginalized at a huge disadvantage. Thus, this book's findings have broader implications in five areas that future research should examine.

First, the racialized legal status framework employed in this book is crucial in demonstrating how pervasively the intersection of race, ethnicity, and legal status shapes the health care and lived experiences of Brazilian, Dominican, and Salvadoran immigrants under shifting policies. This conceptual framework should be used to examine other policy realms and their implications for people of color with various legal statuses within and beyond the United States. At a time when intensified racist, xenophobic, and anti-immigrant rhetoric and policy proposals target those perceived as foreigners in the United States and other immigrant-receiving countries, this framework provides a way to analyze and assess how and why race, ethnicity, and legal status matter in producing inequality.[22] For instance, how does racialized legal status affect those of Asian, Middle Eastern, or Northern African (MENA) heritage in the United States? Like individuals of Latin American heritage, those of Asian and MENA descent represent numerous countries, ethnicities, and languages but are racialized as "forever foreigners," terrorists, and routinely targeted by hate crimes. Similarly, Native Americans, against whom

White settlers committed genocide and whose ancestral lands they stole, continue to be plagued by threats to tribal sovereignty, detrimental social and health outcomes, and environmental damage on and off their reservations.

Second, the concept of racialized legal status deepens our understanding of how citizenship is differentially experienced by immigrants in host societies, particularly because race and ethnicity have been and remain significant for demarcating legal citizenship and social belonging in the United States and other countries. While some of the immigrants I interviewed saw US citizenship as a golden ticket to a better life, I sometimes wondered why they felt this way. As an African American citizen aware of this country's history who was conducting this study and writing this book during an epidemic of police murders of unarmed Black Americans, I knew all too well the limits of legal citizenship without sociocultural membership. Qualitative and quantitative research should build on this framework to understand the connections among policy, socioeconomic stratification, and racial inequality in the 21st century.

Relatedly, this book reveals how racialized legal status differentially shapes immigrant incorporation in US society, from where immigrants live and work to how they navigate social service bureaucracies. Media narratives suggest that immigrants self-segregate and do not want to assimilate. My research shows, however, that limited English proficiency amid entrenched patterns of residential segregation and unaffordable housing pushed Brazilian, Dominican, and Salvadoran immigrants into lower-paying jobs and substandard housing among co-ethnics. In turn, these patterns influenced the social determinants of health that made these communities more vulnerable during the COVID pandemic. Preexisting social inequality and broader structural exclusion that are tied to but extend beyond RLS shape how immigrants are incorporated into their host countries at arrival and throughout the life course, or what sociologist Ken Sun refers to as "temporalities of migration."[23] Additional research should examine the intricacies of this structural exclusion and the multifaceted effects that RLS can have over time and across generations.

The choice of Boston, Massachusetts, was key for illuminating the critical role of place and policy. As a liberal, majority-minority city in a politically blue state, immigrants in principle had access to more state-funded health and other social services than immigrants residing in other states around the country, especially compared with my home state of Tennessee. Although Boston immigrants struggled to navigate the system, many felt fortunate to be living in the commonwealth compared with family and friends in more restrictive locales. Their experiences reveal that where people are geographically situated matters because the policies that govern those localities vary to a surprising extent, and actual practices are even more diverse. As debates over abortion and contraception access, teaching critical race theory in schools, and extending municipal voting rights to immigrants intensify around the country and partisan divides stymie federal legislation, state and local policies shape people's lives more than ever before.

Beyond policy and politics, place matters for health because of the structural discrimination encoded in patterns of residential segregation by race, class, and migration history.[24] People's zip codes are correlated with their life expectancy and specific health outcomes. As the COVID pandemic deepened, the confluence of policy, place, and health became even more apparent. Place, which intersects with race, ethnicity, legal status, and income, makes a significant difference in people's ability to obtain health coverage, use health services, and simply live their lives without unnecessary suffering. More research should center place and policy as intersecting units of analysis for understanding social inequality.

Finally, this book reveals the troubling consequences associated with receiving inadequate health care. Research has documented that having less access to preventive care can result in more serious health outcomes later on.[25] This qualitative study revealed the personal costs in time and effort associated with taking care of one's own health and the health of loved ones, which include lost hours of paid work, fear of detention and deportation in transit to and from appointments, and eventual disability from working through the pain and mental stress of being unable to attend to health matters. Some immigrants and many advocates and providers shared stories of immigrants waiting until their health problems were severe before seeking medical attention.

Across the country, one of the main reasons people forgo care is not having health insurance or being unable to pay premiums, co-pays, and deductibles.[26] Despite its limitations, the ACA took an important step in expanding health coverage to groups of people who were previously uninsured because of their income or being deemed "uninsurable" because of their preexisting conditions. Although this book critiques this federal policy's exclusion of so many immigrants, Obamacare has been effective in reducing the uninsured population of individuals who were eligible for Medicaid and living in states that participated in the program's expansion.

The refusal of legislators in conservative states to expand Medicaid and attempts to dismantle Obamacare under the Trump administration have produced implicit exclusion for income-eligible citizens and qualified immigrants living in states that did not expand Medicaid. This stratification in access to formal coverage has left these populations un- and underinsured and unable to benefit from preventive and specialty health services before, during, and after the COVID pandemic.[27] Even among those with coverage, nearly half have delayed or forgone care.[28] Some did so for similar reasons as the immigrants I interviewed: insufficient health coverage, lack of time, high out-of-pocket costs, or inability to find a provider who accepted their coverage. Furthermore, half of people who had employer-sponsored insurance lost their jobs and coverage during the pandemic.[29] Given that delayed care and lack of coverage are associated with increased healthcare costs and that healthcare costs constitute nearly 20 percent of the gross domestic product, this issue affects the country's fiscal health as well as its rate of preventable deaths.[30]

Although the US population was not as healthy as that of many other wealthy countries before the onset of COVID, individuals with preexisting health conditions—particularly preventable conditions, such as asthma, obesity, and Type II diabetes, that are related to poverty and structural discrimination—were disproportionately likely to contract and die from COVID. Aside from revealing how unequal our society was,

COVID spotlighted the paucity of funding for the public health system, which made it difficult to combat the pandemic. At both the federal and state levels, public health was and remains severely underfunded.[31] At its peak in 1968, the federal government contributed 50 percent of public health expenditures. By 2013, that amount had dropped precipitously, to about 15 percent.[32] At the state level, annual per capita public health expenditures varied, from more than $120 in northeastern and western states to between $59 and $98 in other states.[33] These disparities underline the importance of place and subnational policy in shaping people's access to public health resources as well as health coverage and state-funded social services.

Taken together, this study's findings regarding the health implications of racialized legal status reveal that we need a more expansive notion of citizenship. Even the naturalized citizens I interviewed struggled to receive adequate health care, demonstrating that formal citizenship was insufficient. That is also the case for the millions of un- and underinsured citizens across this country living in states that still have not expanded Medicaid even in the midst of a once-in-a-lifetime public health crisis. Moreover, this country's long and continuing history of socially excluding people based on their race and class has limited access to vital healthcare and other social services. Many disadvantaged and impoverished Americans are deemed undeserving or held responsible for their own position because they failed to work hard enough or made the wrong choices in life. During the COVID pandemic, legal citizenship did not shield the most vulnerable among us from contracting the virus, receiving inadequate care, and dying, leaving many children without a safety net. At the same time, the lack of legal citizenship explicitly excluded many immigrants from COVID relief and workplace protections despite doing the "essential" jobs that kept the country going while the more privileged worked remotely. Racialized legal status is not just about the effects of the intersection of race, ethnicity, and legal status on individuals' lives. This intersection functions at the micro, meso, and macro levels of society and shapes who benefits from citizenship and who does not. Expanding our understanding of citizenship would remove the boundaries defined by formal statuses and help us to ensure that belonging encompasses all who contribute to society. It is in our common interest that everyone—including immigrants—has quality health care, shelter, food, and jobs with dignity and benefits, rather than restricting these rights to those who were born in this country and in more structurally privileged social groups.

The COVID pandemic revealed the strong current of individualism that has long defined American identity, although countervailing models of solidarity have emerged from some ethnocultural and class-based groups at different times and places. The core value of individualism at all costs has been a central tenet of US politics and policy and is reflected in the repeated devolution of powers and funds from the federal to state governments. This devolution also flows from the government to individuals, making them primarily responsible for their life choices and conditions despite the structural inequities that influence their situation. Each chapter of this book has shown how amid major policy implementations, it was the responsibility of individuals, regardless of English proficiency or socioeconomic status, to sign up for health coverage and figure out to use it to obtain care. This is a daunting, sometimes impossible task for everyone who is unfamiliar with the intricacies of health coverage or has limited health literacy. Just as Latinx immigrants in Boston have encountered these challenges, so too have millions of others around the country who try to make healthcare decisions that are constrained by what their insurance covers and whether a specialist is in their insurance network. Despite the complexity of the healthcare system, the pervasive power of individualism has left each of us on our own to figure it out as best we can. That must change. If we want to improve people's health, reduce racial and other social disparities in health, lower healthcare costs, and have quality health care, we have to approach the problem from a collective rather than individualistic perspective and address the racialized legal status and socioeconomic inequities baked into our society and healthcare system at every level.

Policy Recommendations

The COVID pandemic revealed how much inequality matters, in health care and other facets of life. Now is the time to address and remove the structural causes of inequality because they have public health consequences. Given what I observed while conducting this study over the past decade, I offer some policy recommendations that would make the health insurance and healthcare system easier to navigate not only for the immigrants I interviewed but also for all those struggling to obtain adequate coverage and care. These recommendations are organized according to the level of government involved but have some overlap. I recognize that addressing racialized legal status at the macro level is a monumental task that makes people feel as though nothing can be done. Bold and transformative public policies tackling macro-level inequality in housing, employment, and other spheres are vital to ameliorate the social determinants of health that drive health and healthcare disparities. My recommendations aim to address RLS discrimination at the meso and micro levels, where systemic racism translates into institutions and bureaucracies whose staff members interact with people seeking health and social services. These recommendations would make institutions more responsive to the people directly affected by discrimination and create social change from the bottom up. While some of these recommendations sound visionary, others are feasible even under current conditions. I hope that policymakers, healthcare facility administrators, and others will adopt them. As the past has shown, reforms are made when they are urgently advocated by the public.

Federal and National Policies
Make health coverage accessible to all: Remove legal status eligibility requirements

Making affordable health insurance accessible to all would go a long way toward ensuring that everyone can receive preventive care before those conditions become urgent. Obamacare was a start, but much more can be done to provide insurance to those without it. An important reason to remove documentation status barriers to social services and benefits from federal law is that immigrants of various statuses pay taxes. Undocumented immigrants, who are the most structurally excluded, pay an estimated $9 billion in federal payroll taxes and about $11.7 billion in state and local taxes each year.[34] These taxes contribute to the US social welfare, Medicare, and Social Security systems, but most federally ineligible immigrants never receive those benefits. Immigrants use far fewer health services and have lower medical expenditures than the US-born population.[35] Immigrants also typically have better health than US-born individuals. Extending health coverage access to immigrants would both improve their current health and decrease future healthcare costs associated with treating more severe medical conditions.[36]

Some states, such as California and Illinois, are using state funds to extend Medicaid to income-eligible undocumented children and young adults up to age 26 or adults over age 50.[37] Although Massachusetts has inclusive health coverage, its Medicaid program does not yet fully cover undocumented children, and there have been no proposals to include adults over age 50. A practical first step is to remove the legal status restriction in the federal and state government health exchanges, which would assist ineligible immigrants in searching for and purchasing adequate coverage from private insurers. This was done in Massachusetts's initial health reform but ended after the implementation of Obamacare.

Pass and implement immigration reform

There has been no comprehensive immigration reform since 1996 under President Bill Clinton and no amnesty or pathway to citizenship for undocumented immigrants since 1986 under President Ronald Reagan. Immigration reform is needed so that people can "get right with the law," because now there is no "line" that people can get in to regularize their status. To address the millions of people currently living in limbo, that reform should include a clear path to citizenship. By itself, that step would remove the legal status barriers in policy that explicitly discriminate against noncitizens.

Reduce administrative burdens for government services and increase health literacy

The numerous administrative burdens that securing health coverage and care impose are a nightmare. Reducing bureaucratic red tape and rigid documentation requirements would make it easier for people to navigate the system and receive benefits for which they are eligible. More funding should be allocated to health literacy, which should be expanded from educating patients and their caregivers about their health conditions and treatments to include information about how to enroll in coverage, how health insurance works, and where to obtain care. This funding should provide multilingual materials and assistance in applying for coverage on websites or over the phone. Health consumer helplines such as the one at Health Care for All are useful models.[38]

Expand Title VI to all sectors of government and enforce in healthcare settings

Currently, Title VI of the 1964 Civil Rights Act, which includes language access as a civil right, applies to settings that receive federal funds. This includes a wide range of existing healthcare and social services across the country. Enforcement is haphazard, however, relying on complaints rather than proactive measures and regular reviews of federally funded bureaucracies to ensure compliance. Extending this requirement to other sectors of government would make it easier for individuals whose first language is not English to interact more productively with public institutions. Relatedly, official spokespersons in federally funded bureaucracies should convey clear information in multiple languages and settings and disseminate it as widely as possible.

Allocate more funding to English language learning programs

Given the proportion of limited English proficient adults and English language learners in primary and secondary schools, increasing federal and subnational funding to English language learning programs to improve these individuals' English proficiency would enable them to better navigate health and social service bureaucracies. It would also aid their incorporation into the broader society by lowering the language barriers they encounter in their daily lives. For those who rely primarily on medical interpreters, English proficiency would make it easier to communicate with providers and reduce wait times for health services. LEP individuals' attainment of English proficiency would eventually reduce the need for interpretation services.

Allocate more funding to public health infrastructure

Public health experts know what needs to be done to address chronic and acute health problems that affect whole populations and often have environmental or socioeconomic causes, but the public health infrastructure has been starved for lack of funding. Having a more robust public health system would ensure that people are able to get adequate vaccines, testing, and treatment for communicable diseases and other illnesses and help the nation be better prepared for the next pandemic.

Healthcare System Policies

Increase funding and resources for interpretation and education in medical facilities, coverage enrollment sites, and health insurance companies

Beyond federal and state requirements, agencies can tailor their interpretation and information services to the specific needs of the populations they serve. This would ensure not only that no language groups are left out but also that the assistance they are offered addresses the gaps in patients' knowledge of current recommendations for prevention and treatment of conditions that are disproportionately prevalent among them.

Diversify the medical and social service workforce

Healthcare providers and social service employees should more accurately reflect the ethnoracial diversity of those they serve. Physicians, psychiatrists, and staff should have more training on the impact of systemic racism, social determinants of health, and implicit bias in medical encounters and other settings. Medical school curricula must include courses and training on these topics. Students and providers across the full range of health professions should be immersed in settings where ethnoracial minorities and other disadvantaged groups predominate to become accustomed to serving these populations. These students and providers should also participate in group discussions to reflect on their experiences and positionality while working with these populations. Too often, students are taught in settings that are separate from practice that focus on facts or on role-playing among themselves rather than how to effectively interact with patients who are different from them in unexpected and unpredictable ways.

Another way to meet this goal is to leverage the diversity of immigrants with healthcare training in their home country by allowing them to receive certification and practice in the United States. Developing pipeline programs similar to those in STEM (science, technology, engineering, and mathematics) fields and academia to increase the number of Black, Latinx, and Indigenous individuals in health care would also contribute to diversifying the medical workforce.

State and Local Policies: Massachusetts and Metropolitan Boston

End cooperation between federal immigration enforcement and local law enforcement agencies

Agreements to share information have created significant fear in communities of color and disproportionately target Latinx and Black individuals who may be arrested, detained, incarcerated, and deported. Research has shown that these cooperative agreements do not make communities safer or effectively identify immigrants with criminal records as deportation priorities.[39] The Safe Communities Act would limit cooperation between federal immigration and state law enforcement agencies and make Massachusetts a sanctuary state. As of 2023, 12 states had passed similar legislation: California, Colorado, Connecticut, Illinois, Maryland, New Jersey, New York, Oregon, Rhode Island, South Carolina, Vermont, and Washington.[40]

Allocate more funding to the state's Health Safety Net program
Funding for this program has declined over the course of the past decade, even though it is currently the primary program through which most federally ineligible undocumented and documented immigrants can receive comprehensive health coverage. This program also provides vital health services to lower-income citizens. Increasing the funding allocation and restoring income eligibility cutoffs and benefits to pre-2006 levels would furnish more adequate health services to lower-income and immigrant populations in the state.

Pass and implement the Cover All Kids Act and other health reforms
This proposed legislation would ensure that all Massachusetts children are eligible for MassHealth regardless of documentation status. The state should also extend MassHealth to undocumented young adults up to age 26 and elderly adults over age 50 and open the state's health exchange to allow noneligible immigrants to buy better private health insurance.

Final Reflections
This book investigated how racialized legal status constrained immigrants' healthcare access as the health policy landscape shifted, with the aim of figuring out how to improve our healthcare system. My interviews, meetings, and conversations with immigrants and those who work with them opened my eyes to the myriad complications that noncitizens and naturalized citizens with limited English proficiency face. Despite studying health policy for more than a decade, I am still astounded by the complexity of the healthcare system. On the one hand, some factors work in my favor: I am a middle-class, English-speaking US citizen with private health insurance. Yet, like some immigrants I spoke with, I constantly wonder how being a Black woman shapes my own medical encounters and discounts the nonracialized legal status privileges that I have. When I call to schedule a medical appointment, I think about the LEP patients who must go to the office to do so because the tele-robot answering the phone does so in English and does not always have non-English options available.

When I walk through a hospital for lab tests or a radiology scan and follow the English signs to my destination, I consider the confusion that patients who do not read English must feel as they try to find their way around. Although I am healthy, my experience of pregnancy and childbirth while writing this book transformed my experiences with the healthcare system. Having to schedule multiple prenatal and ultrasound appointments and navigating a hospital stay for childbirth made me wonder how less fortunate parents navigated this bureaucratic, burdensome, and costly process. As a Black woman, I also feared that I or my newborn children might suffer complications or even die in or after delivery because of the Black maternal and infant mortality crisis in this country. My own racialized legal status, which in some ways paralleled that of my immigrant respondents, had the potential to put my life at risk in the US healthcare system.

Conducting this study and writing this book fundamentally changed me. While I did not take having access to health insurance and care for granted before, I have become acutely aware of the immense challenges millions of people face as they encounter the healthcare system. It will take a collective effort, judicious use of financial resources, fierce and courageous political will, and herculean efforts to undo implicit and explicit biases in the system and create quality and affordable health care for all.

APPENDIX

The introduction includes an overview of the methods I used to conduct the research for this book. This appendix provides more detailed information about the process of gathering and analyzing the data and reflects on the challenges I encountered while conducting this research. Additional tables present demographic information about the healthcare providers and immigrant and health advocates interviewed for the study. I conclude with more context regarding the federal- and state-level health and immigration policies that shaped the sociopolitical climate for immigrants' healthcare access in Massachusetts before and during the study.

Study Origins

When I started this project, I thought it would be completed during my postdoctoral fellowship with the Robert Wood Johnson Foundation Health Policy Scholars program from 2011 to 2013 at Harvard University. I had recently finished my PhD dissertation, which examined how Brazilians' migration to the United States and subsequent return migration to Brazil transformed their understandings of race, racism, and racial classification in both countries. I had interviewed 49 return migrants in Governador Valadares, a small city in the state of Minas Gerais.[1] Minas Gerais is located in south-central Brazil, with the states of Rio de Janeiro and Espirito Santo to the southeast, Bahia to the northeast, Goias to the northwest, and São Paulo to the southwest. Historically, Governador Valadares has sent larger numbers of immigrants to the United States than any other city in Brazil. Although my project focused on respondents' negotiation of race as they moved between the two countries, the issue of health kept coming up in my interviews. Unprompted, many Brazilians spoke at length about their difficulty accessing health care in the United States as undocumented immigrants, working long hours in physically laborious jobs in housecleaning, construction, and painting and not having enough time to eat a balanced diet or get an adequate amount of sleep. A few said that they returned to Brazil sooner than anticipated because of health conditions that required more consistent health care, which they felt was easier to access in Brazil than in the United States.

As I began my health policy postdoc, those respondents' stories remained with me, particularly because Boston has a sizable Latin American immigrant population and Massachusetts implemented comprehensive health reform in 2006 that extended access to state residents regardless of documentation status. Furthermore, that reform was the model for the federal Affordable Care Act, which had been recently passed in 2010. Given my interest in learning more about the impact of health policy on immigrants, I decided to examine the accessibility of health care from the perspective of Brazilians, Dominicans, and Salvadorans in Boston. This interest culminated into the decade-long research project for this book.

Conceptualizing the Research Design

To conduct a project of this scope, it was vital to include the perspectives of multiple stakeholder groups. Immigrants' experiences were most important, and I included information in the introduction about their demographics and how I recruited that group for the study. In this section, I provide more details and demographic information about the Boston Health Coalition providers and immigrant and health advocates I interviewed.

Providers dedicated to serving marginalized communities understood the major challenges these patients face in trying to maintain their health. Moreover, the shifts in health policy directly affected doctors, nurses, receptionists, medical interpreters, and other health professionals' ability to see and treat their patients. Through my postdoctoral fellowship, I met faculty who described BHC as a suitable research site. As a federally qualified health center with a notable reputation for providing quality care to patients regardless of ethnoracial background and ability to pay, BHC has multiple facilities located throughout the Boston area. These characteristics made BHC an ideal place to recruit healthcare professionals for the study. To include BHC providers, I had to obtain separate human subjects or Institutional Review Board (IRB) approval that had to be renewed each year of the study in addition to the IRB approval from my universities. More detailed information about the BHC providers interviewed for the study is shown in Table A-1. In all three rounds of interviews, the providers I interviewed included more women than men and more individuals who racially classified themselves as White than as people of color. The majority had worked at BHC for more than a decade.

Table A-1. Demographic Characteristics of Boston Health Coalition Providers ($N=52$)

Demographics	2012-2013 ($n=19$)	2015-2016 ($n=19$)	2019 ($n=14$)
Gender (# women)	14	14	9
Average age (years-range)	47 (32-70)	47 (32-70)	45 (31-70)
Number of years at BHC	13	13	13
Number of BHC sites	5	8	5
Occupation categories	Physician, psychiatrist, interpreter, social worker, outreach	Physician, psychiatrist, interpreter, Diversity Affairs	Physician, psychiatrist, interpreter, Diversity Affairs, social worker
Ethnoracial Classification			
- White (#)	9	10	6
- Black (#)	2	1	1
- Latino/Hispanic (#)	7	4	4
- Asian American (#)	0	1	1
- Other (#)	1	3	2

Interviewing immigrant and health advocates shed light on immigrants' perceptions of life in Boston, the experiences of discrimination they encountered, and the challenges they faced in adapting to the city and applying for social services. I recruited employees from organizations that provided support in applying for health coverage or other social services and worked primarily with immigrants. Because I was interviewing Brazilians, Dominicans, and Salvadorans, I also recruited employees from organizations that served or were geographically based in those communities. More information about the advocacy organizations can be found in Table A-2. Like the providers, these respondents included more women than men and more who classified themselves as White than as people of color. Their average age was 45 years.

In addition to conducting interviews, I used publicly available data from state and federal government websites to analyze changes in eligibility under the Massachusetts and ACA reforms and under the Trump administration's immigration policies. I spent countless hours looking up information about health reform and closely reviewing online application forms and eligibility criteria for different types of publicly funded coverage. I read MassHealth member booklets that explained the benefits associated with different types of coverage and where it could be used. Some policies were so confusing that I had to ask advocates who specialized in health coverage and immigration policy whether I was correctly interpreting what I read. This process not only enabled me to understand these developments but also made me realize how difficult this task would be for anyone without these tools and resources at hand.

Through conducting in-depth interviews with stakeholders most affected by these changes, attending health- and immigration-related events, and assessing policy documents, I triangulated this rich data to develop a comprehensive understanding of the concrete social consequences of policy implementation.

Developing a Semilongitudinal Study

When I finished conducting interviews in 2013, I thought the project would end after I analyzed the data and wrote a few articles presenting

Table A-2. Profiles of Advocacy Organizations

Organization focus	2012–2013 (N = 20)		2015–2016 (N = 25)		2019 (N = 30)	
	Staff position	# interviewed	Staff position	# interviewed	Staff position	# interviewed
Brazilian immigrants	Executive director, board member, health educator	6	Executive director, board member, health educator	4	Executive director, health educator and outreach, financial adviser, receptionist	5
Salvadoran immigrants	N/A	0	Executive director, pastor	2	Pastor, executive director	2
Dominican immigrants	Executive director, ESL instructor[a]	2	Executive director	1	Activist	1
Immigration advocacy	Coordinator	3	Coordinator	3	Coordinators, attorney	7
Health advocacy	Health policy, helpline staff, communications	9	Health policy, helpline staff, attorney	11	Health policy, helpline staff, attorneys	7
Miscellaneous advocacy	N/A	0	Policy coordinator, attorney	4	Executive director, attorneys, policy coordinator	8
Local/state government	N/A	N/A	Director	3	City immigrant office, city outreach	3

a. ESL: English as a Second Language

the findings. But numerous healthcare providers and advocates expressed serious concern about how ACA implementation in late 2013 would change the state's health policy and healthcare access for immigrants. After the ACA was implemented, key policy provisions of the Massachusetts reform, particularly its provision of coverage for certain immigrants, had changed, and how the state would address this change and other disparities between the two reforms was not yet clear. I realized that returning to the field to collect data in Boston after ACA implementation would provide a natural social experiment revealing differences in immigrants' access to health coverage and care.

I had not intended to do a third round of interviews for the study. But in my 2015–2016 interviews, respondents had already begun stating concerns that immigrants were disenrolling from social services in response to Donald Trump's emergence as the GOP presidential nominee. When he won the election three months later, I felt it would be important to return and conduct additional interviews in Boston to assess the local impact of Trump's immigration and health policy agenda.

Unintentionally, this research project became a semilongitudinal study, which can be referred to as a "triple prospective cohort research design."[2] This type of design, which is more often used in public health studies or epidemiological surveys than in sociological or policy analyses, allows researchers to follow a similar group of individuals over time to examine how certain factors affect them. Thus, reinterviewing some study participants became essential to understanding the impact of policy changes on Boston Latinx immigrants' healthcare access over time.

I was unable to conduct reinterviews with immigrants due to the shifting sociopolitical climate. The IRB at my various universities did not grant approval to collect their contact information, and I did not want immigrants to feel that our interviews might put them at risk of detention or deportation. Fortunately, I was able to interview 21 BHC providers and advocates at least twice (Table A-3). These interviews enabled me to identify and understand the most salient changes that reconfigured Boston immigrants' healthcare access over time and reinforced the structural barriers to coverage and care that immigrants encountered. Of the

Table A-3. Demographic Characteristics of Advocates and Providers Interviewed at Least Twice Between 2012 and 2019

Advocacy organization employees (N=11)

Pseudonym	Demographic focus of organization	Years interviewed	Sex	Age at first interview	Ethnoracial classification	Education level
Micaela	Brazilians	2012, 2015, 2019	Woman	64	Other: Brazilian	Postgrad
Paola	Health Advocacy	2012, 2019	Woman	40	Hispanic	Postgrad
Carolina	Health Advocacy, Brazilians	2012, 2015, 2019	Woman	46	Latino: Mixed	Some college
Penelope	Health Advocacy	2012, 2015, 2019	Woman	28	White	College
Daniel	Health Advocacy	2012, 2015, 2019	Man	40	Hispanic	Some college
Joshua	Health Advocacy	2015, 2019	Man	34	White	Postgrad
Manuel	Central Americans	2015, 2019	Man	53	Latino	Postgrad
Sebastião	Brazilians	2012, 2015, 2019	Man	37	Other: Brazilian	Postgrad
Lucia	Brazilians	2012, 2015	Woman	36	Other: Brazilian	Postgrad
Rachel	Immigration Advocacy	2015, 2019	Woman	45	White	Postgrad
Jeff	Immigration Advocacy	2015, 2019	Man	71	White	Postgrad

BHC healthcare professionals (N =10)

Pseudonym	Demographic focus of patients	Years interviewed	Sex	Age at first interview	Ethnoracial classification	Education level
Amelia	All[a]	2012, 2019	Woman	41	White	Postgrad
Luisa	All	2015, 2019	Woman	67	Latino: Brazilian	Postgrad
Adriana	Portuguese-speaking	2012, 2015	Woman	54	Latino: Brazilian American	College
Gloria	Spanish-speaking	2012, 2019	Woman	50	Other: Latin American, Honduran	College
Grace	All	2012, 2015	Woman	45	White	Postgrad
Camila	Spanish-speaking	2012, 2015	Woman	29	Latino: Colombian	College
Greg	All	2012, 2015	Man	67	White	Postgrad
Nicholas	All	2015, 2019	Man	50	Black	College
Kevin	All	2012, 2019	Man	42	White: Jewish	Postgrad
Thomas	All	2015, 2019	Man	54	White	Postgrad

a. "All" indicates that these providers see patients of various ethnicities, of whom many are immigrants. Many of these patients are Portuguese- or Spanish-speaking.

21 respondents reinterviewed, 11 were advocates from organizations that primarily served Brazilian immigrants or focused broadly on health and immigration advocacy. They ranged in age from 28 to 71 and ethnoracially classified as White, Brazilian, Latino, or Hispanic. Most had attended college, and some had earned advanced degrees. Women and men were equally represented. The other 10 reinterview respondents were BHC providers. Although they served patients of all racial and ethnic backgrounds, many of their patients were immigrants and spoke Portuguese or Spanish. The providers themselves were predominantly White and Latinx. All had completed college, and some held postgraduate degrees. The providers ranged from age 29 to 67, and women slightly outnumbered men.

Interview Protocols

My interview protocols differed for immigrant, provider, and advocate respondents. In designing them, I had to think carefully about what types of information each group could provide that would be most valuable to reveal the challenges immigrants experience in navigating the healthcare system. The languages in which I conducted the interviews also varied by stakeholder groups. I interviewed immigrants in their preferred language, most often Brazilian Portuguese or Spanish. Of the 82 completed interviews with immigrants, only 5 were conducted in English. Nearly all the provider interviews and the majority of the advocate interviews were conducted in English, but some of those with medical interpreters were done in Brazilian Portuguese or Spanish. With advocates who worked in organizations serving Brazilian, Dominican, or Salvadoran communities, I conducted most interviews in Brazilian Portuguese or Spanish.

Immigrant Protocols

Because of language differences, I developed two identical protocols: one in Brazilian Portuguese for Brazilians and another in Spanish for Dominicans and Salvadorans. I developed the protocol in English and then translated it. Although I am fluent in Portuguese and Spanish, English is my first and primary language of communication. So, I had individuals whose first and primary languages of communication were Portuguese and Spanish review the protocols to ensure that the questions conveyed my meaning accurately. I also did some practice interviews with immigrants to make sure the questions were clear. In constructing this protocol, I considered some of the factors identified in the literature that might shape immigrants' experiences, such as documentation status, ethnoracial identification, income, job type, and knowledge about the US healthcare system. As a researcher who had previously explored the transnational ties of Brazilian immigrants in the US, I knew that individuals' premigration socioeconomic status and healthcare access in the home country relative to the United States would be important. Therefore, I organized my interview protocol for immigrants into four sections.

The first section asked general questions to compile a migration profile of each respondent. I asked a series of closed and open-ended questions about their hometown, reasons for migrating, the number of times they had come to the United States, relatives or friends in the United States who assisted with integration, and their work and income in the home country both before migrating and in the United States. I asked whether respondents sent remittances home, often spoke with relatives at home, and planned to return permanently to their home country. To get a sense of where respondents lived and their degree of comfort in their US communities, I inquired about the demographic makeup of their neighborhoods and their relationships with co-ethnics, Americans, and people of other national origins where they resided.

Two sets of questions in this section were vital to understanding immigrants' healthcare experiences in Boston. The first concerned their English proficiency and the second their documentation status. Rather than asking for this information directly, which might make respondents uncomfortable, I posed two questions. The first asked whether they had arrived in the United States with a visa or employment authorization and, if so, which type they had. The second question inquired whether they had been able to obtain a green card, work permit, or US citizenship during their time in the country. I classified respondents as undocumented if they answered no to both questions or yes to the first question and no to the second. For each wave of the study, I had to change the categories for immigration statuses to account for shifts in the range of documentation status that shaped access to health coverage. For example, when I started the study, I asked only whether respondents arrived with a visa, not which type of visa they had. As I conducted interviews, however, I realized that some immigrant respondents came with specific types of visas that limited their ability to adjust their status. Furthermore, when I added Salvadoran respondents in 2015, some had temporary protected status (TPS), which did not provide a path to citizenship. I also had to revise the question about obtaining a green card, work permit, or citizenship to include Deferred Action for Childhood Arrivals, as that group of childhood arrivals became distinguished from other undocumented immigrants. For respondents with green cards, I also asked how long they had had their green cards, which could limit or extend access to certain federal public benefits given a five-year bar placed on benefits by 1996 legislation.

Because the study focuses on the influence of racialized legal status on immigrants' lives and health care in the US, it was important to understand how immigrants saw themselves in ethnoracial terms and their perceptions of their health and healthcare access. To do so, I included a range of closed and open-ended questions on these topics in the second and third sections of the protocol. The second section focused on immigrants' racial classifications and healthcare experiences in their home countries, and the third explored the same topics in the United States. Including these questions in both sections provided a comprehensive pre- and postmigration profile that allowed me to assess how migration shaped immigrants' perceptions of discrimination associated with race and skin color in their lives and in the healthcare system.

In addition to asking respondents whether they had heard anything about race in the United States before migrating and, if so, what was the source of that information, I asked how they saw themselves with regard to skin color (open-ended) and what factors (i.e., physical features, family background) influenced that classification. I specifically used the Portuguese and Spanish words for "skin color" (*côr de pele* in Portuguese or *color de piel* in Spanish) rather than "race" (*raça* in Portuguese and *raza* in Spanish) because in some Latin American countries people conflate "race" with "racism."[3] Using racial categories from the national censuses in Brazil, the Dominican Republic, and El Salvador, I asked how respondents classified themselves, how they believed others in their country classified them, and how important such a classification was to them. Because of the more fluid boundaries around racial categories and mixed racial heritage in Latin American countries compared with the United States, the categories listed were (1) White, (2) Black, (3) Brown/Pardo(a)/Moreno(a)/Mestizo(a), (4) Asian/Yellow, (5) Indigenous, and (6) other. The "Brown/Pardo/Moreno(a)/Mestizo(a)" category includes various terms used to classify individuals of mixed race. In Brazil, "Pardo/a," which also means Brown, refers to individuals of mixed African, Indigenous, and/or European heritage. "Moreno(a)" is similarly used in the Dominican Republic to refer to individuals of mixed African, Indigenous, and/or European heritage. "Mestizo(a)" typically signifies mixed European and Indigenous heritage in El Salvador. While the former Portuguese and Spanish colonizers in the countries that are now Brazil and the Dominican Republic imported a sizable number of enslaved Africans to work various types of plantations, El Salvador received a considerably smaller number. This colonial history is reflected in the terms used to indicate mixed racial ancestry in these different regions of Latin America.

In addition to their skin color and ethnoracial classifications, respondents were asked whether they had experienced discrimination of any kind and, if so, what they believed was the cause of that discrimination. Next, I asked health-related questions, which consisted of respondents' self-assessment of their physical and mental health (from poor to excellent) and whether they had been professionally diagnosed with any physical or mental health conditions. These questions segued into questions about their premigration health insurance coverage if they had it, whether it was private or public, and their experiences in the healthcare system in their home country.

The questions in the third section were like those in the second section, but I changed the wording to reflect the US context more accurately.

There is no official US census category equivalent to Pardo(a), Moreno(a), or Mestizo(a). The US census treats "Latino" and "Hispanic" as ethnic rather than racial categories and asks individuals to classify their race separately. Furthermore, individuals can denote racially mixed heritage only by checking off more than one racial category. The lack of nuance in US racial categories, particularly its basis in a White/Black binary, creates significant confusion for newly arrived Latin Americans.[4] Although "Latino" and "Hispanic" are often listed together under ethnoracial classification questions on official forms, I chose to separate the two terms when asking respondents how they classify themselves using US ethnoracial categories: (1) White, (2) Black, (3) Hispanic, (4) Latino, (5) Asian, (6) Native American, (7) other. I also asked respondents for their thoughts on the terms "Hispanic" and "Latino," whether they felt those terms applied to them, and whether they regarded certain nationalities as Latino and others as Hispanic. Distinguishing between "Latino" and "Hispanic" was especially important for Brazilians, who may be considered Latino but are not Hispanic. Interestingly, many respondents across stakeholder groups saw Brazilians as different from Latinos, using language such as "Brazilians and Latinos" when discussing Boston immigrants' healthcare access. When asking about the importance of various aspects of social identity in the United States, I added "being an immigrant" to the list of options to see how important being an immigrant was in respondents' lives here. In the second section, I asked a similar question with the following choices about what was most important to respondents' sense of identity: (1) nationality, (2) sex: man or woman, (3) social class, (4) race and skin color, (5) nothing, (6) other, (7) none.

The wording of the health-related questions was like those in the second section but focused on the US context. I included more detailed openended questions about health coverage, whether respondents felt that their physical and mental health had changed since they arrived in the United States, and where they went for medical care when needed. I asked whether they had a regular healthcare provider; about their experiences with that provider; and how language, race or ethnicity, being an immigrant, and other factors such as costs affect their ability to receive care and their interactions with providers. I also asked whether they had heard about health reform and, if so, what they knew about it and whether it had any impact on them. Finally, I asked about their perceptions of life in Boston or Massachusetts and how immigrants are generally treated here as compared with their treatment in other parts of the United States. The last section of the protocol collected demographic information on respondents' age, marital status, education level, and current employment status. On average, most immigrant interviews ranged from 60 to 90 minutes.

Provider Protocol

The protocol for providers inquired about the respondent's title or position, length of time in that position, and overall perceptions of how health reform and the shifting sociopolitical climate affected their ability to care for immigrant patients. I asked about the types of services provided at the specific BHC site and the demographics of the population served according to their type of health coverage. Beyond that, the protocol included questions about language access among staff, the impact of language and cultural differences in shaping patient–provider relationships, and how documentation status shaped immigrants' willingness to obtain care at the respondent's facility. Because I knew that providers likely saw a range of patients, I wanted to know whether particular health issues or healthcare system challenges were common among their immigrant patients. Depending on whether the provider worked with a specific immigrant group, I asked about their familiarity with the culture and whether there were commonalities or differences between these groups in navigating the system. I inquired whether patients disclosed that they had experienced any type of discrimination in their lives outside the healthcare system. I also collected providers' general demographic information. For the providers whom I was able to reinterview, I asked what had changed about their position and in their perceptions of immigrants' healthcare access since the previous interview. On average, these interviews lasted about 60 minutes.

Advocate Protocol

The protocol for advocates started by asking about their title or position and the length of time they had been in that organization. Then, I inquired about the organization's mission, the population it serves, and the types of services it offers. As I did with providers, I asked advocates for their assessment of how health reform and the shifting sociopolitical climate affected their ability to serve immigrant constituents. I asked about particular issues their immigrant constituents faced in accessing health coverage, care, and other social services, as well as in meeting their basic needs. The protocol included more detailed questions about the impact of language and cultural differences in shaping the organization's work with immigrant communities and, most important, about how documentation status along with perceived race and ethnicity shaped immigrants' experiences of discrimination in both health care and their daily lives. If the advocate worked with a specific ethnic group, I asked about their familiarity with the culture and how their positionality shaped their work with the community. For advocates more familiar with immigration and health policy, I asked about how specific policy changes, such as in the public charge rule change, affected their work and immigrants' experiences. Finally, I collected advocates' demographic information. For advocates whom I reinterviewed for a different wave of the study, I specifically asked what had changed about their position and in their perceptions of immigrants' experiences and policy since the previous interview. These interviews lasted about 60 minutes.

Data Transcription and Analysis

All but 2 of the 207 interviews were audio recorded with consent from the respondents. The two people who declined, both in 2019, were an undocumented Brazilian woman and an undocumented Salvadoran woman who feared what might happen to the recording. After conducting each interview, I wrote field notes summarizing major themes, particularly interesting comments, and body language or gestures. In qualitative research, field notes are important for capturing crucial insights about the study's research focus and can provide useful context during data analysis.[5] Given my focus on the potential impact of racialized legal status on individuals' healthcare experiences, I noted their physical characteristics, such as skin color, eye color, and hair color and texture, particularly for immigrant respondents. If participants used certain body language or nonverbal cues when answering specific questions, I recorded these in my field notes.

I used a professional transcription company to transcribe each interview in English, Brazilian Portuguese, or Spanish. Given the large number of interviews, I trained a group of graduate and undergraduate research assistants to correct the transcripts and conduct a preliminary analysis of the interviews. Only those with high reading proficiency in Brazilian Portuguese or Spanish were assigned interviews in those languages. My team of research assistants and I reviewed each transcript while listening to the audio recording to ensure accuracy and consistency between the audio recording and transcript. As different transcribers transcribed the audio recordings using different formatting styles, my team also formatted the transcript in preparation for data analysis in NVivo qualitative software.

For analysis, I used an inductive, grounded theory approach, which is standard in qualitative social scientific research to generate theoretical categories from a systematic analysis of data.[6] I worked with my team of research assistants to code the data. We used open and focused coding, reading each transcript closely and developing an extensive list of recurring themes, with one- to three-word phrases describing various aspects of immigrants' healthcare access related to policy, racialized legal status, and other factors.[7] After this initial open coding process, these themes became part of the codebook for the data. I also had the team do constant comparative coding; every fifth transcript was recoded by a different team member to ensure consistency. Most often, teams of two research assistants were assigned to each stakeholder group to code the interviews in the language of the interview.

I created subcodes that corresponded to each stakeholder group to compare perspectives across the immigrant, healthcare professional, and advocate stakeholder groups. Among the immigrant samples, having separate subcodes for Brazilian, Dominican, and Salvadoran respondents was important for assessing commonalities and differences among the three groups. Each interview was analyzed in the language in which it was conducted, which reduced the likelihood of losing linguistic nuances before the analysis. In writing, I worked with the original materials and translated from Brazilian Portuguese or Spanish interviews only the quotations that appear in the book. Furthermore, to account for the overrepresentation of women in the sample, I first analyzed data of the separate stakeholder groups with women and men together.[8] Then I analyzed the data for women and men separately to identify whether some themes were more central to women than to men and vice versa. This intensive process continued until all interview transcripts, ethnographic observation field notes, and policy data were analyzed.

Protecting Participants

To minimize risks for immigrant respondents, I conducted interviews at a time and in a public location that was convenient and felt safe for them. I asked immigrant respondents not to provide any personal information, even their name, during the interviews to protect their identities. Given that interviews usually lasted at least one hour, I offered most respondents a $25 gift card for their time. BHC providers and advocates who were employees of the municipal or state governments were prohibited from accepting even token compensation.

To protect all respondents' data, I assigned each interview an alphanumeric code to identify it. Typically, this code included the date of the interview and an "F" (female) or an "M" (male) to indicate the sex of the respondent. For immigrant respondents, I also added initials to indicate their national origin ("BR" for Brazilian, "DR" for Dominican, and "SN" for Salvadoran). For providers, I added the initials "BHC" to the alphanumeric code for their interviews. For advocates, I added the initials of their organization to the alphanumeric code. Audio recordings, transcripts, and field notes for each respondent were assigned the same code. Before writing chapters for this book, I used these alphanumeric codes to create culturally appropriate pseudonyms for each respondent that did not overlap with any of the respondents' actual names. I used these pseudonyms to refer to various respondents throughout the book.

The numerous undergraduate and graduate research assistants I worked with to prepare transcripts and analyze data had to complete human subjects research certification training and be added to my IRB approval. Because I felt a huge responsibility to protect the data collected from respondents, I took all these steps to ensure anonymity and confidentiality for each respondent. If some government agency required me to turn over my data for review, I wanted to ensure that none of my respondents could be personally identified.

My Positionality and Other Challenges Conducting the Study

I experienced numerous challenges while conducting this study over a nearly 10-year period. One of the biggest was navigating the fieldwork with immigrants while reconciling my intersectional social positions and identities as a Black US-born middle-class woman and academic. I experienced some major life events over the course of this project that made my own connections with immigrant and health-related issues closer and more personal. These experiences shaped the ways I thought about the project and my own privilege as a US citizen with excellent private health insurance. I started dating the man I eventually married during the second wave of the study; he is originally from Brazil. As our relationship progressed, we discussed the challenges he encountered and the vulnerability he felt because he was an immigrant. As xenophobic rhetoric intensified, he realized that his green card status might not protect him from detention and deportation. Once we got engaged and married, we became a mixed-status couple, which shaped our house-buying experience and limited our travel options, among other life decisions. He was relieved when he became a naturalized citizen after experiencing uncertainty and delays in that process. The fear I felt for him, along with observations from my research over the years, made me realize the vulnerability and structural exclusion that documented immigrants experience as noncitizens. This awareness prompted me to conceptualize documentation status as a continuum of categories between undocumented and citizen that carry different levels of exclusion and deportability.

In the conclusion, I briefly wrote about how conducting this research changed how I engaged with the healthcare system. Beyond those observations, I saw how many of the immigrant enclaves where I began conducting research changed over the course of the study. Neighborhoods in Cambridge, Brighton, Jamaica Plain, and Somerville initially had large concentrations of Brazilian, Dominican, and Salvadoran immigrants, but the high cost of housing, compounded by gentrification, rising rents and housing values, and residential segregation, forced these communities farther away from Boston. I noticed drastic changes in the types of restaurants, shops, and people inhabiting these spaces between 2012 and 2019. Respondents from different stakeholder groups made similar observations. These geographic shifts, alongside the shifting national sociopolitical climate, inhibited my ability to recruit immigrant participants through casual contacts and conversations. As time went on, I had to rely more on Brazilian, Dominican, and Salvadoran organizations as recruitment sites for those groups.

Another challenge I encountered came from using multiple languages to conduct the immigrant interviews. The dialects, accents, and idioms of people vary depending on their country of origin, regional location, and socioeconomic status. Because I studied Brazilian Portuguese and Spanish before living in the Dominican Republic and Brazil, I learned these languages using a formal grammar that is more attuned to reading and writing than to conversation. When conducting interviews, it sometimes took a moment for my brain to click and understand interviewees who spoke in more vernacular ways. In some interviews, I realized that I incorrectly assumed that respondents were literate in their primary languages. When I asked respondents to read a list of racial categories or health statuses to determine which word best applied to them, I noticed that some struggled with the task, so I read the questions and possible answers *to* them. I had failed to consider the possibility that immigrants might be illiterate because in the United States, 88% of adults are literate, and education is free and compulsory, rather than a class privilege.

Although these challenges made conducting the study more difficult, they have made me a better researcher. As I conduct future research, I will be more cognizant of my respondents' experiences and backgrounds so that I can better bridge the structural gaps between us and give voice to their experiences to help create the social change and equitable society I would like to see.

Shifting Policy Landscapes from 2012 to 2019

I had to navigate numerous health and immigration policy shifts while I conducted research for this book. Rather than include that cumbersome level of detail in the book chapters, I have added some of those details to this section of the appendix. They provide more valuable context to better understand how policy shifts shaped the experiences of the immigrants and perspectives of providers and advocates described in the book.

Health Policy

To provide more context about the health policy landscape that shaped Boston Latinx immigrants' health coverage options, I include a timeline outlining relevant Massachusetts and federal health policies from the 1990s to 2019 (Figure A-1). Several more changes have happened in both jurisdictions since then that have continued to shape healthcare access for people in Massachusetts and across the country.

Chapter 2 provides basic information about Chapter 58. See Table 2-1 for the specific coverage programs and eligibility based on documentation status under Chapter 58 (column 1), Massachusetts after ACA Medicaid expansion (column 2), and other states after ACA Medicaid expansion (column 3). Here, I wish to include additional context on that reform, particularly as it related to shaping Massachusetts immigrants' eligibility for health coverage.

CelticCare Debacle in 2009

Though Chapter 58 was important for expanding health coverage to more people in the commonwealth, the costs associated with doing so were

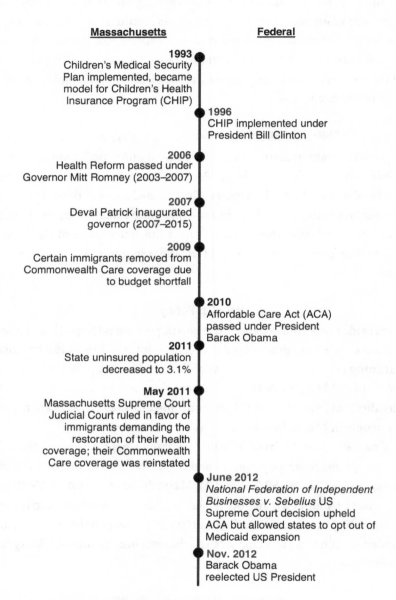

Massachusetts   **Federal**

1993
Children's Medical Security
Plan implemented, became
model for Children's Health
Insurance Program (CHIP)

1996
CHIP implemented under
President Bill Clinton

2006
Health Reform passed under
Governor Mitt Romney (2003–2007)

2007
Deval Patrick inaugurated
governor (2007–2015)

2009
Certain immigrants removed from
Commonwealth Care coverage due
to budget shortfall

2010
Affordable Care Act (ACA)
passed under President
Barack Obama

2011
State uninsured population
decreased to 3.1%

May 2011
Massachusetts Supreme Court
Judicial Court ruled in favor of
immigrants demanding the
restoration of their health
coverage; their Commonwealth
Care coverage was reinstated

June 2012
*National Federation of Independent
Businesses v. Sebelius* US
Supreme Court decision upheld
ACA but allowed states to opt out of
Medicaid expansion

Nov. 2012
Barack Obama
reelected US President

Figure A-1. Timeline of Massachusetts and Federal Health Policy Shifts

Oct. 2013
ACA implementation began and
Massachusetts legislators
reconciled and merged
Massachusetts and ACA reforms

Oct. 2013
ACA implementation
began

Jan. 2015
Charlie Baker inaugurated
governor (2015–2023)

June 2015
US Supreme Court ruled in favor
of allowing tax credits to be used
in state and federal exchanges

June 2016
State removed Health Safety Net (HSN)
from budget; implemented other
changes to HSN program

Nov. 2016
Donald Trump elected US
president; promised to repeal
and replace Obamacare

2017
Massachusetts lawmakers
reviewed and bolstered
health policy infrastructure in
case of ACA repeal

Dec. 2017
Tax Cut and Jobs Act
removed federal tax
penalty for not having
health insurance, removed
ACA individual mandate

2018
Charlie Baker reelected
governor

2018
Proportion of uninsured
adults in the US increased
for the first time since ACA
implementation due to
repeated attempts to
repeal the legislation

2019
Cover All Kids Act, which would
provide coverage to all
Massachusetts children regardless
of documentation status, debated
in State Legislature

Figure A-1. (continued)

high. A few years after implementation, the state's healthcare costs became too high for the annual budget to absorb in 2009 under Governor Deval Patrick. Because of a $130 million budget shortfall, the state removed 30,000 "Aliens with Special Status" (AWSSs)—immigrants who had had their green cards for less than five years and those with PRUCOL status—from Commonwealth Care to balance its budget.[9] Subsequently, these AWSSs were assigned to a lower-cost, substandard health plan called CelticCare that their trusted healthcare providers did not accept.[10] Most Boston-area healthcare providers, including those at BHC, did not accept that plan, which led to a disruption in care for patients.

Massachusetts's decision to remove health coverage for AWSS individuals culminated in a case before the state's Supreme Judicial Court in 2012. The lawsuit was successful, and the Supreme Judicial Court ordered that Commonwealth Care be reinstated for the affected groups of immigrants. But the three-year disruption made it difficult for many to return to their original providers. BHC providers and advocates said that some of the affected patients never returned; their relationships with their physicians were irreparably disrupted.

Federal Health Reform Under the 2010 Affordable Care Act

In Chapter 3, I discussed the most well-known features of the ACA and how federal restrictions limited coverage eligibility based on documentation status. Massachusetts legislators prepared for the reform by redrafting policy to prevent Massachusetts immigrants with coverage under the state reform from losing it under the ACA. Although undocumented immigrants had been able to use the state's health exchange to purchase coverage under the Massachusetts reform, they were not allowed to after ACA implementation. In this section, I outline additional details about how Obamacare complicated applying for coverage for immigrants and for advocates who helped them navigate the (re)enrollment process. Whereas Figure 3-1 showed the state's most common public coverage options after ACA implementation, Figure A-2 is a more complicated flowchart showing the wider range of MassHealth coverage options and how eligibility is shaped by a larger range of ages, documentation and disability statuses, and income levels.

A health advocate I interviewed shared this flowchart with me. Their organization developed it collaboratively with another advocacy organization to guide immigrant and health advocates who assist people in applying for coverage. Despite the disclaimer that "this graphic represents a simplified overview of immigrant eligibility," it is too confusing for most people to comprehend. The categories of documentation statuses include special groups such as lawfully present noncitizens and qualified or nonqualified lawfully present or barred noncitizens, as well as income eligibility ranges based on the federal poverty level. Only people with expert knowledge of immigration and health policy can apply these distinctions to specific cases. This flowchart also exemplifies how racialized legal status generates significant administrative burdens for the people applying for coverage as well as the meso-level bureaucrats and healthcare navigators responsible for managing (re)enrollment processes. It is no wonder some bureaucrats and healthcare navigators inaccurately told immigrants they were ineligible for coverage.

Immigration Policy

To provide more context about the immigration policy landscape that shaped Boston Latinx immigrants' lived experiences and access to public benefits such as health coverage, I include a timeline outlining relevant Massachusetts and federal immigration policies from the 1980s to 2020 (Figure A-3). This section also includes more background on the growth of the immigrant population in Massachusetts and policy responses to that growth during this time. A review of this timeline demonstrates how policies shaping immigrants' eligibility for and access to publicly funded resources for integration and social services became more stringent and limited over time. Immigrants' vulnerability to detention and deportation also increased during this time period.

In the 1970s and 1980s, Massachusetts became home to many refugees who were resettled in the United States after US military intervention in Southeast Asia. The federal Refugee Act of 1980 initially provided

Understanding eligibility of Mass

HEALTH CARE FOR ALL

This is intended to be a preliminary guide.

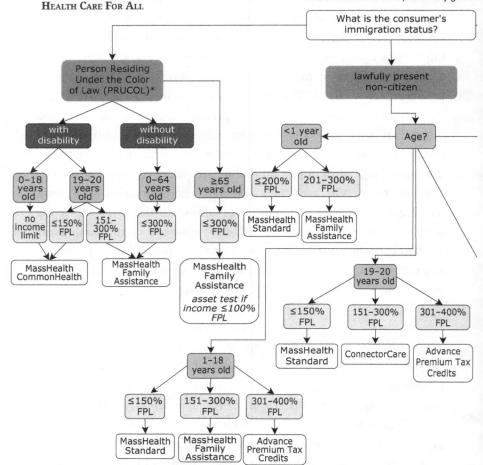

Lawfully present children ages 0–18 with disability and a family income >150% FPL may be eligible for MassHealth CommonHealth

NOTES:
- Definitions of PRUCOL, Lawfully Present, Qualified, and Qualified Barred can be found in regulations at 130 CMR 504.003.
- Pregnant women are eligible for MassHealth Standard regardless of immigration status
- Individuals of all ages with income ≤300% FPL may be be eligible for Health Safety Net benefits regardless of immigration status
- Lawfully present children under age 19 and qualified lawfully present adults age 19 and older who are both disabled and have income too high for MassHealth Standard may qualify for MassHealth CommonHealth. Adults must also be employed if 19 or older or meet a deductible if between the ages of 19 to 64.
- Individuals over age 65 also are subject to an asset test
- Immigrants who have been receiving MassHealth or CommonHealth continuously since June 30, 1997 remain eligible for MassHealth regardless of immigration status

Figure A-2. Immigrant Eligibility for MassHealth and Other Health Programs

Health and other health benefits

For full details, refer to the MassHealth Member Booklet.

immigration status
disability status
income
age

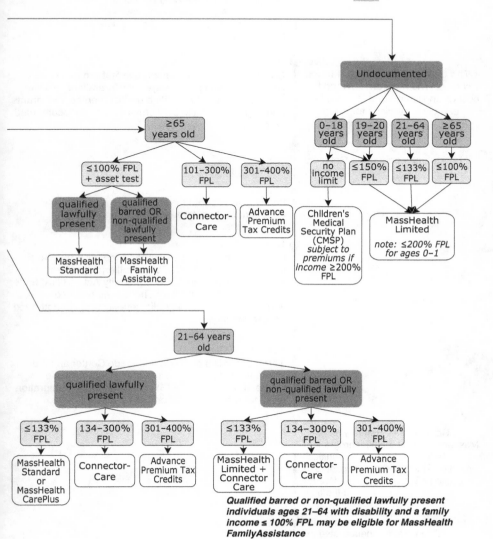

Qualified barred or non-qualified lawfully present individuals ages 21–64 with disability and a family income ≤ 100% FPL may be eligible for MassHealth FamilyAssistance

Massachusetts	Federal
	1980 Congress passed the Refugee Act during the Reagan Administration. It provided three years of cash and medical assistance to refugees.
1986 The Gateway Cities Program was created. The program covered the cost of English classes, translation, and other services for refugees and immigrants.	**1986** Congress passed the Immigration Reform and Control Act (IRCA) during the Reagan administration. This law granted amnesty to qualified undocumented immigrants and imposed penalties on employers of undocumented immigrants.
1989 Budget cuts ended the Gateway Cities Program.	
	1991 Budget cuts reduced the Refugees Act's benefits from three years to eight months.
	1996 Congress passed the Personal Responsibility, Work Opportunity Act (PRWORA) and Illegal Immigration Reform and Immigrant Responsibility Act (IIRIRA) under the Clinton administration. These laws reduced immigrants' access to public benefits and strengthened border security.
	Sept. 11, 2001 Terrorist attacks on the World Trade Center and the Pentagon led to the creation of the Department of Homeland Security (DHS) and heightened immigration enforcement. The "War on Terror" began.
2006 Governor Mitt Romney enrolled Massachusetts in the pilot program of the federal "Secure Communities" program. The program was piloted in Boston / Suffolk County before he left office.	
Jan. 2007 Deval Patrick inaugurated as governor.	

Figure A-3. Timeline of Massachusetts and Federal Immigration Policy Shifts

2008
Federal "Secure Communities" program launched, allowed information sharing between local law enforcement and federal immigration authorities.

2009
Barack Obama inaugurated as president.

2010
Governor Deval Patrick unveiled the New Americans Agenda which allowed funding for citizenship programs and restored health insurance for immigrants who lost it.

2010
DREAM Act failed in Congress.

2011
Governor Patrick objected to Secure Communities Program in Massachusetts, which former Governor Romney had permitted.

2011
Secure Communities expanded nationally, and deportations increased. President Obama dubbed "Deporter in Chief."

Aug. 2012
President Obama signed an executive order creating the Deferred Action for Childhood Arrivals (DACA) Program.

Nov. 2012
President Obama reelected.

Spring 2013
Immigration reform (Border Security, Economic Opportunity, and Immigration Modernization Act) failed.

April 2013
Boston Marathon bombing occurs. The perpetrators were documented immigrants, which led to greater scrutiny of immigrants regardless of legal status or naturalization.

2014
Priority Enforcement Program (PEP) replaced Secure Communities program. PEP prioritized detaining and deporting convicted criminals and others who posed a danger to public safety.

Figure A-3. (continued)

June 2014
Domestic Workers Bill of
Rights passed, which reduced
wage theft and exploitation for
domestic workers, many of whom
are immigrant women.

June 2014
Local sanctuary policies adopted
in Somerville, Boston, and eight
other municipalities.

June 2015
Donald Trump announced bid for US
presidency and ran an explicitly anti-
immigrant campaign.

Jan. 2017
Donald Trump inaugurated
president. He also signed an
executive order known as the
Muslim Travel Ban.

March 2017
ICE started targeting sanctuary cities in
raids.

Sept. 2017
President Trump announced the end of
DACA, leading to state-level court
challenges to the termination of DACA.

Dec. 2017
US Supreme Court granted the Trump
administration's request to temporarily
allow Muslim Travel Ban.

Jan. 2018
President Trump referred to Haiti and
African countries as "shithole" countries
after questioning why the United States
accepts immigrants from those countries.

June 2018
US Supreme Court upheld Muslim Travel
Ban.

Figure A-3. (continued)

April 2019
Boston Judge Shelly Joseph charged
with helping an undocumented
immigrant escape ICE arrest at the
courthouse where she had heard their
legal case on an unrelated charge.

July 2019
President Trump announced ICE raids.

Aug. 2019
El Paso Walmart shooting occurred, where
the shooter targeted Latinx people. DHS
also announced that the public charge rule
change would go into effect; the change
was subsequently challenged in federal
courts. President Trump announced the
end of the Medical Deferred Action
Program for terminally ill immigrants. He
also aimed to abolish birthright citizenship.

Sept. 2019
The Medical Deferred Action Program was
reinstated.

Nov. 2019
Asylum seekers who entered at the US–
Mexico border had to wait in jail in the United
States or Mexico until US immigration
officials could determine their eligibility for
asylum status.

March 2020
COVID lockdowns began. Trump
administration invoked Title 42, which
allowed the United States to reject
migrants at the US–Mexico border.

June 2020
US Supreme Court announced that
President Trump could not immediately
end DACA. President Trump ended
temporary protected status (TPS) for
certain immigrants.

July 2020
Massachusetts state
legislators deliberated on the Safe
Communities Actand Work/Family
Mobility Acts.

Sept. 2020
A federal appeals court stands by
President Trump's decision to end TPS.
President Trump announced that raids of
"sanctuary cities" would continue.

Figure A-3. (continued)

three years of cash and medical assistance. But the period of eligibility and federal funding for assistance was reduced to 18 months in 1982 and to 8 months in 1991, which left local communities with insufficient resources to assist resettled refugees.[11] With many politicians supporting city- and state-level integration policies, Massachusetts created the Gateway Cities Program in 1986. The program allocated state funds to cover the costs of the English language classes, translators, and services to assist refugees and immigrants in towns that had sizable immigrant populations.[12]

As the recession of the late 1980s hit the state budget, funding for Gateway Cities was cut, and then the program was eliminated. Pressure to reduce public health, education, and welfare benefits to unauthorized immigrants took center stage in the 1990 gubernatorial election. Budget constraints also led city officials to end services for newcomers and reduce the availability of translators.[13] Under President Bill Clinton's administration, passage of the 1996 IIRIRA and PRWORA federal legislation limited immigrants' eligibility for public benefits. Massachusetts immigration advocates worked unsuccessfully with state lawmakers and US Senator Ted Kennedy to restore benefits to short-term green card holders, who had lost their eligibility.[14] Most noncitizens, including many who were documented, also faced the prospect of potential deportation.

Under President George W. Bush's administration, enforcement became harsher nationally and in Boston after 9/11, which was followed by a surge of Islamophobia, anti-immigrant rhetoric, and violence toward those perceived as immigrants regardless of their citizenship or documentation status.[15] Raids by government agents from the newly formed Department of Homeland Security (DHS) and Immigration and Customs Enforcement (ICE) generated fear in immigrant and minority communities. In 2006, Governor Mitt Romney enrolled Boston in the pilot program of the federal Secure Communities program. The program collected fingerprints of immigrants who were arrested by local police and forwarded them to the Federal Bureau of Investigation and DHS. Arrested immigrants with potential immigration violations were held in jail and could be turned over to ICE for potential deportation.

By 2010, little progress had been made on immigration reform during President Obama's first term. Legislative efforts to pass the Development, Relief, and Education for Alien Minors Act (DREAM) Act, which would have protected the children of undocumented immigrants from deportation, were unsuccessful. The Obama administration inherited the punitive policies of the Clinton administration and the militarized border enforcement policies of the Bush administration. Consequently, the Obama administration carried out three million deportations, leading the president to be dubbed the "Deporter-in-Chief."[16] In Massachusetts, Governor Patrick announced a "New Americans Agenda" to improve immigrant integration in the state.[17] The agenda included supporting legislation that allowed immigrant students to pay in-state tuition at public universities, finding ways to facilitate the licensing of immigrant medical professionals, funding citizenship education programs, and restoring healthcare coverage for documented immigrants who had lost coverage in the 2010 budget crunch.[18] Despite pressure from immigrant advocates to move the agenda forward, the proposed legislation was not passed.

Nationally, recognizing that Republicans would resist immigration reform efforts, President Obama signed an executive order creating Deferred Action for Childhood Arrivals in August 2012.[19] The program allowed undocumented young adults who had been brought to the country as children to be protected from deportation and given temporary work permits.[20] After winning reelection in November 2012, President Obama expanded the Secure Communities program across the country in 2013.

In the absence of state-level sanctuary legislation, Massachusetts city and county leaders pushed for more inclusive policies for immigrants in their jurisdictions. In 2014, Joseph Curtatone, mayor of Somerville, a densely populated city just west of Boston, decided that local police would no longer hold individuals on behalf of ICE to facilitate their deportation. Somerville became the first city in Massachusetts to call itself a "sanctuary city."[21] That same year, the City of Boston passed the Trust Act, barring local law enforcement from detaining individuals based only on a civil immigration detainer request and from transferring a person to immigration authorities without a court order.[22] By 2017, 49 of the 351 municipalities in the state implemented sanctuary policies in response to harmful Trump administration immigration policies.[23]

Trump Administration Immigration Policy Proposals

In Chapter 4, I discussed some of the most notable Trump administration immigration policies and how Massachusetts legislators, government officials, and advocates attempted to counter those policies in the commonwealth. Here, I provide more detail on some of those policies that dramatically affected the sociopolitical climate for immigrants in Massachusetts and around the country. Most of these were implemented or proposed after Trump was inaugurated through when I conducted interviews in 2019. These policies likely had an impact on the recruitment of immigrants for the last year of my study.

In September 2017, the president rescinded DACA by executive order. Following lower federal court suits challenging the end of the program, the US Supreme Court ruled in June 2020 that the Trump administration had illegally terminated the DACA program, but the justices agreed that the president could end the program if he did so properly.

In June and July 2017, President Trump tweeted proudly that large-scale ICE raids in 10 major cities would detain and deport undocumented immigrants.[24] Although Boston was not one of those cities, local organizations held know-your-rights workshops and provided instructions on what to do if ICE came to people's homes.[25] Locally, there had been an uptick in ICE arrests at courthouses when immigrants showed up for civil hearings. A lawsuit brought by local immigrant advocacy organizations against ICE was successful in stopping such arrests in June.[26] In one infamous case, Middlesex County Judge Shelley Joseph was charged with helping an undocumented immigrant avoid ICE arrest at her courthouse in April 2019.[27]

The summer of 2019 was marked by the escalation of racialized anti-immigrant rhetoric and constant, deliberate denials of the rights of immigrants and asylum seekers. News reports circulated about migrant children being separated from their parents at the US–Mexico border, detained in cages, and held in inhumane conditions for extended periods.[28] In August, there was a mass shooting targeting Mexican shoppers at a Walmart in El Paso, Texas, that killed 22 people. In an online manifesto before going to the store, the perpetrator declared that he aimed to stop the "Hispanic invasion of Texas."[29] His language echoed President Trump's fiery rhetoric, and many Latinx people felt that the shooter acted out Trump's threats. A few days later, the president defended massive ICE raids at Mississippi food processing plants, calling the action a "good deterrent."[30] That day, 680 adults were detained, leaving many of their children with no one to take care of them. Toward the end of August, chronically ill immigrants, many of them children, and their relatives received letters from DHS stating that the medical deferred action program, which allowed people to remain in the country if they demonstrated a severe need for medical treatment, was being terminated.[31] Despite receiving vital health care in the United States that was unavailable in their home countries, they could be deported in 30 days without adjustment in their status. In Boston, lawyers from the American Civil Liberties Union and Lawyers for Civil Rights filed lawsuits on behalf of immigrant advocacy organizations against the Trump administration, challenging the constitutionality of ending the program.[32] After much uproar from both patients and hospitals, the program was reinstated a month later.[33]

Although the Trump administration proposed and implemented additional consequential policies in 2020, the emergence of the COVID pandemic took precedence in national discourse and media, with less focus on immigration policy or the increasing exclusion of immigrants.

Introduction

1. I interchangeably use the terms "immigrants" and "noncitizens" to refer to individuals who migrated to the United States from other countries. Immigrants also include individuals who became naturalized US citizens.

2. I use "Latina" to describe Victoria's ethnicity as it is the term she used. Wherever I mention the ethnoracial classification of respondents, I use the open-ended classification term they provided during our interview. When referring more broadly to individuals with Latin American ancestry in the United States, I use the term "Latinx," as it is more gender inclusive than the terms "Latino" and "Latina" and includes non-Spanish-speaking Latin Americans such as Brazilians. I sometimes use "Hispanic" to refer to Spanish-speaking Latin Americans, particularly in the context of US census categories. Throughout the book, respondents use both terms to identify themselves or others with Latin American ancestry.

3. I capitalize "White" and other ethnoracial categories throughout the book because terms such as "European," "Hispanic," "Latinx," "African American," and "Indigenous" refer to geographic and cultural origins and are proper names.

4. Bailey et al. 2017; Barr 2014; Cuevas, Dawson, and Williams 2016; Geronimus 2023; LaVeist and Isaac 2012; Villarosa 2022.

5. Chapter 1 explains racialized legal status in more detail and outlines the term's use in recent scholarship.

6. Golash-Boza 2015a; Omi and Winant 1994; Joseph and Golash-Boza 2021.

7. Gurrola and Ayon 2018; Krieger 2001, 2013; Palmer et al. 2019.

8. Phelan and Link 2005.

9. Matthew 2022; Bradley and Taylor 2013; Nuila 2022; Schneider et al. 2021.

10. Avendano and Kawachi 2014; Dickman, Himmelstein, and Woolhandler 2017; Hero et al. 2016; Tikkanen and Abrams 2020; Woolf and Aron 2013.

11. Dickman, Himmelstein, and Woolhandler 2017; Hero et al. 2016; Raudenbush 2020; Vargas 2022.

12. Hale et al. 2024.

13. Park, Hoekstra, and Jiménez 2024; Raudenbush 2020; Sangaramoorthy 2023; Van Natta 2023; Vargas 2022; Villarosa 2022.

14. I use the terms "documentation status" and "legal status" interchangeably throughout the book.

15. Beaman 2017; Bloemraad et al. 2019; Calavita 2005; Cheliotis 2017; Joseph 2020c.

16. Alba and Foner 2015; Dines, Montagna, and Vacchelli 2018; Reeves, McKee, and Stuckler 2015; Virdee and McGeever 2018.

17. Asad and Clair 2018; Joseph and Golash-Boza 2021; Negrón-Gonzales 2011.

18. Ward and Batalova 2023.

19. Jones et al. 2021; Ward and Batalova 2023.

20. I use both "Obamacare" and "the Affordable Care Act (ACA)," because "Obamacare" is popular in the media and broader discourse and refers to the plan as it was initially enacted and implemented. Since then, legal challenges have substantially modified the ACA in ways that limited its scope. Breland, Rocco, and Waddan 2016; Dawes 2016; House 2015; McDonough 2011.

21. Davis and Shear 2019; Golash-Boza 2015a. The greatest number of immigrants were deported during the 1930s, when Mexican and Mexican American families were forcibly removed to Mexico. For more on historical deportations, see Molina 2006; Ngai 2004.

22. Rampell 2020; Simmons-Duffin 2019. A "public charge" is a noncitizen who becomes dependent on government assistance. The public charge policy has existed for more than a century, and immigrants' use of certain public benefits has been used to determine whether immigrants are a public charge. For more, see Golash-Boza 2015a and Park 2011. Chapter 4 will discuss the public charge policy in more detail because President Trump changed the long-standing public charge rule to make it more difficult for lower-income immigrants to qualify for lawful permanent residency.

23. The scholarship on intersectionality has been important for assessing how race intersects with other sociopolitical constructions such as gender and how the law has influenced social outcomes among different intersectional demographic groups such as Black women and immigrants of color, for instance. Crenshaw 1991; Collins 2015; Viruell-Fuentes, Miranda, and Abdulrahim 2012.

24. Boston Globe Spotlight Team 2017; Frey 2022; Johnson 2015.

25. The top five countries of origin for immigrants to Boston are China, the Dominican Republic, Brazil, India, and Haiti. Immigrants constitute 17% of the state population. Just over half (54%) of Massachusetts's immigrants are naturalized citizens. Undocumented immigrants are estimated at 3% of the state's population, with around 180,000 living in Boston. See American Immigration Council (AIC) 2020; US Census Bureau 2021; Johnson 2015; Migration Policy Institute, n.d.; Rocheleau 2017.

26. American Immigration Council (AIC) 2020.

27. Kim Janey, a Black woman, served as acting mayor of Boston from March to November 2021 after Mayor Marty Walsh vacated the office to serve as secretary of labor under President Joe Biden.

28. Johnson 2015; Lima and Melnik 2013.

29. Boston Foundation 2019; Johnson 2015.

30. Ward and Batalova 2023.

31. Borrell 2005; Borrell and Crawford 2009; Bustamante et al. 2009; Mora 2014; Rodríguez-Muñiz 2021.

32. Mohl 2023; Russell 2023.

33. Mohl 2023; Russell 2023.

34. Mohl 2023; Russell 2023.

35. Porter 2020.

36. Patel and McDonough 2010.

37. Joseph 2016; Patel and McDonough 2010.

38. Joseph 2016.

39. Among the estimated 528,000 adults in Massachusetts with limited English proficiency, nearly 39% speak Spanish and 7% speak Portuguese. See Boston Planning and Development Agency 2019a; US Census Bureau 2019.

40. Berchick, Hood, and Barnett 2018; Betancourt 2021; Boston Planning and Development Agency 2019a; Garfield, Orgera, and Damico 2019; Karpman et al. 2019.

41. Johnson 2015.

42. Johnson 2015.

43. Boston Planning and Development Agency 2019c.

44. Boston Planning and Development Agency 2019c.

45. Johnson 2015.

46. García Peña 2022; Itzigsohn 2009. Of the 27 Dominicans interviewed in the study, 8 migrated to Puerto Rico or New York City before settling in Boston.

47. Boston Planning and Development Agency 2019c.

48. Abrego and Villalpando 2021; Johnson 2015.

49. Johnson 2015.

50. Granberry and Agarwal 2021.

51. Menjívar 2006.

52. Menjívar 2017; Terrazas 2010. As of July 1, 2024, TPS designations remain in place for El Salvador through March 9, 2025. US Citizenship and Immigration Services (USCIS) 2024.

53. Boston Planning and Development Agency 2019b; Johnson 2015; Joseph 2015.

54. Johnson 2015; Stargardter 2021.

55. Johnson 2015.

56. Johnson 2015.

57. Brazilian immigrants have a notable history of return migration, working in the United States for a few years to earn money and returning home to start a business or purchase a home. Joseph 2015.

58. Rios 2018; Sands 2019; Stargardter 2021.

59. Johnson 2015.

60. Framingham has the highest proportion of Brazilian immigrants in the state and is one of the largest Brazilian enclaves in the United States. Johnson 2015.

61. The increase in the cost of living affected immigrants' access to health care, as well as housing and jobs. Hospital networks centered in downtown Boston incorporated smaller community hospitals and healthcare centers in surrounding suburbs, closing them or transforming them into satellite facilities. Thus, the hyperconcentration of medical resources in the Boston area has recently spread well beyond the urban core.

62. Boston Planning and Development Agency 2019b.

63. Boston Planning and Development Agency 2019b.

64. Johnson 2015; Boston Planning and Development Agency 2019b.

65. Joseph 2015. US embassy officials in Brazil also privilege lighter Brazilians when issuing visas.

66. Joseph 2015.

67. Lorenzi and Batalova 2022.

68. Migration Policy Institute, n.d.

69. Blizzard and Batalova 2019.

70. Joseph 2015.

71. "BHC" is a pseudonym to protect the identity of the hospital network. More demographic information about the providers can be found in the appendix.

72. The state finally passed legislation extending driver's licenses to undocumented residents in June 2022 despite former governor Charlie Baker's veto. A ballot question to repeal or keep the legislation was put before Massachusetts voters, who voted in November 2023 to keep it. Issuing of driver's licenses to undocumented residents began on July 1, 2023. For more, see Drysdale 2023.

73. Beckfield 2018; Bloemraad and Terriquez 2016; Campbell 2014; López-Sanders 2017; Marrow 2011; Small 2006; Watkins-Hayes 2009.

74. Naderifar, Goli, and Ghaljaie 2017; Sadler et al. 2010; Ellard-Gray et al. 2015.

75. Culley, Hudson, and Lohan 2013; Preloran et al. 2001; Slauson-Blevins and Johnson 2016; Ryan et al. 2019.

76. DACA provides recipients with temporary protection from deportation and work permits but does not provide a path to citizenship. The program was rescinded under the Trump administration but reimplemented under the Biden administration. See Alulema 2019; Aranda, Vaquera, and Castañeda 2020; Brindis et al. 2014; Wong and Garcia 2013; Wong et al. 2013.

77. Miles and Huberman 1994; Patton 1999; Wolcott 1994.

78. Cooper-Patrick et al. 1999; Huerto 2020; Nuila 2022; Saha, Arbelaez, and Cooper 2003; Villarosa 2022.

79. Matthew 2022; Cancarevic, Plichtová, and Haider Malik 2021; De Lew et al 1992; Nuila 2022; Villarosa 2022.

80. See Starr 1982 for a detailed history of the development of the US healthcare system.

81. Tomes 1985, 255.

82. A. Cohen et al. 2015.

83. Starr 1982.

84. Robeznieks 2022.

85. Baker 2014; Blackstock 2024; Smith 2016; Matthew 2022; Nuila 2022; Villarosa 2022.

86. Baker 2014; Smith 2016.

87. Smith 2016. These decisions were often not voluntary and were made under duress, with patients not being told the truth about any treatment they could receive. The most well-known cases are the Tuskegee Syphilis Study conducted by the US Public Health Service from 1932 to 1972 and the ongoing use of cell lines derived from the tissues of Henrietta Lacks, who was unaware her cervical cancer cells were cultivated in the lab at Johns Hopkins after she was treated and died there in 1951. For more, see Gray 2002, Reverby 2009, and Skloot 2010.

88. Rice et al. 2013.

89. Cancarevic, Plichtová, and Haider Malik 2021; A. Cohen et al. 2015; De Lew et al 1992.

90. The Children's Health Insurance Program (CHIP) was established in 1997 to ensure that children in families earning too much to qualify for Medicaid have access to low-cost comprehensive coverage. Administered at the state level and separate from Medicaid, the program nonetheless works closely with Medicaid. Eligibility for CHIP varies by state. The program was reauthorized in 2009 under President Obama.

91. Garfield and Rudowitz 2020.

92. Kaiser Family Foundation 2024. The ACA legislation states that the Medicaid expansion eligibility threshold is 133% of the federal poverty level. But the legislation also included a new method for calculating income that makes the minimum threshold 138% of the federal poverty level. Thus, I use the 133% threshold when discussing the ACA in this book. See APHA n.d.

93. Individuals considered to be PRUCOL are noncitizens living in the United States with the knowledge and consent of the Department of Homeland Security, which has not taken action to remove them. In Massachusetts, they are currently covered under the state's ConnectorCare program but are ineligible for long-term care coverage. See Health Care for All 2020.

94. Undocumented children and pregnant women are eligible for some types of Medicaid; the benefits are determined at the state level and vary by state.

95. Bloemraad et al. 2019; Chauvin and Garcés-Mascareñas 2014; Snowden and Graff 2019; Van Natta 2023; Willen 2012.

96. Campbell 2018; Zallman et al. 2013.

97. Rudowitz et al. 2021.

98. Keisler-Starkey and Bunch 2021. In the 10 states that have still not expanded Medicaid under the ACA, an estimated 1.5 million individuals who would be eligible for Medicaid remain uninsured. See Drake et al. 2024.

99. Sainato 2021; CDC 2021. Dental care is generally not included in private health insurance plans, although individuals can purchase separate dental insurance plans. An estimated 74 million Americans do not have access to regular

preventive dental care, which is considered a major health issue in the United States. See Sainato 2021.

100. Cancarevic, Plichtová, and Haider Malik 2021.

101. Hoffman 2006; McKillop et al. 2018; Schoen et al. 2010.

102. Flavin et al. 2018; Zallman et al. 2018.

103. Keisler-Starkey and Bunch 2021.

104. Commonwealth Fund 2022.

105. Rabin et al. 2020; Winters 2022.

106. Berchick, Hood, and Barnett 2018; U.S. Department of Health and Human Services 2021.

107. Garfield and Rudowitz 2020.

108. Hale et al. 2024.

109. Marrow and Joseph 2015; Matthew 2012; Warner 2012.

110. The Emergency Medical Treatment and Labor Act does not prevent hospitals from billing patients for these services. But federal funds under the Disproportionate Share Hospital program (which reached $10 billion in 2009) or state funds can be used to reimburse uncollected emergency care costs. Otherwise, hospitals absorb the loss that results from treating these patients. For more detailed information, see Konczal and Varga 2012; Warner 2012.

111. Wright 2013.

112. Park, Hoekstra, and Jiménez 2024; Portes, Fernández-Kelly, and Light 2012.

113. Jacobs and Skocpol 2010; Spithoven 2016; Wouters 2020.

114. Hero et al. 2016; Reinhart 2018.

115. Breland, Rocco, and Waddan 2016; Campbell 2014; Dawes 2016; Golash-Boza 2015a; House 2015; Illingworth and Parmet 2017; López 2019; McDonough 2011; Molina 2006; Park 2011; Park, Hoekstra, and Jiménez 2024; Van Natta 2023.

116. Intensifying enforcement had a similar chilling effect in other parts of the country. See Orris, Grady, and Mann 2018; Altaf et al. 2021; Raff 2020; Torres-Ardila et al. 2018.

Chapter 1 • Racialized Legal Status and Healthcare Exclusion in Boston

1. Negrón-Gonzales 2011, 4.

2. Asad and Clair 2018.

3. Armenta 2017; Chavez 2013; Garcia 2017; Massey 2012; Menjívar 2021; Provine and Doty 2011.

4. Joseph and Golash-Boza 2021.

5. Armenta 2017; De Genova 2002; Flores and Schachter 2018; Chavez 2013; Garcia 2017; Massey 2012; Menjívar 2021; Provine and Doty 2011; Sáenz and Douglas 2015; Yazdiha 2021.

6. Stumpf 2006.

7. Armenta 2017; Golash-Boza 2015a; Golash-Boza and Hondagneu-Sotelo 2013; Menjívar 2021.

8. People and organizations increasingly use the term "criminal legal system" to describe policing, prosecution, courts, and corrections in the United States, instead

of "criminal justice system," because these systems do not deliver justice. See, for example, Bryant 2021.

9. Bonilla-Silva 1997; Crenshaw 2010; Feagin 2014; Garcia 2017; Golash-Boza 2016; Omi and Winant 1994; Ray 2019.

10. Golash-Boza 2016; Joseph and Golash-Boza 2021; Quisumbing King 2018.

11. Collins 2004; Collins and Bilge 2020; Crenshaw 1991; Valdez 2011.

12. Alba and Nee 2003; Gans 1992; Portes and Rumbaut 2006; Portes and Zhou 1993.

13. Brown 2018; Garcia 2017; Olmos 2019; Sáenz and Douglas 2015; Sanchez and Romero 2010.

14. FitzGerald 2017; FitzGerald and Cook-Martín 2014; Molina 2014; Smith 1997.

15. Bloemraad et al. 2019; Bosniak 2000; Chavez 2013; FitzGerald and Cook-Martín 2014; Marshall 1950; Mettler 1998; Molina 2014; Ong et al. 1996; Smith 1997. These scholars distinguish between social and cultural citizenship, but I combine them because they are closely connected in the impact of racialized legal status on Latinx immigrants.

16. Anderson 2016; Belew and Gutiérrez 2021; Metzl 2019.

17. Flores-Gonzalez 2017; Lee 2019; Lin 2022; Ngai 2004, 2007; Obinna 2021; Schut and Boen 2022; Selod 2018; Tuan 1999.

18. Although state governments had previously decided what groups were forbidden to reside in their territory, the Supreme Court declared that immigration policy was the responsibility of the federal government in 1875. See Bloemraad and De Graauw 2011; Wong et al. 2021; USCIS 2020.

19. Bosniak 2006; De Genova 2002; Joseph 2020a; Menjívar and Lakhani 2016; Zolberg 2006.

20. Golash-Boza 2015b; Mora 2014; Prewitt 2005; Rodriguez 2000.

21. Molina 2014, 11.

22. Calavita 2005; Joseph 2020a; Massey and Bartley 2005; Menjívar 2006; Ngai 2004.

23. Kominers 2016; Menjívar and Lakhani 2016; Zolberg 2006.

24. Fox 2016; Gonzales, Terriquez, and Ruszczyk 2014; Van Natta et al. 2019.

25. Bonilla-Silva 1997; Feagin 2014; Golash-Boza 2015b; Lee 2019; Ngai 2004.

26. Alexander and Stivers 2020; Fox 2012; Jones 2024; Pierson 2018.

27. Fox 2012; Carten 2020; Katznelson 2013.

28. Fox 2012; Robertson 2017.

29. Massey and Denton 1993; Charles 2003; Lacy 2016; Robertson 2017.

30. Oliver and Shapiro 1995; Sullivan et al. 2015.

31. Dyck and Hussey 2008; Gillens 1999; Hero and Preuhs 2007; Metzl 2019; Peffley, Hurwitz, and Sniderman 1997; Reingold and Smith 2012; Soss et al. 2010.

32. Alexander 2010; Hinton 2017.

33. Menjívar and Lakhani 2016; Wong et al. 2021. In Figure 1-1, "other policy domains" include matters, such as eligibility for driver's licenses, that may depend on immigration status.

34. Bloemraad and DeGrauw 2011; Menjívar and Lakhani 2016; Varsanyi et al. 2012; Wong et al. 2021; Zimmerman and Tumlin 1999.

35. De Trinidad Young et al. 2017; Joseph 2016; Marrow 2012; Varsanyi 2010.

36. Jordan 2023; Pillai and Artiga 2023.

37. Armenta 2017; García 2019; Kaufmann 2019; Kuge 2020; Lasch et al. 2018; Roy 2019.

38. Varsanyi et al. 2012.

39. Bosniak 2006; Gonzales 2015; Gonzales and Burciaga 2018; Kominers 2016. The sociological concept of "master status" was originally developed in the study of race, indicating that Blackness trumps class position, education, and other dimensions of social positioning; see Hughes 1945 for the concept's original formulation. This concept has contributed to my theorization of racialized legal status.

40. Amaya 2013; Gomez and Gilkesson 2021; Kreisberg 2019; Rodriguez et al. 2022.

41. Menjívar and Abrego 2012.

42. Abrego and Lakhani 2015; Cervantes and Menjívar 2020; Van Natta 2019, 2023.

43. Feagin 2014.

44. Golash-Boza 2015b.

45. Feagin 2014, 8.

46. Crenshaw et al. 1995; Hing 2002; Jones 2024; Menjívar 2021.

47. Brown and Jackson 2013; Crenshaw 2010; Ray 2022.

48. Ray 2019.

49. Menjívar and Abrego 2012.

50. The "help" Jazmin references is now against the law in Florida, where providing any kind of assistance to undocumented immigrants can be penalized.

51. Herd and Moynihan 2018.

52. Herd and Moynihan 2018, 3.

53. Herd and Moynihan 2018; Link and Phelan 1995; Ray, Herd, and Moynihan 2023.

54. Herd and Moynihan 2018; Kliff 2014; McDonough 2016; Ornstein 2014; Pear, LaFraniere, and Austen 2013.

55. Herd and Moynihan 2018, 4.

56. Ray, Herd, and Moynihan 2023.

57. Ray 2019.

58. Sewell 2016.

59. Whatley and Batalova 2013.

60. Ramos 2016.

61. For more on how time is taxed through interactions with government bureaucracies, see Lowrey 2021; Teles 2013.

62. Armenta and Sarabia 2020; Halim, Moy, and Yoshikawa 2017; Schinkel et al 2018; Shamsi et al. 2020; Ugas et al. 2023.

63. Callagan et al. 2019; Joseph 2020b; Morgante 2021; Parmet 2018; Singh 2020; Van Natta 2023.

64. Chavez-Dueñas, Adames, and Organista 2014; Cuevas, Dawson, and Williams 2016; Espino and Franz 2002; Hall 2011; Monroe and Hall 2018; Murguia and Telles 1996; Santana 2018.

65. Elsewhere, I demonstrate that documentation status exists along a continuum that dramatically shapes individuals' access to public benefits under the Affordable Care Act. See Joseph 2020a.

66. USCIS 2022.

67. Golash-Boza 2015a; Park 2011.

68. USCIS 2023.

69. For more on the 1996 welfare and immigration reforms, see Fox 2016; Menjívar and Lakhani 2016; Park 2011.

70. FitzGerald 2019; Gowayed 2022; USCIS 2015.

71. FitzGerald 2019; Gowayed 2022.

72. Fix and Haskins 2002.

73. Menjívar 2017.

74. Menjívar 2006.

75. The most common nonimmigrant visas are issued for work (H-1B, H-2A/B), tourism (B-1/B-2), and study (F-1/M-1). For more on different types of visas, see E. Cohen 2015; US Department of State 2016.

76. Fox 2016; Viladrich 2012; Capps and Fix 2013. Tourist visa holders (B-1/B-2) cannot receive benefits and have no work authorization, and student visas (F-1/M-1) are issued to those studying in academic or vocational institutions (US Department of State n.d.). Different employment visas provide work authorization: H-1Bs for highly skilled workers in specialized occupations and H-2A/Bs for seasonal workers in agriculture, hospitality, or tourism (US Department of State n.d.). On the documentation status continuum, H-2A/B visa holders are to the right of tourist visa holders and to the left of H-1B and student visa holders, who can more easily obtain sponsors for a green card (Joseph 2020a). As temporary employees, H-2A/B visa holders do not receive employment benefits, an important social boundary distinguishing them from H-1A/B visa holders. Student visa holders have institutional support for visa renewal, unlike H-2A/B visa holders. All visa holders are ineligible for benefits and deportable beyond their visa expiration date.

77. For more on the vulnerability of those who are undocumented, see Armenta 2017; Dreby 2015; García 2019; Gonzales 2015; Silver 2018. High-priority undocumented immigrants, who have criminal records or are recently arrived adults, are targeted first for deportation; low-priority undocumented immigrants include children and Deferred Action for Childhood Arrivals recipients. Yee 2018.

78. Aptekar 2016; Chen 2020.

79. Motomura 2014; Yee 2018.

80. Armenta 2017; Brotherton and Barrios 2011; Epp, Maynard-Moody, and Haider-Markel 2014; Golash-Boza 2015a; Sewell et al. 2020.

81. Alexander 2010; Epp, Maynard-Moody, and Haider-Markel 2014.

82. Brotherton and Barrios 2011; Golash-Boza 2015a.

83. Golash-Boza 2015a. This law is the 1996 Illegal Immigration Reform and Immigration Responsibility Act (IIRIRA).

84. Doty and Wheatley 2013; Eisen 2018; Joseph 2020c.

85. Holloway 2014; Uggen and Manza 2002.

86. Sewell et al. 2020; Vargas, Sanchez, and Juárez 2017.

87. The physical features that align with Whiteness and confer privileges to those considered White in the United States are different from those that align with Whiteness in Brazil, the Dominican Republic, and El Salvador. Whereas racial "purity" has historically been a necessary criterion for the White racial category in the US, the national identity construction of racial mixing (*mestiçagem* in Brazil and *mestizaje* in the Dominican Republic and El Salvador) has meant that individuals with lighter/Whiter physical features in those countries can self-classify and be considered by others as White despite having racially mixed ancestry. Thus, some Brazilians, Dominicans, and Salvadorans who are "White" in their home country are generally not considered White in the United States. For more on this, see Joseph 2015; Telles and PERLA 2014.

Chapter 2 • Included in Coverage but Excluded from Use (2012–2013)

1. R. Cohen, Ward, and Schiller 2011.

2. I use the term "coverage" to refer broadly to public or private plans that provide certain types of benefits associated with paying low or no premiums, deductibles, and co-pays for health services. While health insurance is considered health coverage, some types of health coverage, such as the Health Safety Net Program, are funded directly by the state instead of functioning as insurance.

3. Blue Cross Blue Shield of Massachusetts 2016; Joseph 2018; Long, Goin, and Lynch 2013.

4. For immigrant respondents, I include their age, ethnoracial classification, and documentation status at the time of the interview. Ethnoracial classifications were based on the open-ended categories they provided during our interview as these categories were the best reflection of how immigrants saw themselves in ethnoracial terms. Sometimes these categories overlapped with categories used in the US census. Sometimes they did not, which indicated how individuals' self-classifications do not always align with government-developed categories. It is also important to note that immigrants' ethnoracial classifications in the United States might differ from how they self-classified in their home countries. I do not include similar information for the advocates and providers to prevent them from being identified based on their ethnoracial classification. Some advocates and providers were the only person of color or one of a few people of color employed by their organization.

5. Blue Cross Blue Shield of Massachusetts 2016; Joseph 2018; Long, Goin, and Lynch 2013; Vargas 2022.

6. Gunja and Collins 2019; Sanchez et al. 2017; Terriquez and Joseph 2016; Van Natta 2023; Vargas 2022.

7. Hill, Artiga, and Damico 2024. This number accounts for both US and foreign-born individuals, and the survey lists "Hispanic" as the ethnic category. Brazilians are not included in these data.

8. Blue Cross Blue Shield of Massachusetts 2013; Levy 2013; Long, Goin, and Lynch 2013; Long and Masi 2009; Wilson 2008.

9. Joseph 2017a, 2017b.

10. Joseph 2016.

11. Light 2012.

12. Decker 2012.

13. Massachusetts covered those considered as having Permanent Residence Under Color of Law (PRUCOL) under the original 2006 reform and under the ACA except between 2009 and 2012. They are currently covered under ConnectorCare but are ineligible for long-term care coverage. See Parmet and Sainsbury-Wong 2012 for more on PRUCOL immigrants' exclusion from coverage in Massachusetts from 2009 to 2012.

14. While the ACA uses the term "lawfully present" to assess eligibility, the 1996 Personal Responsibility and Work Opportunity Act uses a different set of terms and criteria.

15. See Joseph 2016 for more on programs and income-level cutoffs.

16. Health Safety Net was known as FreeCare before the 2006 reform.

17. There were seven types of MassHealth coverage under Chapter 58 that were allocated based on income and documentation status. MassHealth Standard, the most comprehensive, provided preventive care, inpatient hospital services, medical services (e.g., lab tests), prescriptions, and behavioral health services. See Massachusetts Executive Office of Health and Human Services 2013 for more detailed information.

18. Before the ACA, Commonwealth Care also covered citizens with incomes higher than the MassHealth income cutoff who could not afford private insurance.

19. Blumenthal 2018; Campbell 2014; R. Cohen, Ward, and Schiller 2015; Patel and McDonough 2010. See the introduction for more on how US health coverage works.

20. Blue Cross Blue Shield of Massachusetts 2016; Blumenthal 2018; Gunja and Collins 2019; Sommers 2019.

21. Joseph 2016.

22. Dawes 2016; Joseph 2017a.

23. Joseph 2017a; Artiga and Damico 2016.

24. Low-income DACA recipients under age 18 are eligible for ACA coverage through the Children's Health Insurance Program.

25. Tourist visa holders are ineligible for all ACA provisions.

26. Danziger 2001; Golash-Boza 2015a; Park 2011.

27. National Academies of Sciences, Engineering, and Medicine 2015.

28. Golash-Boza 2015a; Johnson 2015; Park 2011.

29. Preston 2012. Initiated in 2008 under the Bush administration, the Secure Communities program allowed ICE to join forces with local law enforcement and facilitated the sharing of information about immigration violations.

30. Armenta 2017; Johnson 2015.

31. Preston 2011, 2012.

32. Preston 2012.

33. For more on the Boston Marathon bombings and their aftermath, see Bump 2013; Feyerick 2015; Welsh 2013.

34. Welsh 2013.

35. Abdullah 2013.

36. Associated Press 2012.

37. See the appendix for more on the "2009 CelticCare debacle" and its subsequent impact on some Massachusetts immigrants' healthcare access.

38. Faist et al. 2014; Joseph 2015; Levitt and Jaworsky 2007; Waldinger 2017.

39. There was a similar pattern among the Brazilian, Dominican, and Salvadoran immigrants interviewed in 2015–2016 and 2019. Among the three groups, Brazilians had higher premigration socioeconomic status and were more likely to have had health coverage at home than Dominicans and Salvadorans.

40. There were a total of 21 Brazilian and 10 Dominican respondents. Among the remaining 3 Brazilians, 2 self-classified as Yellow and 1 self-classified as "Other." Among the remaining 5 Dominicans, 1 self-classified as Black, 1 self-classified as White, 1 self-classified as "Other," and 2 did not report a classification.

41. See the Lexicon for more specific definitions of these racial categories.

42. See Candelario 2000; García-Peña 2022; Itzigsohn 2009; Lara 2017; and Roth 2012 for more on race, racism, anti-Blackness, and anti-Haitian sentiment in the Dominican Republic.

43. This was the case for 14 of 21 Brazilians.

44. This was the case for 6 of 10 Dominicans.

45. Ansell 2011; Burton 2013.

46. Bernstein and Dwoskin 2007.

47. Darlington and Londoño 2017; Watts 2017.

48. Gallas and Palumbo 2019; Lima 2020; Moura 2019; Rios 2018; Sands 2019.

49. Grasmuck and Pessar 1991; Hoffnung-Garskof 2008; Itzigsohn 2009.

50. World Bank Group 2020.

51. This was the case for 18 of 21 Brazilians and 9 of 10 Dominicans.

52. US Department of Health and Human Services 2010.

53. Fleary and Ettienne 2019.

54. Apolinario et al. 2013.

55. Lancee and Bol 2017; Toussaint-Comeau 2006.

56. Of the 20 Brazilians and 9 Dominicans who reported having health coverage in the US, 12 Brazilians and 8 Dominicans had public coverage, while 8 Brazilians and 1 Dominican had private coverage.

57. Acevedo-Garcia and Bates 2008; Ortega et al. 2020; Palloni and Arias 2004.

58. Acevedo-Garcia and Bates 2008; Ortega et al. 2020; Palloni and Arias 2004; Viladrich and Tagliaferro 2016.

59. Avendano and Kawachi 2014; Dickman, Himmelstein, and Woolhandler 2017; Hero et al. 2016; Tikkanen and Abrams 2020; Woolf and Aron 2013.

60. Colen et al. 2018; López 2019; Illingworth and Parmet 2017; Nichols, LeBrón, and Pedraza 2018; Van Natta 2023.

61. Van Natta 2023.

62. See the appendix for more on how I collected ethnoracial data in the study.

63. Two Brazilians classified themselves as Asian because they felt it was the US equivalent of Brazil's Yellow category and most closely aligned with their skin tone. Two Brazilians and two Dominicans classified themselves as "Other" rather than any of the listed categories. Compared with their premigration classifications, it appears that some Brazilians moved from the White to the Latino category, and three Brazilians who did not self-classify as Black in Brazil shifted to the Black category in the United States.

64. Among Brazilians, 16 of 21 reported their English proficiency as excellent or good, while 8 of 10 Dominicans rated their English proficiency as good or average.

65. Wilson 2014.

66. Chishti and Botler 2020.

67. This was the case for 19 of 21 Brazilians and 4 of 10 Dominicans.

68. Mercado et al. 2022; Miller et al. 2018; Sangalang et al. 2019.

69. Medical debt in the United States is a major concern that is also considered a social determinant of health. It is highest among people residing in the South and lower-income communities in states that did not expand Medicaid under the ACA. See Kluender et al. 2021; Mendes and Griggs 2021.

70. This direct link to apply for coverage no longer works. The link to apply for coverage at the printing of this book is www.mahealthconnector.org. When websites are restructured, people have trouble finding out where to apply. The application process moved online after ACA implementation in late 2013 and has been primarily online since then. Because computer systems rather than people are reviewing documents for verification, the rate of rejections, often for random reasons, can be very high. These errors can discourage applicants from appealing the decision if they do not know where to get assistance.

71. People who have only HSN do not receive a coverage card. HSN pays for hospital expenses at all acute care hospitals and covers all care delivered at Community Health Centers. People who receive only HSN coverage can get dental care at Community Health Centers that have dental services available. HSN also covers income-eligible children regardless of documentation status.

72. MassHealth Standard was accepted at healthcare facilities that accepted Medicaid. MassHealth Standard recipients could receive dental services if provided at a Community Health Center that offered them. The household income limit for children was 150% of the federal poverty level for MassHealth Standard eligibility under the Massachusetts reform.

73. Given the variation in services provided through different insurance plans, some plans might include dental or other services, and others might not.

74. Zallman et al. 2015.

75. Derose, Escarce, and Lurie 2007; Figuereo and Calvo 2018; Luque et al. 2018; Neufeld et al. 2002.

76. Joseph 2018; Lipsky 1984; Marrow 2012; Schmidt 2019.

77. Lipsky 1984, 3.

78. Bidgood 2012; Blue Cross Blue Shield of Massachusetts 2012.

79. Campbell 2014; Herd and Moynihan 2018; Lipsky 1984.

80. Blue Cross Blue Shield of Massachusetts 2016; Betancourt 2021; Parmet and Sainsbury-Wong 2012.

81. Osborn et al. 2016; Papanicolas, Woskie, and Jha 2018; Woolf and Aron 2013.

82. Davidson 2010; Hero et al. 2016.

83. US Department of Health and Human Services 2010.

84. Becerra, Arias, and Becerra 2016; Calvo 2016; Fernández-Gutiérrez et al. 2017; Fleary and Ettienne 2019; Rikard et al. 2016; Sørensen et al. 2012.

85. Psychiatric services are also difficult to find because most providers take only private coverage, if they accept insurance at all, which makes these services more expensive. See Mastroianni 2021; Peterson 2021.

86. Decker 2012; Hoff 2022; Knight 2019; Zhang et al. 2020.

87. Daly and Mellor 2018; Decker 2012; Hing, Decker, and Jamoom 2015.

88. Solberg et al. 2016.

89. Dental care is not typically included in health insurance coverage but must be purchased separately. Disparities in access to dental care are also shaped by race, ethnicity, documentation status, and socioeconomic status. See Northridge, Kumar, and Kaur 2020; Vujicic and Fosse 2022.

90. Barr 2014; Blackstock 2024; Colen et al. 2018; Matthew 2022; Smedley, Stith, and Nelson 2003.

91. Abramson, Hashemi, and Sánchez-Jankowski 2015; Bleich et al. 2019; Colen et al. 2018; D'Anna et al. 2018; Stepanikova and Oates 2017.

92. Sommers et al. 2016; Swartz 2006.

93. Blue Cross Blue Shield of Massachusetts 2013.

94. Alegría, Hasnain-Wynia, and Ayanian 2012; Asad and Clair 2018; Bustamante et al. 2019; Castañeda et al. 2015; Griffith et al. 2020; Jimenez 2019; Palmer et al. 2019; Park, Hoekstra, and Jiménez 2024; Sanchez et al. 2017; Van Natta et al. 2019; Williams and Cooper 2019.

95. Malat and Hamilton 2006; Smedley, Stith, and Nelson 2003; Stepanikova and Oates 2017; White 2011.

96. Blackstock 2024; Burgess et al. 2014; Hoffman et al. 2016.

97. Artiga et al. 2021; Bustamante et al. 2019.

98. Blackstock 2024; Shavers et al. 2012; Stepanikova and Oates 2017.

99. Hacker et al. 2011; Hacker et al. 2012; Joseph 2020b, 2020c; Nichols, LeBrón, and Pedraza 2018; Sanchez et al. 2017; Van Natta 2019.

100. Jacobs et al. 2006; Schinkel et al. 2018; Steinberg et al. 2016; Whatley and Batalova 2013; Zhao et al. 2019.

101. Schinkel et al. 2018; Terui 2017; Zhao et al. 2019.

102. Brandl, Schreiter, and Schouler-Ocak 2019; Granhagen Jungner et al. 2019; Jacobs et al. 2006.

103. To subsidize the high cost of medical interpretation at BHC, BHC interpreters provide phone interpretation services for healthcare facilities in other states when they are not needed by BHC patients.

104. Finch, Kolody, and Vega 2000; Pérez, Fortuna, and Alegría 2008.

105. Chavez-Dueñas, Adames, and Organista 2014; Cuevas, Dawson, and Williams 2016; Espino and Franz 2002; Murguia and Telles 1996; Santana 2018.

106. López 2019; Nichols, LeBrón, and Pedraza 2018; Vargas, Sanchez, and Juárez 2017.

107. Salsberg et al. 2021; Snyder, Frogner, and Skillman 2018.

108. Armenta 2017; Castañeda 2019; Golash-Boza 2015a; Nichols, LeBrón, and Pedraza 2018; Menjívar, Cervantes, and Alvord 2018; Sanchez et al. 2017.

109. Bogel-Burroughs 2019; Menjívar 2021; Romero et al. 2019a; Villalobos, Hernandez Rodriguez, and Funes 2020; Villazor and Johnson 2019; Wray-Lake et al. 2018.

110. Though the Biden administration has focused primarily on deporting criminals and immigrants who are threats to national security, immigration advocates have accused the administration of having a racist double standard. In 2021, Vice President Kamala Harris told Guatemalans not to come to the United States, while media accounts revealed Border Patrol agents on horseback whipping Haitian migrants at the US southern border. As record levels of migrants attempted to cross the southern border after the COVID public health emergency ended in 2022, (White) Ukrainian refugees escaping war with Russia were allowed to legally cross the border, while Black and Brown migrants were turned away. In October 2023, the Biden administration announced it would resume deporting Venezuelan migrants, who constituted a large percentage of migrants crossing the southern border. In June 2024, the Biden administration issued executive orders that seemed contradictory. The first closed the southern border amid an influx of migrants arriving to seek asylum. The second allowed the undocumented spouses of US citizens to apply for permanent residence without leaving the country. See Aleaziz 2024; Chishti, Bush-Joseph, and Putzel-Kavanaugh 2024; Kanno-Youngs and Aleaziz 2024; Naylor and Keith 2021; Rose 2021; Shoichet 2022.

111. See the appendix for more on Secure Communities in Boston.

112. Beniflah et al. 2013; Gibbs and Hernandez 2014; Hacker et al. 2012; Novak, Geronimus, and Martinez-Cardoso 2017; Rhodes et al. 2015; White et al. 2014.

113. Alexander 2010; Armenta 2017; Golash-Boza 2015a; Joseph 2020c.

114. Chavez 2013; Feagin and Cobas 2014; Flores-Gonzalez 2017; García 2017; Nichols, LeBrón, and Pedraza 2018.

115. Armenta 2017; Golash-Boza 2015a; Nichols, LeBrón, and Pedraza 2018; Sewell et al. 2020.

116. HIPAA refers to the Health Insurance Portability and Accountability Act of 1996, which standardized the protection of patients' sensitive health information so it could not be disclosed without patients' consent or knowledge. See Centers for Disease Control and Prevention 2024.

117. Asad 2020.
118. Menjívar and Abrego 2012.
119. Menjívar and Abrego 2012.
120. Van Natta 2023.

Chapter 3 • The ACA Narrows, Rather than Widens, Healthcare Access (2015–2016)

1. McGowan 2015; Metzger 2018; Norton and Murphy 2020.

2. See the appendix for tables with more demographic information on this set of respondents. Unless otherwise indicated, the quotations in this chapter come from interviews I conducted in 2015–2016 when Democrat Marty Walsh was the mayor of Boston, Republican Charlie Baker was the governor of Massachusetts, and Democrat Barack Obama was president of the United States.

3. See the appendix for more details on ACA reform.

4. Bern, Chrobak, and Dehner 2015; Joseph 2016; Patel and McDonough 2010.

5. Dawes 2016; Joseph 2016.

6. Kaiser Family Foundation 2014. As of 2022, the pattern of states that did and did not expand Medicaid fell along polarized blue–red state lines. In most states, many immigrants remained excluded from any state or federally subsidized coverage. As of October 2021, only nine states had implemented or authorized programs similar to Medicaid or Children's Health Insurance Program (CHIP) for income-eligible residents of any documentation status: Massachusetts, New York, Washington, Maine, Vermont, Connecticut, Illinois, Oregon, and California. Of these, only Massachusetts, New York, and Washington had already implemented such programs using state-level funds. See Kaiser Family Foundation 2022; Manatt Health 2021.

7. Blue Cross Blue Shield of Massachusetts 2016, 2019; Marrow and Joseph 2015.

8. Joseph 2016. Immigrants with the Permanent Residence Under Color of Law (PRUCOL) classification, who were considered "lawfully present" and thus eligible for state-sponsored coverage and subsidies under the Massachusetts reform, were considered "unlawfully present" for federal coverage under Obamacare. Zoe, a health advocate well versed in immigration and health policy, explained that "unfortunately, they were not able to get subsidies through the Affordable Care Act, but we were able to do a state-funded-only program for them under our Medicaid program."

9. See Joseph 2016 for more specifics on these changes.

10. Though I have listed MassHealth Standard in the figure, there are a range of nonstandard MassHealth programs, whose coverage and services differ based on income level and documentation status. Coverage, services, and eligibility criteria also differ for children, pregnant women of any legal status, and disabled individuals. See MassHealth 2022 for more on the other types of MassHealth and age, legal status, and income eligibility for those programs.

11. See Figure 2-1 for public options under the Massachusetts reform. After implementation of the ACA, the income limits were higher for certain populations,

such as pregnant/postpartum people at 200% of the federal poverty level (FPL) or those with breast and cervical cancer at 250% FPL. Eligibility for Health Safety Net changed in 2016: it was reduced from less than 400% FPL to less than 300% FPL.

12. Under ConnectorCare, people with incomes up to 400% FPL could get tax credits without state subsidies. That coverage, however, was regulated differently from Commonwealth Care plans, which accepted those with up to 300% FPL. This coverage was not considered part of the ConnectorCare program. "Lawfully present immigrants" such as short-term green card holders and those with the PRUCOL classification were eligible for ConnectorCare with incomes between 0 and 133% FPL. See Introduction, note 93, for an explanation of the PRUCOL classification.

13. The theme of various documentation statuses generating confusion when applying for coverage was so salient in interviews that I conceptualized "the documentation status continuum" framework to illustrate the range of statuses that exists between undocumented and citizenship and how eligibility for public benefits and level of deportability shifts as one moves along that continuum. See Joseph 2020a.

14. Both the federal and state websites were designed by the CGI Group. When the ACA website was released on October 1, 2013, it crashed as millions of Americans logged on. Much of the blame was laid on the selection of the CGI Group and political fights over adequate funding for this infrastructure. In Massachusetts, many serious errors resulted from state administrators' attempts to link Massachusetts's information technology (IT) system for the state exchange with the ACA's IT system. See Kliff 2014; McDonough 2016; Ornstein 2014; Pear, LaFraniere, and Austen 2013.

15. Graetz et al. 2016; Gray, Joseph, and Olayiwola 2020; Laz and Berenson 2013.

16. McDonough 2016.

17. For corresponding data on immigrants interviewed in 2012–2013, see Chapter 2.

18. Respondents with at least a college degree included 9 of 15 Brazilians, 7 of 14 Dominicans, and 2 of 10 Salvadorans.

19. Fewer among the immigrants interviewed in 2015–2016 reported excellent or good English proficiency than among those interviewed in 2012–2013.

20. Forman, Basma, and Gourley 2020; King and Stucka 2021.

21. Those with coverage (32 of 39) included 13 of 15 Brazilians, 12 of 14 Dominicans, and 7 of 10 Salvadorans. The proportions of both Brazilians and Dominicans with public and private coverage were nearly equal. Those with a regular provider (26 of 39) included 11 Brazilians, 12 Dominicans, and 3 Salvadorans (4 other Salvadorans did not report this information). Before migrating to the United States, a large majority of immigrants, regardless of nationality, rated their health as excellent or good. About half of Brazilians and Dominicans reported having health coverage before migrating. For those who did, their coverage was private—like the Brazilians and different from the Dominican respondents in 2012–2013. Among the 10 Salvadorans, only 2 had coverage before migration, and

in both cases it was public. These health-related data align with the education data and provide some insight into these interviewees' premigration socioeconomic status, which was correlated with their health and access to health coverage. See Chapter 2 for corresponding data on immigrants interviewed in 2012–2013.

22. Barnett and Berchick 2017.

23. Collins et al. 2016. Due to the categories used in this research, it is unclear whether Brazilians were included in this statistic.

24. Silvana is the only immigrant I interviewed who came to the United States after winning the "green card lottery," the formal name for which is the Diversity Immigrant Visa (DVs) Program. Each year, up to 50,000 DVs are issued to citizens of countries with low rates of immigration.

25. Center for Health Information and Analysis 2018; McCluskey 2019; Metzger 2019.

26. Book and Howard 2017; Manchikanti et al. 2017.

27. Dolan 2016.

28. See Lind 2014.

29. National Immigration Forum 2021.

30. Menjívar 2006, 2017.

31. Menjívar 2006.

32. Of the remaining Brazilians, one each self-classified as White, Asian, and "Other," and one did not report a category. The Brazilian who classified himself as Asian was not of Asian descent but chose this term because he felt his skin tone was closer to Yellow than to White. Of the remaining Dominicans, one classified as "Other" and one did not report. See Chapter 2 for corresponding data on immigrants interviewed in 2012–2013.

33. Some Brazilians who live near national borders with neighboring Latin American countries speak Spanish or a mix of Portuguese and Spanish known as *Portunhol*. I did not ask Brazilian respondents whether they spoke Spanish.

34. Mora 2014; Oboler 1992, 1995; Rodríguez-Muñiz 2021.

35. For more on the racial classification and conceptions of Brazilian immigrants in the United States, see Joseph 2015; McDonnell and Lourenço 2009; Zubaran 2008.

36. I also collected this data for immigrants in 2012–2013 and 2019. I chose to highlight it for the 2015–2016 immigrants because this group included Brazilians, Dominicans, and Salvadorans, unlike in 2012–2013, and enough immigrants to make the data worth discussing in relation to these immigrants' US ethnoracial self-classifications, unlike in 2019.

37. One Brazilian immigrant chose "Other, Brazilian" when required to pick among a set of ethnoracial categories but described herself as European in response to the open-ended question. She thought that others in the United States classify her as Latina but was classified as White in Brazil. I thought that she would be perceived as White in both the United States and Brazil due to her very fair skin; brownish-red, straight, shoulder-length hair; and dark eyes.

38. Doer 2017; Jones 2020.

39. Horowitz, Igielnik, and Kochhar 2020.

40. Clauss 2016; Holmes and Berube 2016.

41. Fujiwara and Prignano 2022.

42. Hermann, Luberoff, and McCue 2019; McGloin 2018.

43. Bryant et al. 2017; Hermann, Luberoff, and McCue 2019; McGloin 2018.

44. Muñoz et al. 2015.

45. Ebbert 2021; Reilly 2021.

46. Bowden 2020; Parker and Eder 2016; Struyk 2016.

47. Milligan 2016.

48. Bobo 2017; Joseph 2020c; Lamont, Park, and Ayala-Hurtado 2017.

49. I first asked immigrant respondents whether or not they thought they had experienced discrimination at any time in the United States. Then I asked what they perceived as the cause of the discrimination. Although this was an open-ended question, I tabulated the results from all immigrant respondents to derive the data presented in this paragraph.

50. Andrea, a Dominican quoted in Chapter 1, also experienced what could be described as racialized legal status discrimination. I refer to her here to indicate that women and men shared an awareness of how this intersection affected their lives.

51. Haywood 2017; Sanchez, Masuoka, and Abrams 2019; Sanchez and Espinosa 2016; Uzogara 2019.

52. Jiménez 2010; Ochoa 2000; Sanchez and Espinosa 2016.

53. Asad 2020.

54. Bloemraad et al. 2019; Castañeda 2019; Flores-Gonzalez 2017; Joseph and Golash-Boza 2021; Selod 2018; Valle 2018.

55. Flores-Gonzalez 2017; Valle 2018.

56. For more on these raids, which primarily affected women and children, see Edwards 2016.

57. Bauder 2017; Houston 2019; Houston et al. 2022; Lasch et al. 2018; Roy 2019; Wong et al 2019.

58. Those reporting good or excellent physical health included 12 of 15 Brazilians, 8 of 14 Dominicans, and 8 of 10 Salvadorans. Three Brazilians reported their physical health as average. Those reporting good or excellent mental health included 15 Brazilians, 11 Dominicans, and 9 Salvadorans. Those diagnosed with the conditions listed were distributed across the three nationalities.

59. Becerra et al. 2020; Ortega et al. 2018; Park, Hoekstra, and Jiménez 2024.

60. Van Natta 2023.

61. Asad 2023.

62. Asad 2020; Makhlouf 2021; Patler and Gonzalez 2020.

63. Kline 2019; Nichols, LeBrón, and Pedraza 2018; Novak, Geronimus, and Martinez-Cardoso 2017; Vargas, Sanchez, and Juárez 2017.

64. Geronimus et al. 2006; Nichols, LeBrón, and Pedraza 2018; Novak, Geronimus, and Martinez-Cardoso 2017; Vargas, Sanchez, and Juárez 2017; Williams et al. 2010.

65. Armenta and Sarabia 2020; Castañeda 2019; Cervantes and Menjívar 2020; Nichols, LeBrón, and Pedraza 2018; Van Natta 2019; Vargas, Sanchez, and Juárez 2017.

66. DeCosta-Klipa 2020; Mehta 2020; Porter 2020.

67. Bedford 2017; Mohl 2020; Schoenberg 2017.

68. Mass Legal Services 2016.

69. Mass Legal Services 2016.

70. Massachusetts Executive Office of Health and Human Services 2016.

71. Asad 2020; Makhlouf 2021; Patler and Gonzalez 2020.

Chapter 4 • *Deterring Immigrants from Using Services Under Trump (2019)*

1. See Chapter 2, "Premigration Racial Identification, Health, and Health Care," for the demographic information on immigrants interviewed in 2012–2013, and Chapter 3, "Introduction," for the demographic information on immigrants interviewed in 2015–2016.

2. Three Brazilians rated their physical health as excellent, one as good, and four as average. One Salvadoran rated their physical and mental health as excellent, and the other rated theirs as good. One Dominican rated their physical and mental health as good, and the other rated both as average. In terms of mental health, four Brazilians rated theirs as excellent, two as good, and two as average.

3. Only one respondent, a Brazilian, reported not having health coverage. Brazilians were nearly evenly split in terms of public ($n = 3$) and private ($n = 4$) coverage. The two Salvadoran respondents had public coverage, and the two Dominican respondents had private coverage. Five Brazilians reported having a regular provider, while three Brazilians did not. The two Dominicans had a regular provider. One Salvadoran reported having a regular provider, while the other did not.

4. As for English language proficiency, one Brazilian, one Salvadoran, and two Dominicans reported excellent proficiency, and one Brazilian reported good proficiency. Three Brazilians reported average proficiency, and one Salvadoran did not speak English. For education, seven Brazilians, one Dominican, and two Salvadorans had attended or completed college. One Dominican completed a postgraduate education, and one Brazilian completed high school.

5. See the appendix for more on the reinterview sample.

6. Kenney, Haley, and Wang 2018; Orris, Grady, and Mann 2018; Shear and Jordan 2021; Torres-Ardila et al. 2018.

7. After the Department of Justice announced the proposed rule change on October 10, 2018, 226,000 public comments were received during the next 60 days. The rule change was initially set to be implemented on October 15, 2019, but federal court injunctions delayed it until February 24, 2020. See Department of Homeland Security 2018, 2019; Immigrant Legal Resource Center 2021; Miller 2019; and Pillai and Artiga 2022.

8. Immigrants' actual or suspected future use of the following public benefits would cause them to be considered a "public charge" under the Trump administra-

tion's proposed rule: cash assistance programs such as Temporary Assistance for Needy Families (TANF) or Supplementary Security Income (SSI); the Supplemental Nutritional Assistance Program (SNAP); and Section 8 housing, if received for 12 consecutive months or if the value of the benefit exceeded more than 15% of federal policy guidelines. Immigrants also would be considered a "public charge" under the rule change if they used any of the following benefits for at least 12 months during a 36-month period: nonemergency Medicaid, any benefit for long-term institutional care, subsidies under Medicare Part D, and subsidized housing. See Sekhavat 2019.

9. Artiga, Garfield, and Damico 2019; Kenney, Haley, and Wang 2018; Orris, Grady, and Mann 2018; Shaw and Barraza 2020; Torres-Ardila et al. 2018; Valencia 2020.

10. Cathey 2021; Spocchia 2021.

11. Blue Cross Blue Shield of Massachusetts 2019. As of 2021, the state's uninsured rate was 2.4%. See Center for Health Information and Analysis 2021.

12. Anthony et al. 2021; Blue Cross Blue Shield of Massachusetts 2019.

13. Blue Cross Blue Shield of Massachusetts 2019; Massachusetts Medical Society 2017.

14. Blue Cross Blue Shield of Massachusetts 2019.

15. Anthony et al. 2021.

16. "Un-DACA-mented" is a term sometimes used to refer to undocumented immigrants who have DACA status.

17. Lloyd and Heflin 2016; Seifert and Love 2018; WBUR Newsroom 2018.

18. Originally established as a Medicare payment model in 2012, state Medicaid plans and commercial health insurance companies have adopted ACOs in the last decade. Since that time, the number of ACOs has increased to more than 700; ACOs currently exist in all 50 states and provide care to more than 23 million individuals. See Tu et al. 2015; Lloyd and Heflin 2016.

19. Joseph and Marrow 2017; Obama 2016.

20. Joseph and Marrow 2017.

21. Eibner and Nowak 2018.

22. Jost 2018.

23. Simmons-Duffin 2019; Tolbert et al. 2019.

24. Ennen, de León, and Maney 2023.

25. Kuge 2020.

26. Bauder 2017; Houston et al. 2022; Lasch et al. 2018; Villazor 2010.

27. Abraham 2019; Anderson and Murphy 2020; Valencia 2019.

28. Valencia 2019.

29. Gulasekaram et al. 2019; Miroff and Barrett 2020; Paik 2017; Pierce and Selee 2017.

30. Blackburn and Sierra 2021; Parmet 2018; Pham and Van 2019; Rhodan and Dias 2017.

31. Massachusetts Supreme Judicial Court 2017.

32. Fox 2020; Gartsbeyn 2020. Maura Healey was elected governor of Massachusetts in 2022.

33. De Graauw 2021; García 2019; Marrow and Joseph 2015; Marrow 2012.

34. García 2019.

35. Marrow and Joseph 2015; De Graauw 2021; Tully and Gold 2019.

36. Callagan et al. 2019; Edwards and Rushin 2018; Edyburn and Meek 2021; Johnson 2019; Morgante 2021; Rodriguez et al. 2019.

37. Anderson and Murphy 2020; Ellement 2020.

38. Anderson and Murphy 2020.

39. Alanez 2022.

40. See Valle 2018 for more on Puerto Ricans' stratified citizenship.

41. Arevalo 2018; Mata-Greve and Torres 2019; Politi et al. 2021.

42. Du Bois 1903; Joseph and Golash-Boza 2021.

43. In December 2020, Attorney General Maura Healey filed suit to force Homeland Security to terminate its contracts with Bristol County. See Dooling 2020a; Fortier 2021; Montoya-Galvez 2020.

44. Ahmed 2019; Eisen 2018; Jefferis 2019; Tartaglia 2014.

45. Dooling 2020b; Gavin 2020; McKanders 2020.

46. Brown, et al. 2000; Colen et al. 2018; Geronimus 2023; Krieger et al. 2011.

47. Nichols, LeBrón, and Pedraza 2018; Novak, Geronimus, and Martinez-Cardoso 2017; Williams and Cooper 2019.

48. Nichols, LeBrón, and Pedraza 2018; Novak, Geronimus, and Martinez-Cardoso 2017; Williams and Cooper 2019.

49. Some providers may view appointment delays or cancellations as patient noncompliance. Beyond racialized legal status, inability to comply with physicians or being perceived as noncompliant by physicians could also have negative physical and mental health consequences for patients. See Chan et al. 2020; Gerber et al. 2010; and Nguyen et al. 2009.

Conclusion

1. Kruzel 2021; Montoya-Galvez 2021.

2. Decker, Varsanyi, and Lewis 2016; Marrow and Joseph 2015; Pierson 2018; Sparer, France, and Clinton 2011; Thompson 2015; Varsanyi 2010.

3. Bustamante et al. 2019; Dietz et al. 2019; Kluender et al. 2021; Ortega, Rodriguez, and Bustamante 2015.

4. Gorman 2021; Gutierrez 2021.

5. Bruce 2021.

6. García 2019; Jirmanus et al. 2022; Tuohy 2020; Van Natta 2019.

7. See Chapters 2, 3, and 4 for more on these changes over time.

8. Grunder 2021; García 2020; Page et al. 2020; Suro and Findling 2020; Tracy 2021.

9. In addition, after a 20-year struggle, in August 2023 Massachusetts legislators passed a state budget that finally extended eligibility for in-state tuition and state-funded financial aid to undocumented students.

10. Asad 2023; Jiménez 2021; López 2019; Nuila 2022; Park, Hoekstra, and Jiménez 2024; Sangaramoorthy 2023; Van Natta 2023.

11. Gee et al. 2019; Lowrey 2021; Ray, Herd, and Moynihan 2023; Teles 2013.

12. Teles 2013.

13. Hoekstra and Jiménez 2022; Park, Hoekstra, and Jiménez 2024; Van Natta 2023.

14. Gee et al. 2019; Ray, Herd, and Moynihan 2023; Link and Phelan 1995.

15. Brinkerhoff et al. 2019; Colen et al. 2018; Cuevas, Dawson, and Williams 2016; Halim, Moy, and Yoshikawa 2017; Hamilton 2019; Williams and Mohammed 2009.

16. Armenta 2017; Chavez 2013; Flores-Gonzalez 2017; Flores and Schachter 2018; Menjívar 2021.

17. Panikkar et al. 2012.

18. Armenta 2017; Asad 2023; Jimenez 2021; López 2019; Nuila 2022; Sangaramoorthy 2023; Van Natta 2023.

19. Fortuna, Porche, and Alegria 2008; Sangalang et al. 2019; Vesely, Bravo, and Guzzardo 2019.

20. Castañeda 2019; López 2019; Nichols, LeBrón, and Pedraza 2018; Novak, Geronimus, and Martinez-Cardoso 2017; Vargas, Sanchez, and Juárez 2017.

21. According to some BHC physicians, immigrants sometimes showed up in emergency rooms with complications from surgery or side effects from prescription medications obtained abroad.

22. Armenta 2017; Alba and Foner 2015; Bloemraad et al. 2019; Joseph 2020c; Joseph and Golash-Boza 2021; Virdee and McGeever 2018; Selod 2018; Yazdiha 2018.

23. Sun 2021.

24. Chen and Krieger 2021; Mehra, Boyd, and Ickovics 2017; Williams and Collins 2001; Wu et al. 2019.

25. Maciosek et al. 2010; Musich et al. 2016; Salkeld 1998.

26. Butkus et al. 2020; Lazar and Davenport 2018; Shamsi et al. 2020; Wolfe, McDonald, and Holmes 2020.

27. Artiga, Stephens, and Damico 2015; Artiga and Damico 2016; Artiga et al. 2021.

28. Kearney et al. 2021.

29. Commonwealth Fund 2021.

30. Centers for Medicaid and Medicare Services 2020.

31. Maani and Galea 2020; Himmelstein and Woolhandler 2016; Trust for America's Health 2021.

32. Himmelstein and Woolhandler 2016.

33. Maani and Galea 2020.

34. Campbell 2018; Gee et al. 2017; Zallman et al. 2015.

35. Flavin et al. 2018; Sarría-Santamera et al. 2016; Wilson et al. 2020; Zallman et al. 2013, 2015.

36. Kolstad and Kowalski 2012; Marcozzi et al. 2018; Miller 2012; Sommers et al. 2017.

37. Bruce 2021; Gorman 2021; Gutierrez 2021.

38. Health Care for All n.d.

39. Armenta and Alvarez 2017; Becerra et al. 2017; Casellas and Wallace 2020; Nguyen and Gill 2016; Wong et al. 2021.

40. Immigrant Legal Resource Center 2023.

Appendix

1. Joseph 2015.

2. Boston University School of Public Health (n.d.); Vandenbroucke et al. 2007.

3. When conducting research with Brazilians in Governador Valadares for my last book, participants initially thought I was asking them if they were racist when I asked how they racially classified themselves using the term *raça*.

4. Joseph 2015; Montalvo 2005; Pedraza 2000; Rodriguez 2000; Roth 2012.

5. Emerson, Fretz, and Shaw 1995.

6. Creswell 2007; Emerson, Fretz, and Shaw 1995; Glaser and Strauss 1967; Harding 2013; Strauss and Corbin 1998.

7. Strauss and Corbin 1998.

8. In Latin American immigrant families, as in the United States and other societies, women are more likely to be engaged in and seeking health care for their families.

9. Bidgood 2012; Goodnough 2009; Parmet and Sainsbury-Wong 2012.

10. Bidgood 2012; Goodnough 2009; Parmet and Sainsbury-Wong 2012.

11. Johnson 2015.

12. Johnson 2015.

13. Johnson 2015.

14. Johnson 2015.

15. Johnson 2015; Selod 2018.

16. Garza 2018.

17. Johnson 2015.

18. Boston.com 2010; Sacchetti and Lang 2010.

19. Through an executive order, the Obama administration also created DAPA, Deferred Action for Parental Accountability, to deprioritize certain undocumented immigrants for removal, but this program was held up in federal courts and never implemented.

20. Gonzales 2015; Wong et al. 2013.

21. While there is no official designation, and the term covers a wide range of measures that vary depending on where they are proposed or adopted, sanctuary cities typically use local policy to limit cooperation with federal immigration enforcement. See Bauder 2017; Rose and Rotolo 2014; Roy 2019.

22. Walsh 2019.

23. Ennen, de León, and Maney 2023.

24. Kanno-Youngs and Dickerson 2019; Dickerson, Del Real, and Bosman 2019.

25. Cramer and Kuznitz 2019.

26. Dooling 2019b.
27. Dooling 2019a.
28. Holpuch 2019; Kanno-Youngs 2019; Romero et al. 2019b.
29. Arango, Bogel-Burroughs, and Benner 2019; Bogel-Burroughs 2019; Romero et al. 2019a.
30. Bernal 2019; Tamborrino 2019.
31. Dooling 2019c; Jordan and Dickerson 2019.
32. Anderson 2019; Dooling 2019d.
33. Montoya-Galvez 2019.

BIBLIOGRAPHY

Abdullah, Halimah. "Boston Marathon Bombings Cast Shadow on Immigration Debate." *CNN.com*, April 22, 2013. https://www.cnn.com/2013/04/22/politics /immigration-boston/index.html.

Abraham, Yvonne. "Is Boston Truly Looking Out for Immigrants? Not in This Case." *Boston Globe*, March 6, 2019. https://www.bostonglobe.com/metro/2019 /03/06/boston-truly-looking-out-for-immigrants-not-this-case/YgAvgeue6fYZx C7h3wJJ9J/story.html.

Abramson, Corey, Manata Hashemi, and Martín Sánchez-Jankowski. "Perceived Discrimination in U.S. Healthcare: Charting the Effects of Key Social Characteristics Within and Across Racial Groups." *Preventive Medicine Reports* 2 (2015): 615–21. https://www.sciencedirect.com/science/article/pii/S2211335515 000972.

Abrego, Leisy, and Sarah Lakhani. "Incomplete Inclusion: Legal Violence and Immigrants in Liminal Legal Statuses." *Law & Policy* 37, no. 4 (2015): 265–93.

Abrego, Leisy, and Alejandro Villalpando. "Racialization of Central Americans in the United States." In *Precarity and Belonging: Labor, Migration, and Noncitizenship*, edited by Catherine Ramírez, Sylvanna Falcón, Juan Poblete, Steven McKay, and Felicity Schaeffer, 51–66. New Brunswick, NJ: Rutgers University Press, 2021.

Acevedo-Garcia, Dolores, and Lisa Bates. "Latino Health Paradoxes: Empirical Evidence, Explanations, Future Research, and Implications." In *Latinas/os in the United States: Changing the Face of América*, edited by Havidán. Rodríguez, Rogelio Sáenz and Cecilia Menjívar, 101–13. New York: Springer, 2008.

Ahmed, Hauwa. *How Private Prisons Are Profiting Under the Trump Administration*. Center for American Progress, August 30, 2019. https://www.americanprogress .org/article/private-prisons-profiting-trump-administration/.

Alanez, Tonya. "Woman in East Boston Assault That Was Called a Hate Crime Gets Probation, Drawing Criticism." *Boston Globe*, February 23, 2022. https://www .bostonglobe.com/2022/02/23/metro/racially-motivated-east-boston-crime

-garners-probation-sentence-civil-rights-group-laments-leniency/?event
=event12.

Alba, Richard, and Nancy Foner. *Strangers No More: Immigration and the Challenges of Integration in North America and Western Europe*. Princeton, NJ: Princeton University Press, 2015.

Alba, Richard, and Victor Nee. *Remaking the American Mainstream: Assimilation and Contemporary Immigration*. Cambridge, MA: Harvard University Press, 2003.

Aleaziz, Hamed. "How Biden's New Immigration Policy Works." *New York Times*, June 18, 2024. https://www.nytimes.com/2024/06/18/us/politics/biden -immigration-policy.html.

Alegría, Margarita, Romana Hasnain-Wynia, and John Z. Ayanian. "Taking the Measure of Health Care Disparities." *Health Services Research* 47, no. 3 (2012): 1225–31.

Alexander, Jennifer, and Camilla Stivers. "Racial Bias: A Buried Cornerstone of the Administrative State." *Administration and Society* 52, no. 10 (2020): 1470–90.

Alexander, Michelle. *The New Jim Crow: Mass Incarceration in the Age of Colorblindness*. New York: New Press, 2010.

Altaf, Saadi, Sophia Taleghani, Kathryn Hampton, and Michele Heisler. "Clinicians' Perspectives on the Impacts of Post-2016 Immigration Enforcement on Immigrant Health and Health Care Use." *Journal of Health Care for the Poor and Underserved* 32, no. 4 (2021): 1778–97. https://doi.org/10.1353/hpu.2021.0166.

Alulema, Daniela. *DACA and the Supreme Court: How We Got to This Point, a Statistical Profile of Who Is Affected, and What the Future May Hold for DACA Beneficiaries*. Center for Migration Studies, 2019. https://cmsny.org /publications/daca-and-the-supreme-court/.

Amaya, Hector. *Citizenship Excess: Latino/as, Media, and the Nation*. New York: New York University Press, 2013.

American Immigration Council. *Immigrants in Massachusetts*. August 6, 2020. https://www.americanimmigrationcouncil.org/research/immigrants-in -massachusetts.

American Public Health Association. "ACA Frequently Asked Questions." n.d., accessed December 12, 2023. https://www.apha.org/topics-and-issues/health -reform/aca-frequently-asked-questions.

Anderson, Carol. *White Rage: The Unspoken Truth of Our Racial Divide*. New York: Bloomsbury, 2016.

Anderson, Travis. "Mass. Groups Sue to Stop Policy Change That Would Deport Families of Seriously Ill Children." *Boston Globe*, September 5, 2019. https:// www.bostonglobe.com/metro/2019/09/05/mass-civil-rights-groups-file -lawsuit-stop-policy-change-that-would-deport-families-seriously-ill-children /AO26lYq3wjEF8d3xlLrnnO/story.html.

Anderson, Travis, and Shelley Murphy. "'We Were Attacked Based on Our Race, Our Language, and Our Identity,' Victim of East Boston Attack Says." *Boston Globe*, February 24, 2020. https://www.bostonglobe.com/2020/02/24/metro

/woman-15-year-old-daughter-brutally-attacked-speaking-spanish-east-boston
-group-says/.

Ansell, Aaron. "Brazil's Social Safety Net Under Lula." *NACLA Report on the
Americas*, May 12, 2011. https://nacla.org/article/brazil%E2%80%99s-social
-safety-net-under-lula.

Anthony, Stephanie, Patricia Boozang, Linda Elam, Kevin McAvey, Adam Striar,
and Mannat Health. *Racism and Racial Inequities in Health: A Data-Informed
Primer on Health Disparities in Massachusetts.* Blue Cross Blue Shield of Massachusetts Foundation, December 2021. https://www.bluecrossmafoundation
.org/sites/g/files/csphws2101/files/2021-12/Health_Equity_Primer_Dec%20
2021_final_0.pdf.

Apolinario, Daniel, Leticia Lessa Mansur, Maria Teresa Carthery-Goulart, Sonia
Maria Dozzi Brucki, and Ricardo Nitrini. "Detecting Limited Health Literacy in
Brazil: Development of a Multidimensional Screening Tool." *Health Promotion
International* 29, no. 1 (2013): 5–14. https://doi.org/10.1093/heapro/dat074.

Aptekar, Sofya. "Constructing the Boundaries of U.S. Citizenship." In *The Era of
Enforcement and Securitization*, edited by Nicole Stokes-Dupass and Ramona
Fruja, 1–31. New York: Palgrave-Macmillan, 2016.

Aranda, Elizabeth, Elizabeth Vaquera, and Heide Castañeda. "Shifting Roles in
Families of Deferred Action for Childhood Arrivals (DACA) Recipients and
Implications for the Transition to Adulthood." *Journal of Family Issues* 42,
no. 9 (2020), 2111–32. https://journals.sagepub.com/doi/full/10.1177
/0192513X20967977.

Arango, Tim, Nicholas Bogel-Burroughs, and Katie Benner. "Minutes Before El Paso
Killing, Hate-Filled Manifesto Appears Online." *New York Times*, August 3, 2019.

Arevalo, Christian. "Ethnic Identity, Self-Esteem and Intra Group Conflicts
Amongst Latinos." *McNair Research Journal SJSU* 14, (2018): Article 4. https://
doi.org/10.31979/mrj.2018.1404.

Armenta, Amada. "Racializing Crimmigration: Structural Racism, Colorblindness,
and the Institutional Production of Immigrant Criminality." *Sociology of Race and
Ethnicity* 3, no. 1 (2017): 82–95. https://journals.sagepub.com/doi/10.1177
/2332649216648714.

Armenta, Amada, and Isabela Alvarez. "Policing Immigrants or Policing Immigration?
Understanding Local Law Enforcement Participation in Immigration Control."
Sociology Compass 11, no. 2 (2017): 1–10. https://doi.org/10.1111/soc4.12453.

Armenta, Amada, and Heidy Sarabia. "Receptionists, Doctors, and Social Workers:
Examining Undocumented Immigrant Women's Perceptions of Health Services."
Social Science & Medicine 246 (2020): 1–7. https://doi.org/10.1016/j.socscimed
.2020.112788.

Artiga, Samantha, and Anthony Damico. *Health and Health Coverage in the South: A
Data Update.* Kaiser Family Foundation, February 10, 2016. https://www.kff.org
/racial-equity-and-health-policy/issue-brief/health-and-health-coverage-in-the
-south-a-data-update/.

Artiga, Samantha, Rachel Garfield, and Anthony Damico. *Estimated Impacts of Final Public Charge Inadmissibility Rule on Immigrants and Medicaid Coverage*. Kaiser Family Foundation, September 18, 2019. https://www.kff.org/racial-equity -and-health-policy/issue-brief/estimated-impacts-of-final-public-charge -inadmissibility-rule-on-immigrants-and-medicaid-coverage/.

Artiga, Samantha, Jessica Stephens, and Anthony Damico. *The Impact of the Coverage Gap in States Not Expanding Medicaid by Race and Ethnicity*. Kaiser Family Foundation, October 26, 2015. http://kff.org/disparities-policy/issue-brief/the-impact-of -the-coverage-gap-in-states-not-expanding-medicaid-by-race-and-ethnicity/.

Asad, Asad. "On the Radar: System Embeddedness and Latin American Immigrants' Perceived Risk of Deportation." *Law & Society Review* 54 (2020): 133–67. https://onlinelibrary.wiley.com/doi/10.1111/lasr.12460.

Asad, Asad. *Engage and Evade: How Latino Immigrant Families Manage Surveillance in Everyday Life*. Princeton, NJ: Princeton University Press, 2023.

Asad, Asad, and Matthew Clair. "Racialized Legal Status as a Social Determinant of Health." *Social Science and Medicine* 199 (2018): 19–28. https://www .sciencedirect.com/science/article/abs/pii/S0277953617301508.

Associated Press. "Romney Had Mixed Record on Immigration in Mass." *Telegram*, July 23, 2012. https://www.telegram.com/story/news/state/2012/07/23 /romney-had-mixed-record-on/49554231007/.

Avendano, Mauricio, and Ichiro Kawachi. "Why Do Americans Have Shorter Life Expectancy and Worse Health Than Do People in Other High-Income Countries?" *Annual Review of Public Health* 35, no. 1 (2014): 307–25. https://www .annualreviews.org/doi/abs/10.1146/annurev-publhealth-032013-182411.

Bailey, Zinzi, Nancy Krieger, Madina Agénor, Jasmine Graves, Natalia Linos, and Mary Bassett. "Structural Racism and Health Inequities in the USA: Evidence and Interventions." *The Lancet* 389, no. 10077 (2017): 1453–63. https://doi.org /10.1016/S0140-6736(17)30569-X.

Baker, Robert. "The American Medical Association and Race." *AMA Journal of Ethics* 16, no. 6 (2014): 479–88. https://journalofethics.ama-assn.org/article /american-medical-association-and-race/2014-06.

Barnett, Jessica, and Edward Berchick. *Health Insurance Coverage in the United States: 2016*. United States Census Bureau, September 12, 2017. https://www .census.gov/library/publications/2017/demo/p60-260.html.

Barr, Donald. *Health Disparities in the United States: Social Class, Race, Ethnicity, and Health*. Baltimore: Johns Hopkins University Press, 2014.

Bauder, Harald. "Sanctuary Cities: Policies and Practices in International Perspective." *International Migration* 55, no. 2 (2017): 174–87. https://onlinelibrary .wiley.com/doi/abs/10.1111/imig.12308.

Beaman, Jean. *Citizen Outsider: Children of North African Immigrants in France*. Berkeley: University of California Press, 2017.

Becerra, Benjamin, Devin Arias, and Monideepa Becerra. "Low Health Literacy Among Immigrant Hispanics." *Journal of Racial and Ethnic Health Disparities* 4, no. 3 (2016): 480–83.

Becerra, David, Gladys Hernandez, Francisca Porchas, Jason Castillo, Van Nguyen, and Raquel Perez González. "Immigration Policies and Mental Health: Examining the Relationship Between Immigration Enforcement and Depression, Anxiety, and Stress Among Latino Immigrants." *Journal of Ethnic & Cultural Diversity in Social Work* 29, no. 1–3 (2020): 43–59. https://doi.org/10.1080/15313204.2020.1731641.

Becerra, David, Alex Wagaman, David Androff, Jill Messing, and Jason Castillo. "Policing Immigrants: Fear of Deportations and Perceptions of Law Enforcement and Criminal Justice." *Journal of Social Work* 17, no. 6 (2017): 715–31.

Beckfield, Jason. *Political Sociology and the People's Health.* New York: Oxford University Press, 2018.

Bedford, Tori. "Gov. Baker: Trump's Travel Ban, Budget 'Bad for Massachusetts.'" *WGBH News*, March 16, 2017. https://www.wgbh.org/news/2017/03/16/local-news/gov-baker-trumps-travel-ban-budget-bad-massachusetts.

Belew, Kathleen, and Ramon A. Gutiérrez, eds. *A Field Guide to White Supremacy.* Oakland: University of California Press, 2021.

Beniflah, Jacob, Wendalyn Little, Harold Simon, and Jesse Sturm. "Effects of Immigration Enforcement Legislation on Hispanic Pediatric Patient Visits to the Pediatric Emergency Department." *Clinical Pediatrics* 52, no. 12 (2013): 1122–26.

Berchick, Edward, Emily Hood, and Jessica Barnett. *Health Insurance Coverage in the United States: 2017.* United States Census Bureau, 2018. https://www.census.gov/content/dam/Census/library/publications/2018/demo/p60-264.pdf.

Bern, Jaimie, Stephanie Chrobak, and Tom Dehner. *Implementing the Affordable Care Act in Massachusetts: Changes in Subsidized Coverage Programs.* Blue Cross Blue Shield of Massachusetts Foundation, August 2015. https://www.bluecrossmafoundation.org/sites/g/files/csphws2101/files/2020-10/Changes%20in%20Subsidized%20Coverage%20Programs_final.pdf.

Bernal, Rafael. "Trump Praises ICE Raids in Mississippi, Calls Them 'a Very Good Deterrent.'" *The Hill*, August 9, 2019. https://thehill.com/latino/456857-trump-praises-ice-raids-in-mississippi-calls-them-a-very-good-deterrent/.

Bernstein, Nina, and Elizabeth Dwoskin. "Brazilians Giving Up Their American Dream." *New York Times*, December 4, 2007. https://www.nytimes.com/2007/12/04/nyregion/04brazilians.html.

Betancourt, Sarah. "Black and Hispanic Mass. Residents Face Disparities with Health Care Access, Report Finds." *WGBH News*, December 16, 2021. https://www.wgbh.org/news/local-news/2021/12/16/black-and-hispanic-mass-residents-face-disparities-with-health-care-access-report-finds.

Bidgood, Jess. "Massachusetts Health Plan Extended to Immigrants." *New York Times*, January 5, 2012. https://www.nytimes.com/2012/01/06/health/policy/massachusetts-health-plan-extended-to-immigrants.html.

Blackburn, Christine Crudo, and Lidia Azurdia Sierra. "Anti-Immigrant Rhetoric, Deteriorating Health Access, and COVID-19 in the Rio Grande Valley." *Health Security* 19, no. S1 (2021): 1–7. https://doi.org/10.1089/hs.2021.0005.

Blackstock, Uché. *Legacy: A Black Physician Reckons with Racism in Medicine*. New York: Penguin Random House, 2024.

Bleich, Sara, Mary Findling, Logan Casey, Robert Blendon, John Benson, Gillian Steel Fisher, Justin Sayde, and Carolyn Miller. "Discrimination in the United States: Experiences of Black Americans." *Health Services Research* 54, no. S2 (2019): 1399–408. https://onlinelibrary.wiley.com/doi/abs/10.1111/1475-6773.13220.

Blizzard, Brittany, and Jeanne Batalova. *Brazilian Immigrants in the United States in 2017*. Migration Policy Institute, August 29, 2019. https://www.migrationpolicy.org/article/brazilian-immigrants-united-states-2017.

Bloemraad, Irene, and Els De Graauw. "Immigrant Integration and Policy in the United States: A Loosely Stitched Patchwork." UC Berkeley: Institute for Research on Labor and Employment (2011). https://escholarship.org/uc/item/2nc0m8bm#main.

Bloemraad, Irene, Will Kymlicka, Michéle Lamont, and Leanne Son Hing. "Membership Without Social Citizenship? Deservingness and Redistribution as Grounds for Equality." *Daedalus* 148, no. 3 (2019): 73–104. https://www.amacad.org/publication/membership-without-social-citizenship-deservingness-redistribution-grounds-equality.

Bloemraad, Irene, and Veronica Terriquez. "Cultures of Engagement: The Organizational Foundations of Advancing Health in Immigrant and Low-Income Communities of Color." *Social Science & Medicine* 165 (2016): 214–22. https://www.sciencedirect.com/science/article/pii/S0277953616300582.

Blue Cross Blue Shield of Massachusetts. *Sick in Massachusetts: Views on Health Care Costs and Quality*. June 12, 2012. https://www.bluecrossmafoundation.org/sites/g/files/csphws2101/files/2020-09/Sick%20in%20MA.pdf.

Blue Cross Blue Shield of Massachusetts. *Health Reform in Massachusetts: Expanding Access to Health Insurance Coverage Accessing the Results, March 2013*. 2013. https://www.bluecrossmafoundation.org/sites/g/files/csphws2101/files/2020-10/Monitoring%20MA%20Reform%20March%202013_0.pdf.

Blue Cross Blue Shield of Massachusetts. *The Remaining Uninsured in Massachusetts: Experiences of Individuals Living Without Health Insurance Coverage*. February 18, 2016. https://www.bluecrossmafoundation.org/publication/remaining-uninsured-massachusetts-experiences-individuals-living-without-health.

Blue Cross Blue Shield of Massachusetts. *MassHealth: The Basics*. December 29, 2019. https://www.mamh.org/assets/files/MassHealthBasics_Jul2019update.pdf.

Blumenthal, David. "Americans Can't Afford to Get Sick—and Limited Plans Could Make Things Worse." *The Hill*, November 1, 2018. https://thehill.com/opinion/healthcare/413960-americans-cant-afford-to-get-sick-and-limited-plans-could-make-things.

Bobo, Lawrence, "Racism in Trump's America: Reflections on Culture, Sociology, and the 2016 US Presidential Election." *British Journal of Sociology* 68, no. S1 (2017): S85–S104. https://doi.org/10.1111/1468-4446.12324.

Bogel-Burroughs, Nicholas. "'I'm the Shooter': El Paso Suspect Confessed to Targeting Mexicans, Police Say." *New York Times*, August 9, 2019. https://www.nytimes.com/2019/08/09/us/el-paso-suspect-confession.html.

Bonilla-Silva, Eduardo. "Rethinking Racism." *American Sociological Review* 62, no. 3 (1997): 465–80.

Book, Robert, and Paul Howard. "Yes, It Was the 'Affordable' Care Act That Increased Premiums." *Forbes*, March 22, 2017. https://www.forbes.com/sites/theapothecary/2017/03/22/yes-it-was-the-affordable-care-act-that-increased-premiums/?sh=648a408c11d2.

Borrell, Luisa. "Racial Identity Among Hispanics: Implications for Health and Well-Being." *American Journal of Public Health* 95, no. 3 (2005): 379–81. https://ajph.aphapublications.org/doi/abs/10.2105/AJPH.2004.058172.

Borrell, Luisa, and Natalie D. Crawford. "All-Cause Mortality Among Hispanics in the United States: Exploring Heterogeneity by Nativity Status, Country of Origin, and Race in the National Health Interview Survey-Linked Mortality Files." *Annals of Epidemiology* 19, no. 5 (2009): 336–43. https://www.sciencedirect.com/science/article/pii/S1047279708003621.

Bosniak, Linda. "Citizenship Denationalized." *Indiana Journal of Global Legal Studies* 7, no. 2 (2000): 447–92. http://www.repository.law.indiana.edu/cgi/viewcontent.cgi?article=1185&context=ijgls.

Bosniak, Linda. *The Citizen and the Alien: Dilemmas of Contemporary Membership.* Princeton, NJ: Princeton University Press, 2006.

Boston.com. "Patrick's Pledge to Immigrants." July 22, 2010. http://archive.boston.com/news/local/massachusetts/articles/2010/07/22/governor_patricks_pledge_to_immigrants.

Boston Foundation. *Changing Faces of Greater Boston: A Report from Boston Indicators, the Boston Foundation, UMass Boston and the UMass Donahue Institute.* May 2019. https://www.bostonindicators.org/-/media/indicators/boston-indicators-reports/report-files/changing-faces-2019/indicators-changing-facesf2web.pdf.

Boston Globe Spotlight Team. "Boston. Racism. Image. Reality." *Boston Globe*, December 5, 2017. https://www.bostonglobe.com/metro/2017/12/05/boston-racism-image-reality/FHxuoVw4zOcRlorBiDT97K/story.html?event=event12.

Boston Planning and Development Agency. *Imagine All the People: Dominicans.* 2016. http://www.bostonplans.org/getattachment/f2812291-6aa9-4fa1-9d0b-3f41354acaaa.

Boston Planning and Development Agency. *Brazilians in Boston.* 2017a. http://www.bostonplans.org/getattachment/ad985146-c34a-4f51-8c6e-b277d4cda498.

Boston Planning and Development Agency. *Salvadorans in Boston.* June 2017b. https://www.slideshare.net/alvaroelima/salvadorans-in-boston-2017.

Boston Planning and Development Agency. *Demographic Profile of Adult Limited English Speakers in Massachusetts.* 2019a. https://www.bostonplans.org/getattachment/dfe1117a-af16-4257-b0f5-1d95dbd575fe.

Boston Planning and Development Agency. *Imagine All the People: Brazilians.* 2019b.

Boston Planning and Development Agency. *A Prosperous Boston for All: Dominicans.* 2019c.

Boston University School of Public Health. "Prospective and Retrospective Cohort Studies." n.d., accessed November 15, 2021. https://sphweb.bumc.bu.edu/otlt /mph-modules/ep/ep713_analyticoverview/ep713_analyticoverview3.html.

Bowden, John. "Woodward: Trump Insulted Obama's Intelligence, Called Him 'Overrated.'" *The Hill*, September 9, 2020. https://thehill.com/homenews /administration/515670-woodward-trump-insulted-obamas-intelligence-called -him-overrated.

Bradley, Elizabeth, and Lauren Taylor. *The American Health Care Paradox: Why Spending More Is Getting Us Less.* New York: Public Affairs, 2013.

Brandl, Eva, Stefanie Schreiter, and Meryam Schouler-Ocak. "Are Trained Medical Interpreters Worth the Cost? A Review of the Current Literature on Cost and Cost-Effectiveness." *Journal of Immigrant and Minority Health* 22, no. 1 (2019): 175–81.

Breland, Daniel, Philip Rocco, and Alex Waddan. *Obamacare Wars: Federalism, State Politics, and the Affordable Care Act.* Lawrence: University of Kansas Press, 2016.

Brindis, Claire, Max Hadler, Laurel Lucia, Nadereh Pourat, Marissa Raymond-Flesch, Rachel Siemons, and Efrain Talamantes. *Realizing the Dream for Californians Eligible for Deferred Action for Childhood Arrivals (DACA): Demographics and Health Coverage.* UC Berkeley Labor Center, February 2014. https:// laborcenter.berkeley.edu/pdf/2014/DACA_health_coverage.pdf.

Brinkerhoff, Cristina Araujo, C. Eduardo Siqueira, Rosalyn Negrón, Natalicia Tracy, Magalis Troncoso Lama, and Linda Sprague Martinez. "'There You Enjoy Life, Here You Work': Brazilian and Dominican Immigrants' Views on Work and Health in the U.S." *International Journal of Environmental Research and Public Health* 16, no. 20 (2019): 4025. https://www.mdpi.com/1660-4601/16 /20/4025.

Brooks, Anthony. "Boston's 2 Sides: How the City Can Have a Booming Innovation Economy and Widening Inequality." *WBUR*, June 9, 2016. https://www.wbur .org/news/2016/06/09/innovation-economy-inequality.

Brotherton, David, and Luis Barrios. *Banished to the Homeland: Dominican Deportees and Their Stories of Exile.* New York: Columbia University Press, 2011.

Brown, Kevin, and Darrell Jackson. "The History and Conceptual Elements of Critical Race Theory." In *Handbook of Critical Race Theory in Education*, edited by Adrienne D. Dixson and Marvin Lynn, 29–42. New York: Routledge, 2013.

Brown, Tony N., David R. Williams, James S. Jackson, Harold W. Neighbors, Myriam Torres, Sherrill L. Sellers, and Kendrick T. Brown. "'Being Black and Feeling Blue': The Mental Health Consequences of Racial Discrimination." *Race and Society* 2, no. 2 (2000): 117–31.

Brown, Tyson H. "Racial Stratification, Immigration, and Health Inequality: A Life Course-Intersectional Approach." *Social Forces* 96, no. 4 (2018): 1507–40.

Bruce, Giles. "Illinois Is First in the Nation to Extend Health Coverage to Undocumented Seniors." *Kaiser Health News*, January 7, 2021. https://khn.org/news

/article/illinois-is-first-in-the-nation-to-extend-health-coverage-to
-undocumented-seniors/.

Bryant, David, Ginger Haggerty, Cynthia Parker, Mimi Turchinetz, and Esther
Schlorholtz. *Reducing Racial Wealth Inequalities in Greater Boston: Building a
Shared Agenda.* Federal Reserve Bank of Boston, May 31, 2017. https://www
.bostonfed.org/publications/one-time-pubs/reducing-racial-wealth-inequalities
-in-greater-boston.aspx.

Bryant, Erica. "Why We Say 'Criminal Legal System,' Not 'Criminal Justice
System.'" *Vera Institute of Justice*, December 1, 2021. https://www.vera.org
/news/why-we-say-criminal-legal-system-not-criminal-justice-system.

Bump, Philip. "How the Boston Bombing Suspect Became a U.S. Citizen." *The
Atlantic*, April 19, 2013. https://www.theatlantic.com/national/archive/2013
/04/how-boston-bombing-suspects-became-us-citizens/316082/.

Burgess, Diana, Sean Phelan, Michael Workman, Emily Hagel, David Nelson,
Steven Fu, Rachel Widome, and Michelle Ryn. "The Effect of Cognitive Load
and Patient Race on Physicians' Decisions to Prescribe Opioids for Chronic Low
Back Pain: A Randomized Trial." *Pain Medicine* 15, no. 6 (2014): 965–74.

Burton, Guy. "An End to Poverty in Brazil? An Assessment of the Lula and Rousseff
Governments' Poverty Reduction and Elimination Strategies." *Journal of Policy
Practice* 12, no. 3 (2013): 194–215. https://doi.org/10.1080/15588742.2013
.796203.

Bustamante, Arturo Vargas, Jie Chen, Ryan McKenna, and Alexander Ortega.
"Health Care Access and Utilization among U.S. Immigrants Before and After
the Affordable Care Act." *Journal of Immigrant and Minority Health* 21, no. 2
(2019): 211–18. https://doi.org/https://doi.org/10.1007/s10903-018-0741-6.

Bustamante, Arturo Vargas, H. Fang, John Rizzo, and Alexander Ortega. "Heterogeneity in Health Insurance Coverage among US Latino Adults." *Journal of
General Internal Medicine* 24 (2009): 561–66.

Butkus, Renee, Katherine Rapp, Thomas Cooney, and Lee Engel. "Envisioning a
Better US Health Care System for All: Reducing Barriers to Care and Addressing
Social Determinants of Health." *Annals of Internal Medicine* 172 (2020): S50–S59.

Calavita, Kitty. *Immigrants at the Margins: Law, Race, and Exclusion in Southern
Europe.* Cambridge, UK: Cambridge University Press, 2005.

Callagan, Timothy, David Washburn, Katharine Nimmons, Delia Duchicela, Anoop
Gurram, and James Burdine. "Immigrant Health Access in Texas: Policy,
Rhetoric, and Fear in the Trump Era." *BMC Health Services Research* 19, no. 342
(2019): 1–8. https://doi.org/10.1186/s12913-019-4167-1.

Calvo, Rocío. "Health Literacy and Quality of Care Among Latino Immigrants in the
United States." *Health & Social Work* 41, no. 1 (2016): e44–e51.

Campbell, Alexia Fernandez. "Trump Says Undocumented Immigrants Are an
Economic Burden. They Pay Billions in Taxes." *Vox*, October 25, 2018. https://
www.vox.com/2018/4/13/17229018/undocumented-immigrants-pay-taxes.

Campbell, Andrea. *Trapped in America's Safety Net: One Family's Struggle.* Chicago:
University of Chicago Press, 2014.

Cancarevic, Ivan, Lucia Plichtová, and Bilal Haider Malik. "Healthcare Systems Around the World." In *International Medical Graduates in the United States*, edited by H. Tohid and H. Maibach, 45–79. New York: Springer, 2021. https://doi.org/10.1007/978-3-030-62249-7_3.

Candelario, Ginetta. "Hair Race-ing: Dominican Beauty Culture and Identity Production." *Meridians* 1, no. 1 (2000): 128–56.

Capps, Randy, and Michael Fix. "Immigration Reform: A Long Road to Citizenship and Insurance Coverage." *Health Affairs* 32, no. 4 (2013): 639–42.

Carten, Alma. "How Racism Has Shaped Welfare Policy in America." In *The State of Families: Law, Policy, and the Meaning of Relationships*, edited by Jennifer Katznelson Reich, 368–71. New York: Routledge, 2020.

Casellas, Jason, and Sophia Jordan Wallace. "Sanctuary Cities: Public Attitudes toward Enforcement Collaboration Between Local Police and Federal Immigration Authorities." *Urban Affairs Review* 56, no. 1 (2020): 32–64.

Castañeda, Heide. *Borders of Belonging: Struggle and Solidarity in Mixed-Status Immigrant Families*. Palo Alto, CA: Stanford University Press, 2019.

Castañeda, Heide, Seth Holmes, Daniel Madrigal, Maria-Elena De Trinidad Young, Naomi Beyeler, and James Quesada. "Immigration as a Social Determinant of Health." *Annual Review of Public Health* 36 (2015): 375–92. https://doi.org/10.1146/annurev-publhealth-032013-182419.

Cathey, Libby. "Legacy of Lies: How Trump Weaponized Mistruths During His Presidency." *ABC News*, January 20, 2021. https://abcnews.go.com/Politics/legacy-lies-trump-weaponized-mistruths-presidency/story?id=75335019.

Center for Health Information and Analysis. *Health Care Costs in Massachusetts Are Growing Slowly as Out-of-Pocket Costs Rise*. September 12, 2018. https://www.chiamass.gov/report-health-care-costs-in-massachusetts-are-growing-slowly-as-out-of-pocket-costs-rise/.

Center for Health Information and Analysis. *Findings from the 2021 Massachusetts Health Insurance Survey*. July 2021. https://www.chiamass.gov/massachusetts-health-insurance-survey/.

Centers for Disease Control and Prevention. "Disparities in Oral Health." February 2021. https://www.cdc.gov/oral-health/health-equity/?CDC_AAref_Val=https://www.cdc.gov/oralhealth/oral_health_disparities/index.html.

Centers for Disease Control and Prevention. *Health Insurance Portability and Accountability Act of 1996: U.S. Department of Health & Human Services*. Last updated July 10, 2024. https://www.cdc.gov/phlp/php/resources/health-insurance-portability-and-accountability-act-of-1996-hipaa.html.

Centers for Medicaid and Medicare Services. *NHE Fact Sheet, Historical NHE 2020. 2020*, updated December 15, 2021. https://www.cms.gov/Research-Statistics-Data-and-Systems/Statistics-Trends-and-Reports/NationalHealthExpendData/NHE-Fact-Sheet.

Cervantes, Andrea Gómez, and Cecilia Menjívar. "Legal Violence, Health, and Access to Care: Latina Immigrants in Rural and Urban Kansas." *Journal of Health and Social Behavior* 61, no. 3 (2020): 307–23.

Chan, Amy Hai Yan, Vanessa Cooper, Helen Lycett, and Rob Horne. "Practical Barriers to Medication Adherence: What Do Current Self- or Observer-Reported Instruments Assess?" *Frontiers in Pharmacology* 11 (2020): 572–72. https://doi .org/10.3389/fphar.2020.00572.

Charles, Camille Zubrinsky. "The Dynamics of Racial Residential Segregation." *Annual Review of Sociology* 29 (2003): 167–207.

Chauvin, Sébastien and Blanca Garcés-Mascareñas. "Becoming Less Illegal: Deservingness Frames and Undocumented Migrant Incorporation." *Sociology Compass* 8, no. 4 (2014): 422–32. https://compass.onlinelibrary.wiley.com/doi /abs/10.1111/soc4.12145.

Chavez, Leo. *The Latino Threat: Constructing Immigrants, Citizens, and the Nation.* 2nd ed. Palo Alto, CA: Stanford University Press, 2013.

Chavez-Dueñas, Nayeli, Hector Adames, and Kurt Organista. "Skin-Color Prejudice and Within-Group Racial Discrimination: Historical and Current Impact on Latino/a Populations." *Hispanic Journal of Behavioral Sciences* 36, no. 1 (2014): 3–26.

Cheliotis, L. "Punitive Inclusion: The Political Economy of Irregular Migration in the Margins of Europe." *European Journal Criminology* 14, no. 1 (2017): 78–99. https://journals.sagepub.com/doi/10.1177/1477370816640137.

Chen, Jarvis, and Nancy Krieger. "Revealing the Unequal Burden of COVID-19 by Income, Race/Ethnicity, and Household Crowding: US County Versus Zip Code Analyses." *Journal of Public Health Management Practice* 27, no. 1 (2021): S43–S56.

Chen, Ming Hsu. *Pursuing Citizenship in the Enforcement Era.* Palo Alto, CA: Stanford University Press, 2020.

Chishti, Muzaffar, and Jessica Bolter. *Vulnerable to COVID-19 and in Frontline Jobs, Immigrants Are Mostly Shut Out of U.S. Relief.* Migration Policy Institute, April 24, 2020. https://www.migrationpolicy.org/article/covid19-immigrants -shut-out-federal-relief.

Chishti, Muzaffar, Kathleen Bush-Joseph, and Colleen Putzel-Kavanaugh. *Biden at the Three-Year Mark: The Most Active Immigration Presidency Yet Is Mired in Border Crisis Narrative.* Migration Policy Institute, January 19, 2024. https://www .migrationpolicy.org/article/biden-three-immigration-record.

Clauss, Kyle Scott. "Gentriwatch: Boston, Big-City Inequality Capital of the United States." *Boston Magazine*, January 15, 2016. https://www.bostonmagazine.com /news/2016/01/15/gentriwatch-boston-income-inequality/.

Cohen, Alan, David Colby, Keith Wailoo, and Julian Zelizer, eds. *Medicare and Medicaid at 50: America's Entitlement Programs in the Age of Affordable Care.* New York: Oxford University Press, 2015.

Cohen, Elizabeth. "The Political Economy of Immigrant Time: Rights, Citizenship, and Temporariness in the Post-1965 Era." *Polity* 47, no. 3 (2015): 337–51.

Cohen, Robin, Brian Ward, and Jeannine Schiller. *Health Insurance Coverage: Early Release of Estimates from the National Health Interview Survey, 2010.* National Center for Health Statistics, Centers for Disease Control and Prevention, June 2011. https://www.cdc.gov/nchs/data/nhis/earlyrelease/insur201106.htm.

Colen, Cynthia, David Ramey, Elizabeth Cooksey, and David Williams. "Racial Disparities in Health Among Nonpoor African Americans and Hispanics: The Role of Acute and Chronic Discrimination." *Social Science & Medicine* 199 (2018): 167–80. https://doi.org/10.1016/j.socscimed.2017.04.051.

Collins, Patricia Hill. *Black Sexual Politics: African Americans, Gender, and the New Racism.* New York: Routledge, 2004.

Collins, Patricia Hill. "Intersectionality's Definitional Dilemmas." *Annual Review of Sociology* 41 (2015): 1–20.

Collins, Patricia Hill, and Sirma Bilge. *Intersectionality.* Medford, MA: John Wiley & Sons, 2020.

Collins, Sara R., Munira Z. Gunja, Michelle M. Doty, and Sophie Beutel. *Who Are the Remaining Uninsured and Why Haven't They Signed Up for Coverage? Findings from the Commonwealth Fund Affordable Care Act Tracking Survey, February–April 2016.* Commonwealth Fund, August 18, 2016. https://www.commonwealthfund.org /publications/issue-briefs/2016/aug/who-are-remaining-uninsured-and-why -havent-they-signed-coverage.

Commonwealth Fund. "Update: How Many Americans Have Lost Jobs with Employer Health Coverage During the Pandemic?" January 11, 2021. https:// www.commonwealthfund.org/blog/2021/update-how-many-americans-have -lost-jobs-employer-health-coverage-during-pandemic.

Commonwealth Fund. "New State-by-State Report: In 37 States, Workers' Health Insurance Premiums and Deductibles Take up 10 Percent or More of Median Income." January 12, 2022. https://www.commonwealthfund.org/press-release /2022/new-state-state-report-37-states-workers-health-insurance-premiums-and.

Cooper-Patrick, Lisa, Joseph Gallo, Jinius Gonzales, Hong Thi Vu, Neil Powe, Christine Nelson, and Daniel E. Ford. "Race, Gender, and Partnership in the Patient-Physician Relationship." *JAMA* 282, no. 6 (1999): 583–89. https://doi .org/10.1001/jama.282.6.583.

Cramer, Maria, and Alison Kuznitz. "As Threat of Raids Loom, Immigrants in Boston Brace for the Worst." *Boston Globe*, July 12, 2019. https://www .bostonglobe.com/metro/2019/07/12/threat-raids-loom-immigrants-boston -brace-for-worst/660t57FxYobeUNlANjtGfI/story.html.

Crenshaw, Kimberlé Williams. "Mapping the Margins: Intersectionality, Identity Politics, and Violence Against Women of Color." *Stanford Law Review* 43, no. 6 (1991): 1241–99.

Crenshaw, Kimberlé Williams. "Twenty Years of Critical Race Theory: Looking Back to Move Forward." *Connecticut Law Review* 43 (2010): 1253.

Crenshaw, Kimberlé Williams, Neil Gotanda, and Gary Peller. *Critical Race Theory: The Key Writings That Formed the Movement.* New York: New Press, 1995.

Creswell, John. *Qualitative Inquiry and Research Design: Choosing Among Five Approaches.* 2nd ed. London: Sage Publications, 2007.

Cuevas, Adolfo, Beverly Araujo Dawson, and David Williams. "Race and Skin Color in Latino Health: An Analytic Review." *American Journal of Public Health* 106, no. 12 (2016): 2131–36. https://doi.org/https://doi.org/10.2105/AJPH.2016.303452.

Culley, Lorraine, Nicky Hudson, and Maria Lohan. "Where Are All the Men? The Marginalization of Men in Social Scientific Research on Infertility." *Reproductive Biomedicine Online* 27, no. 3 (2013): 225–35.

Daly, Michael, and Jennifer Mellor. "Racial and Ethnic Differences in Medicaid Acceptance by Primary Care Physicians: A Geospatial Analysis." *Medical Care Research and Review* 77, no. 1 (2020): 85–95.

D'Anna, Laura Hoyt, Marissa Hansen, Brittney Mull, Carol Canjura, Esther Lee, and Stephanie Sumstine. "Social Discrimination and Health Care: A Multidimensional Framework of Experiences Among a Low-Income Multiethnic Sample." *Social Work in Public Health* 33, no. 3 (2018): 187–201. https://doi.org/10.1080/19371918.2018.1434584.

Danziger, Sheldon. "Welfare Reform Policy from Nixon to Clinton: What Role for Social Science?" In *Social Science and Policy Making*, edited by D. Featherman and M. Vinovskis, 137–64. Ann Arbor: University of Michigan Press, 2001.

Darlington, Shasta, and Ernesto Londoño. "Brazilian Corruption Case Ensnares Ex-Presidents Da Silva and Rousseff." *New York Times*, September 5, 2017. https://www.nytimes.com/2017/09/05/world/americas/brazil-dilma-rousseff-lula-corruption-workers-party.html.

Davidson, Stephen. *Still Broken: Understanding the U.S. Health Care System*. Palo Alto, CA: Stanford University Press, 2010.

Davis, Julie Hirschfield and Michael Shear. *Border Wars: Inside Trump's Assault on Immigration*. New York: Simon & Schuster, 2019.

Dawes, Daniel. *150 Years of ObamaCare*. Baltimore, MD: John Hopkins University Press, 2016.

Decker, Sandra L. "In 2011 Nearly One-Third of Physicians Said They Would Not Accept New Medicaid Patients, but Rising Fees May Help." *Health Affairs* 31, no. 8 (2012): 1–14. https://doi.org/10.1377%2Fhlthaff.2012.0294.

Decker, Scott, Monica Varsanyi, and Paul G. Lewis. "The Problematic Patchwork of Immigration Federalism." In *Policing Immigrants: Local Law Enforcement on the Front Lines*, edited by Doris Provine, Monica W. Varsanyi, Paul G. Lewis, and Scott H. Decker, 40–61. Chicago: University of Chicago Press, 2016.

DeCosta-Klipa, Nik. "Charlie Baker's Long Reign as America's Most Popular Governor Is Over." *Boston.com*, January 17, 2020. https://www.boston.com/news/politics/2020/01/17/charlie-baker-not-so-popular-but-still-pretty-popular/.

De Genova, Nicholas. "Migrant 'Illegality' and Deportability in Everyday Life." *Annual Review of Anthropology* 31 (2002): 419–47.

De Graauw, Els. "City Government Activists and the Rights of Undocumented Immigrants: Fostering Urban Citizenship Within the Confines of US Federalism." *Antipode* 53, no. 2 (2021): 379–98. https://doi.org/https://doi.org/10.1111/anti.12660.

De Lew, Nancy, George Greenberg, and Kraig Kinchen. "A Layman's Guide to the U.S. Health Care System." *Health Care Financing Review* 14, 1 (1992): 151–69. https://www.ncbi.nlm.nih.gov/pmc/articles/PMC4193322/.

Department of Homeland Security. "Inadmissibility on Public Charge Grounds." *Federal Register*, October 10, 2018. https://www.federalregister.gov/documents /2018/10/10/2018-21106/inadmissibility-on-public-charge-grounds.

Department of Homeland Security. "Inadmissibility on Public Charge Grounds." *Federal Register*, August 14, 2019. https://www.federalregister.gov/documents /2019/08/14/2019-17142/inadmissibility-on-public-charge-grounds.

Derose, Kathryn Pitkin, José J. Escarce, and Nicole Lurie. "Immigrants and Health Care: Sources of Vulnerability." *Health Affairs* 26, no. 5 (2007): 1258–68.

De Trinidad Young, Maria-Elena, Gabriela Leon-Perez, Steven Wallace, and Christine Wells. "Inclusive State Immigrant Policies and Health Insurance Among Latino, Asian/Pacific Islander, Black, and White Noncitizens in the United States." *Ethnicity & Health* 24 (2017): 960–72. https://doi.org/10.1080 /13557858.2017.1390074.

Dickerson, Caitlin, Jose Del Real, and Julie Bosman. "With ICE Raids Looming, Immigrants Worry: 'Every Time Someone Knocks, You Get Scared.'" *New York Times*, July 13, 2019. https://www.nytimes.com/2019/07/13/us/ice-raids. html.

Dickman, Samuel, David Himmelstein, and Steffie Woolhandler. "Inequality and the Health-Care System in the USA." *The Lancet* 389 (2017): 1431–41.

Dietz, Miranda, Laurel Lucia, Xiao Chen, Dave Graham-Squire, Hanqing Yao, Petra Rasmussen, Gregory Watson, Dylan Roby, Ken Jacobs, Srikanth Kadiyala, and Gerald Kominski. *California's Steps to Expand Health Coverage and Improve Affordability: Who Gains and Who Will Be Uninsured*. UC Berkeley Labor Center, November 19, 2019. https://laborcenter.berkeley.edu/ca-steps-to-expand -health-coverage-and-improve-affordability/.

Dines, Nick, Nicola Montagna, and Elena Vacchelli. "Beyond Crisis Talk: Interrogating Migration and Crises in Europe." *Sociology* 52, no. 3 (2018): 439–47. https://journals.sagepub.com/doi/full/10.1177/0038038518767372.

Doer, Kristen. "4 Economists Evaluate Obama's Economic Legacy." *PBS NewsHour*, January 12, 2017. https://www.pbs.org/newshour/economy/4-economists -evaluate-obamas-economic-legacy.

Dolan, Rachel. "Health Policy Brief: High-Deductible Health Plans." *Health Affairs*, February 4, 2016. https://www.healthaffairs.org/do/10.1377/hpb20160204 .950878/full/.

Dooling, Shannon. "Mass. Judge, Retired Court Officer Face Federal Charges for Allegedly Helping Defendant Evade ICE." *WBUR*, April 25, 2019a. https://www .wbur.org/news/2019/04/25/joseph-macgregor-obstruction-conspiracy -charges-ice.

Dooling, Shannon. "Judge Halts Immigration Arrests at Massachusetts Courts." *WBUR*, June 10, 2019b. https://www.wbur.org/news/2019/06/20/ice -courthouse-arrests-judge-decision.

Dooling, Shannon. "Trump Administration Ends Protection for Migrants' Medical Care." *NPR*, August 27, 2019c. https://www.npr.org/2019/08/27/754634022 /trump-administration-ends-protection-for-migrants-medical-care.

Dooling, Shannon. "Civil Rights Advocates Sue Trump Administration over Medical Deferred Action." *WBUR*, September 5, 2019d. https://www.wbur.org /news/2019/09/05/aclu-lawsuit-medical-deferred-action.

Dooling, Shannon. "57 Inmates to a Unit, Bunk Beds 3 Feet Apart; ICE Detainees in Bristol County Cite Overcrowding Amid COVID-19 Fears." *WBUR*, March 20, 2020a. https://www.wbur.org/news/2020/03/20/bristol-county-sheriff -immigration-covid-19-coronavirus.

Dooling, Shannon. "ICE Confirms Immigration Officials Stopped Black Man Jogging in West Roxbury." *WBUR*, October 7, 2020b. https://www.wbur.org /news/2020/10/07/ice-officers-west-roxbury-unexplained-stop-jogger.

Doty, Roxanne Lynne, and Elizabeth Shannon Wheatley. "Private Detention and the Immigration Industrial Complex." *International Political Sociology* 7, no. 4 (2013): 426–43. https://doi.org/10.1111/ips.12032.

Drake, Patrick, Jennifer Tolbert, Robin Rudowitz, and Anthony Damico. *How Many Uninsured Are in the Coverage Gap and How Many Could Be Eligible If All States Adopted the Medicaid Expansion?* Kaiser Family Foundation, February 26, 2024. https://www.kff.org/medicaid/issue-brief/how-many-uninsured-are-in-the -coverage-gap-and-how-many-could-be-eligible-if-all-states-adopted-the-medicaid -expansion/.

Dreby, Joanna. *Everyday Illegal: When Policies Undermine Immigrant Families.* Berkeley: University of California Press, 2015.

Drysdale, Sam. "What It Will Cost to Issue Drivers Licenses to Undocumented Immigrants in Massachusetts." *WBUR*, March 16, 2023. https://www.wbur.org /news/2023/03/16/drivers-license-immigrants-massachusetts-registry-motor -vehicles.

Du Bois, W. E. B. *The Souls of Black Folk.* Chicago: A.C. McClurg and Company, 1903.

Ebbert, Stephanie. "How Underrepresented Candidates in Mass. Communities Can Be Squelched by Electoral Systems." *Boston Globe*, January 26, 2021. https:// www.bostonglobe.com/2021/01/26/metro/how-underrepresented-candidates -mass-communities-can-be-squelched-by-electoral-systems/?event=event12.

Edwards, Griffin Sims, and Stephen Rushin. "The Effect of President Trump's Election on Hate Crimes." *Social Science Research Network* (2018). https://dx.doi .org/10.2139/ssrn.3102652.

Edwards, Julia. "Exclusive: U.S. Plans New Wave of Immigrant Deportation Raids." *Reuters*, May 12, 2016. https://www.reuters.com/article/us-usa-immigration -deportation-exclusive/exclusive-u-s-plans-new-wave-of-immigrant-deportation -raids-idUSKCN0Y32J1.

Edyburn, Kelly, and Shantel Meek. "Seeking Safety and Humanity in the Harshest Immigration Climate in a Generation: A Review of the Literature on the Effects of Separation and Detention on Migrant and Asylum-Seeking Children and Families in the United States During the Trump Administration." *Social Policy Report* 34, no. 1 (2021): 1–46. https://doi.org/10.1002/sop2.12.

Eibner, Christine, and Sarah Nowak. *The Effect of Eliminating the Individual Mandate Penalty and the Role of Behavioral Factors.* Commonwealth Fund, 2018. https://

www.commonwealthfund.org/publications/fund-reports/2018/jul/eliminating
-individual-mandate-penalty-behavioral-factors.

Eisen, Lauren-Brooke. *Inside Private Prisons*. New York: Columbia University Press, 2018.

Ellard-Gray, Amy, Nicole Jeffrey, Melisa Choubak, and Sara Crann. "Finding the Hidden Participant: Solutions for Recruiting Hidden, Hard-to-Reach, and Vulnerable Populations." *International Journal of Qualitative Methods* 14, no. 5 (2015): 1–10. https://doi.org/https://doi.org/10.1177/1609406915621420.

Ellement, John. "Two Women Charged with Attack on Hispanic Mother and Daughter in East Boston." *Boston Globe*, February 28, 2020. https://www .bostonglobe.com/2020/02/28/metro/2-women-charged-with-attack-hispanic -mother-daughter-east-boston/.

Emerson, Robert, Rachel Fretz, and Linda Shaw. *Writing Ethnographic Fieldnotes*. Chicago: University of Chicago, 1995.

Ennen, Elizabeth, Andra Lehotay de León, and Colleen Maney. *Safe Communities in Massachusetts: The Response of Massachusetts Municipalities to the Immigration Enforcement Policies of the Trump Administration*. Northeastern Law Program on Human Rights and the Global Economy and Partnership for Immigrants' Rights, October 2023. https://law.northeastern.edu/wp-content/uploads/2023 /10/phrge-safe-communities-report.pdf.

Epp, Charles, Steven Maynard-Moody, and Donald Haider-Markel. *Pulled Over: How Police Stops Define Race and Citizenship*. Chicago: University of Chicago Press, 2014.

Espino, Rodolfo, and Michael Franz. "Latino Phenotypic Discrimination Revisited: The Impact of Skin Color on Occupational Status." *Social Science Quarterly* 83, no. 2 (2002): 612–24.

Faist, Thomas, Başak Bilecen, Karolina Barglowski, and Joanna Jadwiga Sienkie-wicz. "Transnational Social Protection: Migrants' Strategies and Patterns of Inequalities." *Population, Space, and Place* 21 (2014): 193–202.

Feagin, Joe. *Racist America: Roots, Current Realities, and Future Reparations*. 4th ed. New York: Routledge, 2014.

Feagin, Joe, and José A. Cobas. *Latinos Facing Racism: Discrimination, Resistance, and Endurance*. Boulder, CO: Paradigm Publishers, 2014.

Fernández-Gutiérrez, Martina, Pilar Bas-Sarmiento, Maria-Jesus Albar-Marín, Olga Paloma-Castro, and José Manuel Romero-Sánchez. "Health Literacy Interventions for Immigrant Populations: A Systematic Review." *International Nursing Review* 65, no. 1 (2017): 54–64.

Feyerick, Deborah. "Tsarnaev's Connections: Who's Who." *CNN.com*, March 4, 2015. https://www.cnn.com/2015/03/04/us/tsarnaev-trial-people/index.html.

Figuereo, Victor, and Rocío Calvo. "Latinx Use of Traditional Health Care: The Social Network Effect." *Health & Social Work* 43, no. 4 (2018): 217–25.

Finch, B. K., B. Kolody, and W. Vega. "Perceived Discrimination and Depression among Mexican-Origin Adults in California." *Journal of Health and Social Behavior* 41, no. 3 (2000): 295–313.

FitzGerald, David Scott. "The History of Racialized Citizenship." In *The Oxford Handbook of Citizenship*, edited by Ayelet Shachar, Rainer Brubeck, Irene Bloemraad, and Maarten Vink, chapter 7. Oxford: Oxford University Press, 2017.

FitzGerald, David Scott. *Refuge Beyond Reach: How Rich Democracies Repel Asylum Seekers*. New York: Oxford University Press, 2019.

FitzGerald, David Scott, and David Cook-Martín. *Culling the Masses: The Democratic Origins of Racist Immigration Policy in the Americas*. Cambridge, MA: Harvard University Press, 2014.

Fix, Michael, and Ron Haskins. "Welfare Benefits for Non-citizens." Brookings Institution, February 2, 2002. https://www.brookings.edu/research/welfare -benefits-for-non-citizens/.

Flavin, Lila, Leah Zallman, Danny McCormick, and J. Wesley Boyd. "Medical Expenditures on and by Immigrant Populations in the United States: A Systematic Review." *International Journal of Health* 48, no. 4 (2018): 601–21. https://doi.org/10.1177/0020731418791963.

Fleary, Sasha, and Reynolette Ettienne. "Social Disparities in Health Literacy in the United States." *Health Literacy Research and Practice* 3, no. 1 (2019): E47–E52. https://doi.org/https://doi.org/10.3928/24748307-20190131-01.

Flores, René, and Ariela Schachter. "Who Are the 'Illegals'? The Social Construction of Illegality in the United States." *American Sociological Review* 83 (2018): 839–68. https://www.jstor.org/stable/48588674.

Flores-Gonzalez, Nilda. *Citizens but Not Americans: Race and Belonging Among Latino Millennials*. New York: New York University Press, 2017.

Forman, Ben, Zayna Basma, and Kelly Gourley. *Going for Growth: Promoting Digital Equity in Massachusetts Gateway Cities*. MassInc Gateway Cities Innovation Institute, November 2020. https://www.latinosforeducation.org /wp-content/uploads/2020/12/Promoting-Digital-Equity-in-MA-Gateway -Cities-MassINC.pdf.

Fortier, Marc. "ICE to Close Detention Center in Massachusetts Accused of Mistreatment." *NBC Boston*, May 20, 2021. https://www.nbcboston.com/news /local/ice-to-close-detention-center-in-massachusetts-after-allegations-of -mistreatment/2385676/.

Fortuna, Lisa, Michelle Porche, and Margarita Alegria. "Political Violence, Psychosocial Trauma, and the Context of Mental Health Services Use Among Immigrant Latinos in the United States." *Ethnicity & Health* 13, no. 5 (2008): 435–63.

Fox, Bethanne. *New Report: Affordable Care Act Has Narrowed Racial and Ethnic Gaps in Access to Health Care, but Progress Has Stalled*. Commonwealth Fund, January 16, 2020. https://www.commonwealthfund.org/press-release/2020/new -report-affordable-care-act-has-narrowed-racial-and-ethnic-gaps-access-health.

Fox, Cybelle. *Three Worlds of Relief: Race, Immigration, and the American Welfare State from the Progressive Era to the New Deal*. Princeton, NJ: Princeton University Press, 2012.

Fox, Cybelle. "Unauthorized Welfare: The Origins of Immigrant Status Restrictions in American Social Policy." *Journal of American History* 102, no. 4 (2016): 1051–74.

Frey, William. *A 2020 Census Portrait of America's Largest Metro Areas: Population Growth, Diversity, Segregation, and Youth*. Brookings Institution, April 21, 2022. https://digitalscholarship.unlv.edu/brookings_policybriefs_reports/11.

Fujiwara, Daigo, and Christina Prignano. "Charts: How Much Did Housing Costs Go Up in Your Town?" *Boston Globe*, March 29, 2022. https://www.bostonglobe .com/2022/03/29/metro/new-census-data-confirms-massachusetts-has-some -highest-housing-costs-us/?event=event12.

Gallas, Daniel, and Daniele Palumbo. "What's Gone Wrong with Brazil's Economy?" *BBC News*, May 26, 2019. https://www.bbc.com/news/business-48386415.

Gans, Herbert J. "Second-Generation Decline: Scenarios for the Economic and Ethnic Futures of the Post-1965 American Immigrants." *Ethnic and Racial Studies* 15, no. 2 (1992): 173–92.

García, Angela. *Legal Passing: Navigating Undocumented Life and Local Immigration Law*. Berkeley: University of California Press, 2019.

Garcia, Marcela. "Chelsea, City of the Working Latino Immigrant, Emerges as a COVID-19 Hotspot." *Boston Globe*, April 7, 2020. https://www.bostonglobe.com /2020/04/07/opinion/chelsea-city-working-latino-immigrant-emerges-covid-19 -hotspot.

García, San Juanita. "Racializing 'Illegality': An Intersectional Approach to Understanding How Mexican-Origin Women Navigate an Anti-Immigrant Climate." *Sociology of Race and Ethnicity* (2017): 474–90. https://journals .sagepub.com/doi/10.1177/2332649217713315.

Garfield, Rachel, Kendal Orgera, and Anthony Damico. *The Uninsured and the ACA: A Primer—Key Facts About Health Insurance and the Uninsured Amidst Changes to the Affordable Care Act*. Kaiser Family Foundation, January 25, 2019. https:// www.kff.org/report-section/the-uninsured-and-the-aca-a-primer-key-facts -about-health-insurance-and-the-uninsured-amidst-changes-to-the-affordable -care-act-how-many-people-are-uninsured.

Garfield, Rachel, and Robin Rudowitz. *Eliminating the ACA: What Could It Mean for Medicaid Expansion?* Kaiser Family Foundation, 2020. https://www.kff.org/policy -watch/eliminating-the-aca-what-could-it-mean-for-medicaid-expansion/.

Gartsbeyn, Mark. "'State A.G.s Became the De Facto U.S. Department of Justice': 6 Key Takeaways from Maura Healey's Vanity Fair Interview." *Boston.com*, December 19, 2020. https://www.boston.com/news/politics/2020/12/09 /maura-healey-vanity-fair-interview-takeaways.

Garza, Ronnie. "Immigration Policy Timeline (1994–2018)." *Medium*, June 28, 2018. https://medium.com/@ronniegarzatx/immigration-policy-timeline-1994 -2018-11d4cbeb8268.

Gavin, Christopher. "Boston Leaders Demand Answers After Black Man Is Stopped by ICE While Jogging in West Roxbury." *Boston.com*, October 7, 2020. https:// www.boston.com/news/local-news/2020/10/07/black-man-stopped-by-ice -jogging-west-roxbury/.

Gee, Gilbert, Anna Hing, Selina Mohammed, Derrick Tabor, and David Williams. "Racism and the Life Course: Taking Time Seriously." *American Journal of Public Health* 109, no. S1 (2019): S43–S47. https://ajph.aphapublications.org/doi/pdf/10.2105/AJPH.2018.304766.

Gee, Lisa, Matthew Gardner Christensen, Misha Hill, and Meg Wiehe. *Undocumented Immigrants' State and Local Tax Contributions*. Institute on Taxation and Economic Policy, March 2017. https://itep.sfo2.digitaloceanspaces.com/ITEP-2017-Undocumented-Immigrants-State-and-Local-Contributions.pdf.

Gerber, Ben, Ik Cho Young, Ahsan Arozullah, and Shoou-Yih D Lee. "Racial Differences in Medication Adherence: A Cross-Sectional Study of Medicare Enrollees." *American Journal of Geriatric Pharmacotherapy* 8, no. 2 (2010): 136–45.

Geronimus, Arline. *Weathering: The Extraordinary Stress of Ordinary Life in an Unjust Society*. New York: Little, Brown Spark, 2023.

Geronimus, Arline, Margaret Hicken, Danya Keene, and John Bound. "Weathering and Age Patterns of Allostatic Load Scores Among Blacks and Whites in the United States." *American Journal of Public Health* 96, no. 5 (2006): 826–33. https://www.ncbi.nlm.nih.gov/pmc/articles/PMC1470581/.

Gibbs, Virginia, and Luz Maria Hernandez. *Shattered Dreams: The Story of a Historic ICE Raid in the Words of the Detainees*. Moorpark, CA: Floricanto Press, 2014.

Gillens, Martin. *Why Americans Hate Welfare: Race, Media, and the Politics of Antipoverty Policy*. Chicago: University of Chicago Press, 1999.

Glaser, Barney, and Anselm Strauss. *The Discovery of Grounded Theory: Strategies for Qualitative Research*. New York: Aldine Publishing Company, 1967.

Golash-Boza, Tanya. *Deported: Immigrant Policing, Disposable Labor and Global Capitalism*. New York: New York University Press, 2015a.

Golash-Boza, Tanya. *Race and Racism: A Critical Approach*. New York: Oxford University Press, 2015b.

Golash-Boza, Tanya. "A Critical and Comprehensive Sociological Theory of Race and Racism." *Sociology of Race and Ethnicity* 2, no. 2 (2016): 129–41.

Golash-Boza, Tanya, and Pierrette Hondagneu-Sotelo. "Latino Immigrant Men and the Deportation Crisis: A Gendered Racial Removal Program." *Latino Studies* 11, no. 3 (2013): 271–92.

Gomez, Juan, and Parker Gilkesson. *25 Years of Immigrant Exclusion from Public Benefits. Center for Law and Social Policy*, 2021. https://www.clasp.org/blog/25-years-immigrant-exclusion-public-benefits/.

Gonzales, Roberto. *Lives in Limbo: Undocumented and Coming of Age in America*. Berkeley: University of California Press, 2015.

Gonzales, Roberto, and Edelina M. Burciaga. "Segmented Pathways of Illegality: Reconciling the Coexistence of Master and Auxiliary Statuses in the Experiences of 1.5-Generation Undocumented Young Adults." *Ethnicities* 18, no. 2 (2018): 178–91.

Gonzales, Roberto, Veronica Terriquez, and Stephen Ruszczyk. "Becoming DACA-mented: Assessing the Short-Term Benefits of Deferred Action for Childhood Arrivals (DACA)." *American Behavioral Scientist* 58, no. 14 (2014): 1852–72.

Goodnough, Abby. "Massachusetts Adjusts a Cut, Providing Some Health Care for 30,000 Immigrants." *New York Times*, July 30, 2009. https://www.nytimes.com /2009/07/30/us/30immigrant.html.

Gorman, Steve. "California Expands State Healthcare to Undocumented Residents 50 and Up." *Reuters*, July 27, 2021. https://www.reuters.com/world/us/california -expands-state-healthcare-undocumented-residents-50-up-2021-07-28/.

Gowayed, Heba. *Refuge: How the State Shapes Human Potential.* Princeton, NJ: Princeton University Press, 2022.

Graetz, Ilana, Nancy Gordon, Vick Fung, Courtnee Hamity, and Mary E. Reed. "The Digital Divide and Patient Portals: Internet Access Explained Differences in Patient Portal Use for Secure Messaging by Age, Race, and Income." *Medical Care* 54, no. 8 (2016): 772–79.

Granberry, Phillip, and Vishakha Agarwal. "Latinos in Massachusetts: Boston." *Gastón Institute Publications* 267 (2021). https://scholarworks.umb.edu/gaston _pubs/267/.

Granhagen Jungner, Johanna, Elisabet Tiselius, Klas Blomgren, Kim Lützén, and Pernilla Pergert. "Language Barriers and the Use of Professional Interpreters: A National Multisite Cross-Sectional Survey in Pediatric Oncology Care." *Acta Oncologica* 58, no. 7 (2019): 1015–20. https://doi.org/https://doi.org/10.1080 /0284186X.2019.1594362.

Grasmuck, Sherri, and Patricia Pessar. *Between Two Islands: Dominican International Migration.* Berkeley: University of California Press, 1991.

Gray, Darrell M., II, Joshua J. Joseph, and J. Nwando Olayiwola. "Strategies for Digital Care of Vulnerable Patients in a COVID-19 World—Keeping in Touch." *JAMA Health Forum* 1, no. 6 (2020): e200734–e34. https://doi.org/10.1001 /jamahealthforum.2020.0734.

Gray, Fred. *The Tuskegee Syphilis Study.* Montgomery, AL: NewSouth Books, 2002.

Griffith, Kevin, David Jones, Jacob Bor, and Benjamin Sommers. "Changes in Health Insurance Coverage, Access to Care, and Income-Based Disparities Among US Adults 2011–17." *Health Affairs* 39, no. 2 (2020): 319–26. https:// www.healthaffairs.org/doi/10.1377/hlthaff.2019.00904.

Grunder, Amy. "The Impact of COVID-19 in Massachusetts Immigrant Community Survey." Supporting Immigrant Communities in the COVID Pandemic Panel, MIRA Coalition, June 1, 2021.

Gulasekaram, Pratheepan, Rick Su, and Cuison Rose Villazor. "Anti-sanctuary and Immigration Localism." *Columbia Law Review* 119, no. 3 (2019): 837–94.

Gunja, Munira, and Sara Collins. *Who Are the Remaining Uninsured, and Why Do They Lack Coverage?* Commonwealth Fund, August 28, 2019. https://www .commonwealthfund.org/publications/issue-briefs/2019/aug/who-are -remaining-uninsured-and-why-do-they-lack-coverage.

Gurrola, Maria, and Cecilia Ayón. "Immigration Policies and Social Determinants of Health: Is Immigrants' Health at Risk?" *Race and Social Problems* 10 (2018): 209–20. https://doi.org/10.1007/s12552-018-9239-z.

Gutierrez, Melody. "California Expands Medi-Cal, Offering Relief to Older Immigrants Without Legal Status." *Los Angeles Times*, July 27, 2021. https://www.latimes.com/california/story/2021-07-27/medi-cal-expansion-immigrants-budget-california-newsom-legislature.

Hacker, Karen, Jocelyn Chu, Lisa Arsenault, and Robert Marlin. "Provider's Perspectives on the Impact of Immigration and Customs Enforcement (ICE) Activity on Immigrant Health." *Journal of Health Care for the Poor and Underserved* 23 (2012): 651–65.

Hacker, Karen, Jocelyn Chu, Carolyn Leung, Robert Marra, Alex Pirie, Mohamed Brahimi, Margaret English, Joshua Beckmann, Dolores Acevedo-Garcia, and Robert Marlin. "The Impact of Immigration and Customs Enforcement on Immigrant Health: Perceptions of Immigrants in Everett, Massachusetts, USA." *Social Science & Medicine* 73, no. 4 (2011): 1–9.

Hale, Jessica, Nianyi Hong, Ben Hopkins, Sean Lyons, Eamon Molloy, and The Congressional Budget Office Coverage Team. "Health Insurance Coverage Projections for the US Population and Sources of Coverage, by Age, 2024–34." *Health Affairs* 43, no. 7 (2024): 922–32. https://doi.org/10.1377/hlthaff.2024.00460.

Halim, May Ling, Keith Moy, and Hirokazu Yoshikawa. "Perceived Ethnic and Language-Based Discrimination and Latina Immigrant Women's Health." *Journal of Health Psychology* 22, no. 1 (2017): 68–78. https://doi.org/10.1177/1359105315595121.

Hall, Ronald. "Eurocentrism and the Postcolonial Implications of Skin Color Among Latinos." *Hispanic Journal of Behavioral Sciences* 33 (2011): 105–17.

Hamilton, Tod. *Immigration and the Remaking of Black America*. New York: Russell Sage Foundation, 2019.

Harding, Jamie. *Qualitative Analysis from Start to Finish*. London: Sage Publications Ltd., 2013.

Hassan, Adeel. "Hate-Crime Violence Hits 16-Year High, F.B.I. Reports." *New York Times*, November 12, 2019. https://www.nytimes.com/2019/11/12/us/hate-crimes-fbi-report.html.

Haywood, Jasmine M. "'Latino Spaces Have Always Been the Most Violent': Afro-Latino Collegians' Perceptions of Colorism and Latino Intragroup Marginalization." *International Journal of Qualitative Studies in Education* 30, no. 8 (2017): 759–82.

Health Care for All. *Introduction to PRUCOL*. 2020. https://hcfama.org/wp-content/uploads/2020/11/itl-ma_prucol_fact_sheet.pdf.

Health Care for All. *How to Get Covered*. n.d., accessed January 3, 2022. https://hcfama.org/health-insurance-help/.

Herd, Pamela, and Donald Moynihan. *Administrative Burden: Policymaking by Other Means*. New York: Russell Sage Foundation, 2018.

Hermann, Alexander, David Luberoff, and Daniel McCue. *Mapping over Two Decades of Neighborhood Change in the Boston Metropolitan Area*. Joint Center for Housing Studies of Harvard University, January 2019. https://www.jchs

.harvard.edu/sites/default/files/Harvard_JCHS_mapping_neighborhood
_change_boston_january_2019.pdf.

Hero, Joachim, Robert Blendon, Alan Zaslavsky, and Andrea Campbell. "Understanding What Makes Americans Dissatisfied with Their Health Care System: An International Comparison." *Health Affairs* 35, no. 3 (2016). https://doi.org/https://doi.org/10.1377/hlthaff.2015.0978.

Hero, Rodney, and Robert Preuhs. "Immigration and the Evolving American Welfare State: Examining Policies in the U.S. States." *American Journal of Political Science* 51, no. 3 (2007): 498–517.

Hill, Latoya, Samantha Artiga, and Anthony Damico. *Health Coverage by Race and Ethnicity, 2010–2022*. Kaiser Family Foundation, 2024. https://www.kff.org/racial-equity-and-health-policy/issue-brief/health-coverage-by-race-and-ethnicity/.

Himmelstein, David, and Steffie Woolhandler. "Public Health's Falling Share of US Health Spending." *American Journal of Public Health* 106, no. 1 (2016): 56–57. https://doi.org/10.2105/AJPH.2015.302908.

Hing, Bill Ong. "Institutional Racism, ICE Raids, and Immigration Reform." *University of San Francisco Law Review* 44, no. 197 (2009): 1–49. https://papers.ssrn.com/sol3/papers.cfm?abstract_id=1525578.

Hing, Esther, Sandra Decker, and Eric Jamoom. "Acceptance of New Patients with Public and Private Insurance by Office-Based Physicians: United States, 2013." *National Center for Health Statistics Data Brief*, no. 195 (2015):1–8. https://pubmed.ncbi.nlm.nih.gov/25932895/.

Hinton, Elizabeth. *From the War on Poverty to the War on Crime: The Making of Mass Incarceration in America*. Cambridge, MA: Harvard University Press, 2017.

Hoekstra, Erin, and Anthony Michael Jiménez. "Versatile Brokerage: Migrant-Provider Relationships in the Third Net of the U.S. Healthcare System." *Journal of Ethnic and Migration Studies* (2022): 3132–51. https://doi.org/10.1080/1369183X.2022.2161494.

Hoff, Timothy. *Searching for the Family Doctor: Primary Care on the Brink*. Baltimore, MD: Johns Hopkins University Press, 2022.

Hoffman, Beatrix. "Restraining the Health Care Consumer: The History of Deductibles and Co-Payments in U.S. Health Insurance." *Social Science History* 30, no. 4 (2006): 501–28. https://www.cambridge.org/core/journals/social-science-history/article/abs/restraining-the-health-care-consumer/7DBF541C18ACCE37FDA26DFEFC7F0B02.

Hoffman, Kelly, Sophie Trawalter, Jordan Axt, and Norman Oliver. "Racial Bias in Pain Assessment and Treatment Recommendations, and False Beliefs About Biological Differences Between Blacks and Whites." *Proceedings of the National Academy of Sciences* 113 (2016): 4296–301.

Hoffnung-Garskof, Jesse. *A Tale of Two Cities: Santo Domingo and New York After 1950*. Princeton, NJ: Princeton University Press, 2008.

Holloway, Pippa. *Living in Infamy: Felon Disfranchisement and the History of American Citizenship*. New York: Oxford University Press, 2014.

Holmes, Natalie, and Alan Berube. *City and Metropolitan Inequality on the Rise, Driven by Declining Incomes.* Brookings Institution, 2016. https://www .brookings.edu/research/city-and-metropolitan-inequality-on-the-rise-driven -by-declining-incomes/.

Holpuch, Amanda. "Migrant Children Held in Texas Facility Need Access to Doctors, Says Attorney." *The Guardian*, July 8, 2019. https://www.theguardian .com/us-news/2019/jul/08/migrant-children-detention-center-texas-attorney -health-crisis.

Horowitz, Juliana Menasce, Ruth Igielnik, and Rakesh Kochhar. *Most Americans Say There Is Too Much Economic Inequality in the U.S., but Fewer Than Half Call It a Top Priority.* Pew Research Center, January 9, 2020. https://www.pewsocial trends.org/2020/01/09/trends-in-income-and-wealth-inequality/.

House, James. *Beyond Obamacare: Life, Death, and Social Policy.* New York: Russell Sage Foundation, 2015.

Houston, Ashley, Tibrine Da Fonseca, Tiffany Joseph, and Alisa Lincoln. "Challenging Federal Exclusion: Immigrant Safety, Health, and Healthcare Access in Sanctuary Cities." *Health & Place* 75 (2022): 102822. https://doi.org/10.1016/j .healthplace.2022.102822.

Houston, Serin. "Conceptualizing Sanctuary as a Process in the United States." *Geographical Review* 109, no. 4 (2019): 562–79.

Huerto, Ryan. "Minority Patients Benefit from Having Minority Doctors, But That's a Hard Match to Make." *University of Michigan Health Lab*, March 31, 2020. https://labblog.uofmhealth.org/rounds/minority-patients-benefit-from -having-minority-doctors-but-thats-a-hard-match-to-make-0.

Hughes, Everett Cherrington. "Dilemmas and Contradictions of Status." *American Journal of Sociology* 50, no. 5 (1945): 353–59.

Illingworth, Patricia, and Wendy Parmet. *The Health of Newcomers: Immigration, Health Policy, and the Case for Global Solidarity.* New York: New York University Press, 2017.

Immigrant Legal Resource Center. *Public Charge Timeline.* 2021. https://www.ilrc .org/sites/default/files/resources/2020.01.08_public_charge_timeline.pdf.

Immigrant Legal Resource Center. *State Map on Immigration Enforcement.* 2023. https://www.ilrc.org/state-map-immigration-enforcement.

Itzigsohn, Jose. *Encountering American Fault Lines: Race, Class, and the Dominican Experience in Providence.* New York: Russell Sage Foundation, 2009.

Jacobs, Elizabeth, Alice Chen, Leah Karliner, Niels Agger-Gupta, and Sunita Mutha. "The Need for More Research on Language Barriers in Health Care: A Proposed Research Agenda." *Milbank Quarterly* 84, no. 1 (2006): 111–33.

Jacobs, Lawrence, and Theda Skocpol. *Health Care Reform and American Politics: What Everyone Needs to Know.* New York: Oxford University Press, 2010.

Jefferis, Danielle. "Private Prisons, Private Governance: Essay on Developments in Private-Sector Resistance to Privatized Immigration Detention." *Northwestern Journal of Law and Social Policy* 15, no. 82 (2019): 1–17. https://papers.ssrn.com /sol3/papers.cfm?abstract_id=3399833.

Jiménez, Anthony. "The Legal Violence of Care: Navigating the US Healthcare System While Undocumented and Illegible." *Social Science & Medicine* 270 (2021). https://doi.org/https://doi.org/10.1016/j.socscimed.2021.113676.

Jiménez, Tomás. *Replenished Ethnicity: Mexican Americans, Immigration, and Identity*. Berkeley: University of California Press, 2010.

Jirmanus, Lara, Lynsie Ranker, Sharon Touw, Rumel Mahmood, Sarah Kimball, Amresh Hanchate, and Karen Lasser. "Impact of United States 2017 Immigration Policy Changes on Missed Appointments at Two Massachusetts Safety-Net Hospitals." *Journal of Immigrant and Minority Health* 24 (2022): 807–18. https://doi.org/10.1007/s10903-022-01341-9.

Johnson, Kevin. "Trump's Latinx Repatriation." *UCLA Law Review* 66 (2019): 1444–1501. https://www.uclalawreview.org/trumps-latinx-repatriation/.

Johnson, Marilynn. *The New Bostonians: How Immigrants Have Transformed the Metro Area Since the 1960s*. Amherst: University of Massachusetts Press, 2015.

Jones, Chuck. "Obama's 2009 Recovery Act Kicked Off Over 10 Years of Economic Growth." *Forbes*, February 17, 2020. https://www.forbes.com/sites/chuckjones/2020/02/17/obamas-2009-recovery-act-kicked-off-over-10-years-of-economic-growth/?sh=1d860d1768b7.

Jones, James. *The Last Plantation: Racism and Resistance in the Halls of Congress*. Princeton, NJ: Princeton University Press, 2024.

Jones, Nicholas, Rachel Marks, Roberto Ramirez, and Merarys Rios-Vargas. *2020 Census Illuminates Racial and Ethnic Composition of the Country*. United States Census Bureau, August 12, 2021. https://www.census.gov/library/stories/2021/08/improved-race-ethnicity-measures-reveal-united-states-population-much-more-multiracial.html.

Jordan, Miriam. "DeSantis Pushes Toughest Immigration Crackdown in the Nation." *New York Times*, April 10, 2023. https://www.nytimes.com/2023/04/10/us/florida-desantis-immigration.html.

Jordan, Miriam, and Caitlin Dickerson. "Sick Migrants Undergoing Lifesaving Care Can Now Be Deported." *New York Times*, August 29, 2019. https://www.nytimes.com/2019/08/29/us/immigrant-medical-treatment-deferred-action.html.

Joseph, Tiffany. *Race on the Move: Brazilian Migrants and the Global Reconstruction of Race*. Palo Alto, CA: Stanford University Press, 2015.

Joseph, Tiffany. "What Healthcare Reform Means for Immigrants: A Comparison of the Affordable Care Act and Massachusetts Health Reforms." *Journal of Health Policy, Politics, and Law* 41, no. 1 (2016): 101–16.

Joseph, Tiffany. "Falling Through the Coverage Cracks: How Documentation Status Minimizes Immigrants' Access to Health Care." *Journal of Health Policy, Politics, and Law* 42, no. 5 (2017a): 961–84. https://doi.org/10.1215/03616878-3940495.

Joseph, Tiffany. "Still Left Out: Health Care Stratification Under the Affordable Care Act." *Journal of Ethnic and Migration Studies* 43, no. 12 (2017b): 2089–107. https://doi.org/http://dx.doi.org/10.1080/1369183X.2017.1323453.

Joseph, Tiffany. "Stratification and 'Universality': Immigrants and Barriers to Coverage in Massachusetts." In *Unequal Coverage: The Experience of Health Care Reform in the United States*, edited by Heide Castañeda and Jessica Mulligan, chapter 3. New York: New York University Press, 2018.

Joseph, Tiffany. "The Documentation Status Continuum: Citizenship and Increasing Stratification in American Life." *SocArXiv Papers* (2020a). https://osf.io/preprints/socarxiv/2x6hq/.

Joseph, Tiffany. "Trump's Immigration Policies Are Making the Coronavirus Pandemic Worse." Opinion, *Newsweek*, April 24, 2020b. https://www.newsweek.com/trumps-immigration-policies-are-making-coronavirus-pandemic-worse-opinion-1500129.

Joseph, Tiffany. "Whitening Citizenship: Race, Ethnicity, and Documentation Status as Brightened Boundaries of Exclusion in the U.S. and Europe." In *International Handbook of Contemporary Racisms*, edited by John Solomos, chapter 4. New York: Routledge Press, 2020c.

Joseph, Tiffany, and Tanya Golash-Boza. "Double Consciousness in the 21st Century: Du Boisian Theory and the Problem of Racialized Legal Status." *Social Sciences* 10, no. 9 (2021): 345. https://www.mdpi.com/2076-0760/10/9/345.

Joseph, Tiffany, and Helen Marrow. "Health Care, Immigrants and Minorities: Lessons from the Affordable Care Act in the United States." *Journal of Ethnic and Migration Studies* 43, no. 12 (2017): 1965–84. https://doi.org/10.1080/1369183X.2017.1323446.

Jost, Timothy. "Court Decision to Invalidate the Affordable Care Act Would Affect Every American." *Commonwealth Fund*, December 17, 2018. https://www.commonwealthfund.org/blog/2018/court-decision-invalidate-affordable-care-act-would-affect-every-american.

Kaiser Family Foundation. "Current Status of State Medicaid Expansions, 2014." https://www.kff.org/medicaid/issue-brief/status-of-state-medicaid-expansion-decisions-interactive-map/.

Kaiser Family Foundation. *Medicaid Income Eligibility Limits for Other Non-disabled Adults 2011–2024*. 2024. https://www.kff.org/medicaid/state-indicator/medicaid-income-eligibility-limits-for-other-non-disabled-adults/?currentTimeframe=0&sortModel=%7B%22colId%22:%22Location%22,%22sort%22:%22asc%22%7D.

Kaiser Family Foundation. *Status of State Medicaid Expansions: Interactive Map*. 2024. https://www.kff.org/medicaid/issue-brief/status-of-state-medicaid-expansion-decisions-interactive-map/.

Kanno-Youngs, Zolan. "Squalid Conditions at Border Detention Centers, Government Report Finds." *New York Times*, July 2, 2019. https://www.nytimes.com/2019/07/02/us/politics/border-center-migrant-detention.html.

Kanno-Youngs, Zolan, and Hamed Aleaziz. "In Shift, Biden Issues Order Allowing Temporary Border Closure to Migrants." *New York Times*, June 4, 2024. https://www.nytimes.com/2024/06/04/us/politics/biden-executive-order-border-asylum.html.

Kanno-Youngs, Zolan, and Caitlin Dickerson. "Trump Again Threatens 'Major Operation' Against Undocumented Migrants." *New York Times*, July 12, 2019. https://www.nytimes.com/2019/07/12/us/ice-raids-migrant-families.html.

Karpman, Michael, Hamutal Bernstein, Dulce Gonzalez, Sara McTarnaghan, and Stephen Zuckerman. "Five Ways the 'Public Charge' Rule Is Affecting Immigrants in America." *Urban Wire*, August 19, 2019. https://www.urban.org/urban-wire/five-ways-public-charge-rule-affecting-immigrants-america.

Katznelson, Ira. *Fear Itself: The New Deal and the Origins of Our Time.* New York: W. W. Norton & Company, 2013.

Kaufmann, David. "Comparing Urban Citizenship, Sanctuary Cities, Local Bureaucratic Membership, and Regularizations." *Public Administration Review* 79, no. 3 (2019): 443–46.

Kearney, Audrey, Liz Hamel, Meillisha Stokes, and Mollyann Brodie. "Americans' Challenges with Health Care Costs." Kaiser Family Foundation, December 14, 2021. https://www.kff.org/health-costs/issue-brief/americans-challenges-with-health-care-costs/.

Keisler-Starkey, Katherine, and Lisa Bunch. *Health Insurance Coverage in the United States: 2020.* United States Census Bureau, September 14, 2021. https://www.census.gov/library/publications/2021/demo/p60-274.html.

Kenney, Genevieve, Jennifer Haley, and Robin Wang. "Proposed Public Charge Rule Could Erode Health Insurance Coverage Gains Among Citizen Children with Noncitizen Parents." *Urban Wire*, December 4, 2018. https://www.urban.org/urban-wire/proposed-public-charge-rule-could-erode-health-insurance-coverage-gains-among-citizen-children-noncitizen-parents.

King, Ledyard, and Mike Stucka. "In Massachusetts, Many Still Lack Broadband Access." *Herald News*, July 7, 2021. https://www.heraldnews.com/story/news/2021/07/07/gda-broadband-local-ma-nher/47205505/.

Kliff, Sarah. "How Massachusetts Screwed up Obamacare." *Vox*, May 13, 2014. https://www.vox.com/2014/5/12/5691934/how-massachusetts-screwed-up-obamacare.

Kline, Nolan. *Pathogenic Policing: Immigration Enforcement and Health in the U.S. South.* New Brunswick, NJ: Rutgers University Press, 2019.

Kluender, Raymond, Neale Mahoney, Francis Wong, and Wesley Yin. "Medical Debt in the US, 2009–2020." *JAMA* 326, no. 3 (2021): 250–56. https://doi.org/10.1001/jama.2021.8694.

Knight, Victoria. "America to Face Shortage of Primary Care Physicians Within a Decade or So." *Daily Courier*, July 28, 2019. http://web.thedailycourier.com/eedition/2019/07/28/Health_and_Wellness/11.pdf.

Kolstad, Jonathan, and Amanda Kowalski. "The Impact of Health Care Reform on Hospital and Preventive Care: Evidence from Massachusetts." *Journal of Public Economics* 96, no. 11–12 (2012): 909–29.

Kominers, Sara. "Caught in the Gap Between Status and No-Status: Lawful Presence Then and Now." *Rutgers Race and the Law Review* 17, no. 1 (2016): 57–83.

Konczal, Lisa, and Leah Varga. "Structural Violence and Compassionate Compatriots: Immigrant Health Care in South Florida." *Ethnic and Racial Studies* 35 (2012): 88–103.

Krieger, Nancy. "Theories for Social Epidemiology in the 21st Century: An Ecosocial Perspective." *International Journal of Epidemiology* 30 (2001): 668–77.

Krieger, Nancy. "Methods for the Scientific Study of Discrimination and Health: An Ecosocial Approach." *American Journal of Public Health* 102, no. 5 (2013): 936–45.

Krieger, Nancy, Anna Kosheleva, Pamela D. Waterman, Jarvis T. Chen, and Karestan Koenen. "Racial Discrimination, Psychological Distress, and Self-Rated Health among US-Born and Foreign-Born Black Americans." *American Journal of Public Health* 101, no. 9 (2011): 1704–13.

Kreisberg, A. Nicole. "Starting Points: Divergent Trajectories of Labor Market Integration among US Lawful Permanent Residents." *Social Forces* 98, no. 2 (2019): 849–84.

Kruzel, John. "Biden Rescinds Trump's 'Public Charge' Rule." *The Hill*, March 11, 2021. https://thehill.com/regulation/court-battles/542860-biden-rescinds-trumps-public-charge-rule/.

Kuge, Janika. "Countering Illiberal Geographies Through Local Policy? The Political Effects of Sanctuary Cities." *Territory, Politics, Governance* 8, no. 1 (2020): 43–59.

Lacy, Karyn. "The New Sociology of Suburbs: A Research Agenda for Analysis of Emerging Trends." *Annual Review of Sociology* 42 (2016): 369–84.

Lamont, Michele, Bo Yun Park, and Elena Ayala-Hurtado. "Trump's Electoral Speeches and His Appeal to the American White Working Class." *British Journal of Sociology* 68 (2017): S153–S80. https://onlinelibrary.wiley.com/doi/full/10.1111/1468-4446.12315.

Lancee, Bram, and Thijs Bol. "The Transferability of Skills and Degrees: Why the Place of Education Affects Immigrant Earnings." *Social Forces* 96, no. 2 (2017): 691–716.

Lara, Ana-Maurine. "A Smarting Wound: Afro-Dominicanidad and the Fight Against Ultranationalism in the Dominican Republic." *Feminist Studies* 43, no. 2 (2017): 468–84. https://doi.org/10.15767/feministstudies.43.2.0468.

Lasch, Christopher, Linus Chan, Ingrid Eagly, Dina Francesca Haynes, Annie Laj, Elizabeth McCormick, and Juliet Stumpf. "Understanding 'Sanctuary Cities.'" *Boston College Law Review* 59, no. 5 (2018): 1703–74.

LaVeist, T., and L. Isaac. *Race, Ethnicity, and Health: A Public Health Reader.* Hoboken, NJ.: John Wiley and Sons, 2012.

Laz, Tabassum, and Abbey B. Berenson. "Racial and Ethnic Disparities in Internet Use for Seeking Health Information Among Young Women." *Journal of Health Communication* 18, no. 2 (2013): 250–60.

Lazar, Malerie, and Lisa Davenport. "Barriers to Health Care Access for Low Income Families: A Review of Literature." *Journal of Community Health Nursing* 35, no. 1 (2018): 28–37.

Lee, Erika. *America for Americans: A History of Xenophobia in the United States.* New York: Basic Books, 2019.

Levitt, Peggy, and B. Nadya Jaworsky. "Transnational Migration Studies: Past Developments and Future Trends." *Annual Review of Sociology* 33 (2007): 129–56.

Levy, Helen. "Health Reform: Learning from Massachusetts." *Inquiry* 49 (2013): 300–302.

Light, Donald. "Categorical Inequality, Institutional Ambivalence, and Permanently Failing Institutions: The Case of Immigrants and Barriers to Health Care in America." *Ethnic and Racial Studies* 35, no. 1 (2012): 23–39.

Lima, Alvaro, and Mark Melnik. *Boston: Measuring Diversity in a Changing City.* Boston Planning & Development Agency, December 13, 2013. https://www.bostonplans.org/getattachment/32e9b68a-ce1b-41c7-808c-0395cb4f4d19.

Lima, Rômulo. "Bolsonaro and the Current Stage of the Brazilian Social Crisis." In *Democracy and Brazil: Collapse and Regression,* edited by Bernardo Bianchi, Jorge Chaloub, Patricia Rangel, and Frieder Otto Wolf, chapter 7. New York: Routledge, 2020.

Lin, Shen Lamson. "Access to Health Care Among Racialised Immigrants to Canada in Later Life: A Theoretical and Empirical Synthesis." *Ageing & Society* 42, no. 8 (2022): 1735–59.

Lind, Dara. "The 2014 Central American Migrant Crisis." *Vox,* October 11, 2014. https://www.vox.com/2014/10/10/18088638/child-migrant-crisis-unaccompanied-alien-children-rio-grande-valley-obama-immigration.

Link, Bruce, and Jo Phelan. "Social Conditions as Fundamental Causes of Disease." *Health and Social Behavior* 35 (1995): 80–94.

Lipsky, Michael. "Bureaucratic Disentitlement in Social Welfare Programs." *Social Service Review* 58, no. 1 (1984): 3–27.

Lloyd, Jim, and Katherine Heflin. "Massachusetts' Medicaid ACO Makes a Unique Commitment to Addressing Social Determinants of Health." *Center for Health Care Strategies* (blog), December 19, 2016. https://www.chcs.org/massachusetts-medicaid-aco-makes-unique-commitment-addressing-social-determinants-health/.

Long, Sharon, Dana Goin, and Victoria Lynch. *Reaching the Remaining Uninsured in Massachusetts: Challenges and Opportunities.* Urban Institute, 2013. https://www.urban.org/research/publication/reaching-remaining-uninsured-massachusetts-challenges-and-opportunities.

Long, Sharon, and Paul B. Masi. *Access to Affordability of Care in Massachusetts as of Fall 2008: Geographic and Racial/Ethnic Differences.* Urban Institute, 2009. https://www.urban.org/research/publication/access-and-affordability-care-massachusetts-fall-2008-geographic-and-racialethnic-differences.

López, William. *Separated: Family and Community in the Aftermath of an Immigration Raid.* Baltimore, MD: Johns Hopkins Press, 2019.

López-Sanders, Laura. "Navigating Health Care: Brokerage and Access for Undocumented Latino Immigrants Under the 2010 Affordable Care Act." *Journal of Ethnic and Migration Studies* 43 (2017): 2072–88. https://doi.org/10.1080/1369183X.2017.1323452.

Lorenzi, Jane, and Jeanne Batalova. "South American Immigrants in the United States." *Migration Information Source*, February 16, 2022. https://www.migrationpolicy.org/article/south-american-immigrants-united-states.

Lowrey, Annie. "The Time Tax." *The Atlantic*, July 27, 2021. https://www.theatlantic.com/politics/archive/2021/07/how-government-learned-waste-your-time-tax/619568/.

Luque, John, Grace Soulen, Caroline Davila, and Kathleen Cartmell. "Access to Health Care for Uninsured Latina Immigrants in South Carolina." *BMC Health Services Research* 18, no. 310 (2018): 1–12. https://doi.org/10.1186/s12913-018-3138-2.

Maani, Nason, and Sandro Galea. "COVID-19 and Underinvestment in the Public Health Infrastructure of the United States." *Millbank Quarterly* 98 (2020). https://www.milbank.org/quarterly/articles/covid-19-and-underinvestment-in-the-public-health-infrastructure-of-the-united-states/.

Maciosek, Michael, Ashley Coffield, Thomas Flottemesch, Nichol Edwards, and Leif Solberg. "Greater Use of Preventive Services in U.S. Health Care Could Save Lives at Little or No Cost." *Health Affairs* 29 (2010): 1656–60.

Makhlouf, Medha. "Health Care Sanctuaries." *Yale Journal of Health Policy, Law and Ethics* 20 (2021). http://dx.doi.org/10.2139/ssrn.3915570.

Malat, Jennifer, and Mary Ann Hamilton. "Preference for Same-Race Health Care Providers and Perceptions of Interpersonal Discrimination in Health Care." *Journal of Health and Social Behavior* 47, no. 2 (2006): 173–87.

Manatt Health. *Supporting Health Equity and Affordable Health Coverage for Immigrant Populations: State-Funded Affordable Coverage Programs for Immigrants*. State Health and Value Strategies, Robert Wood Johnson Foundation, October 2021. https://www.shvs.org/wp-content/uploads/2021/10/State-Funded-Affordable-Coverage-Programs-for-Immigrants.pdf.

Manchikanti, Laxmaiah, Standiford Helm li, Ramsin Benyamin, and Joshua Hirsch. "A Critical Analysis of Obamacare: Affordable Care or Insurance for Many and Coverage for Few?" *Pain Physician* 20, no. 3 (2017): 111–38. https://pubmed.ncbi.nlm.nih.gov/28339427/.

Marcozzi, David, Brendan Carr, Aisha Liferidge, Nicole Baehr, and Brian Browne. "Trends in the Contribution of Emergency Departments to the Provision of Hospital-Associated Health Care in the USA." *International Journal of Health Services* 48, no. 2 (2018): 267–88.

Marrow, Helen. *New Destination Dreaming: Immigration, Race, and Legal Status in the Rural American South*. Palo Alto, CA: Stanford University Press, 2011.

Marrow, Helen. "Deserving to a Point: Unauthorized Immigrants in San Francisco's Universal Access Healthcare Model." *Social Science and Medicine* 74, no. 6 (2012): 846–54.

Marrow, Helen, and Tiffany Joseph. "Excluded and Frozen Out: Unauthorized Immigrants' (Non) Access to Care After Healthcare Reform." *Journal of Ethnic and Migration Studies* 41, no. 14 (2015): 2253–73. http://www.tandfonline.com/doi/full/10.1080/1369183X.2015.1051465#.Va_hn_lVhBc.

Marshall, T. H. *Citizenship and Social Class*. Cambridge, UK: Cambridge University Press, 1950.

Mass Legal Services. "Alert: Health Safety Net Cuts: Public Hearing Feb. 26, 2016," https://www.masslegalservices.org/content/alert-health-safety-net-cuts-public -hearing-feb-26-2016.

Massachusetts Executive Office of Health and Human Services. *MassHealth Member Booklet*, 2013.

Massachusetts Executive Office of Health and Human Services. *Health Safety Net Annual Report, Fiscal Year 2016*. December 1, 2016. https://www.mass.gov/lists /health-safety-net-hsn-annual-reports#fiscal-year-2016-.

Massachusetts Medical Society. *High Deductibles: What They Mean for Patients and Physicians*. 2017. https://www.massmed.org/Templates/Article.aspx?id =4294980232.

Massachusetts Supreme Judicial Court. *Sreynuon Lunn vs. Commonwealth and Another*. 477 Mass. 517 (Suffolk County, 2017). http://masscases.com/cases/sjc /477/477mass517.html.

Massey, Douglas. *The New Latino Underclass: Immigration Enforcement as a Race-Making Institution*. Stanford Center on Poverty and Inequality, 2012. https:// inequality.stanford.edu/sites/default/files/media/_media/working_papers /massey_new-latino-underclass.pdf.

Massey, Douglas, and Katherine Bartley. "The Changing Legal Status Distribution of Immigrants: A Caution." *International Migration Review* 39, no. 2 (2005): 469–84. http://www.jstor.org/stable/27645505.

Massey, Douglas, and Nancy Denton. *American Apartheid: Segregation and the Making of the Underclass*. Cambridge, MA: Harvard University Press, 1993.

MassHealth. *Member Booklet for Health and Dental Coverage and Help Paying Costs*. Commonwealth of Massachusetts, 2022.

Mastroianni, Brian. "Why It's Not Easy to Access Mental Health Care When You're Covered by Medicaid." *Healthline*, August 19, 2021. https://www.kropro.law /article.cfm?ArticleNumber=104.

Mata-Greve, Felicia, and Lucas Torres. "Rejection and Latina/o Mental Health: Intragroup Marginalization and Intragroup Separation." *American Journal of Orthopsychiatry* 89, no. 6 (2019): 716–26.

Matthew, Dayna Bowen. "Applying Lessons from Social Psychology to Repair the Health Care Safety Net for Undocumented Immigrants." In *The Health Care "Safety Net" in a Post-Reform World*, edited by Mark A. Hall and Sara Rosenbaum, 91–107. New Brunswick, NJ: Rutgers University Press, 2012.

Matthew, Dayna Bowen. *Just Health: Treating Structural Racism to Heal America*. New York: New York University Press, 2022.

McCluskey, Priyanka Dayal. "Massachusetts Contains Health Care Costs, but Consumers Keep Paying More." *Boston Globe*, October 8, 2019. https://www .bostonglobe.com/business/2019/10/08/massachusetts-contains-health-care -costs-but-consumers-keep-paying-more/fLtpd430o1FwOrCCmcxJaM/story. html.

McDonnell, Judith, and Cileine De Lourenço. "You're Brazilian, Right? What Kind of Brazilian Are You? The Racialization of Brazilian Immigrant Women." *Journal of Ethnic and Racial Studies* 32, no. 2 (2009): 239–56.

McDonough, John. *Inside National Health Reform.* Berkeley: University of California Press, 2011.

McDonough, John. "Behind the Massachusetts Health Connector's Rehab." *Commonwealth Magazine,* April 11, 2016. https://commonwealthmagazine.org /health-care/behind-the-massachusetts-health-connectors-rehab/.

McGloin, Catherine. "Wealth Gap Widens as Boston Booms." *Bay State Banner,* October 17, 2018. https://www.baystatebanner.com/2018/10/17/wealth-gap -widens-as-boston-booms/.

McGowan, Amanda. "Governor Baker Would Veto In-State Tuition for Undocumented Immigrants." *WGBH News,* July 16, 2015. https://www.wgbh.org/news /post/governor-baker-would-veto-state-tuition-undocumented-immigrants.

McKanders, Karla. "Immigration and Racial Justice: Enforcing the Borders of Blackness." *Georgia State University Law Review* 37, no. 4 (2021): 1139–75. https://readingroom.law.gsu.edu/gsulr/vol37/iss4/6/.

McKillop, Caitlin, Teresa Waters, Cameron Kaplan, Erin Kaplan, Michael Thompson, and Ilana Graetz. "Three Years in—Changing Plan Features in the U.S. Health Insurance Marketplace." *BMC Health Services Research* 18, no. 450 (2018): 1–14. https://doi.org/10.1186/s12913-018-3198-3.

Mehra, Renee, Lisa Boyd, and Jeannette Ickovics. "Racial Residential Segregation and Adverse Birth Outcomes: A Systematic Review and Meta-Analysis." *Social Science & Medicine* 191 (2017): 237–50. https://pubmed.ncbi.nlm.nih.gov/28942206/.

Mehta, Dhrumil. "Most Americans Like How Their Governor Is Handling the Coronavirus Outbreak." *FiveThirtyEight,* April 10, 2020. https://fivethirtyeight .com/features/most-americans-like-how-their-governor-is-handling-the -coronavirus-outbreak/.

Mendes de Leon, Carlos, and Jennifer Griggs. "Medical Debt as a Social Determinant of Health." *JAMA* 326, no. 3 (2021): 228–29. https://doi.org/10.1001 /jama.2021.9011.

Menjívar, Cecilia. "Liminal Legality: Salvadoran and Guatemalan Immigrants' Lives in the United States." *American Journal of Sociology* 111, no. 4 (2006): 999–1037.

Menjívar, Cecilia. "Immigrant Criminalization in Law and the Media: Effects on Latino Immigrant Workers' Identities in Arizona." *American Behavioral Scientist* 60 (2016): 597–616. https://journals.sagepub.com/doi/10.1177/0002764216 632836.

Menjívar, Cecilia. *Temporary Protected Status in the United States: The Experiences of Honduran and Salvadoran Immigrants.* Center for Migration Research, University of Kansas, May 2017. https://www.wola.org/wp-content/uploads/2017/06/TPS _REPORT_FINAL.pdf.

Menjívar, Cecilia. "The Racialization of Illegality." *Daedalus* 150, no. 2 (Spring 2021). https://doi.org/https://doi.org/10.1162/DAED_a_01848.

Menjívar, Cecilia, and Leisy Abrego. "Legal Violence: Immigration Law and the Lives of Central American Immigrants." *American Journal of Sociology* 117, no. 5 (2012): 1380–421.

Menjívar, Cecilia, Andrea Cervantes, and Daniel Alvord. "The Expansion of 'Crimmigration,' Mass Detention, and Deportation." *Sociology Compass* (2018). https://doi.org/https://doi.org/10.1111/soc4.12573.

Menjívar, Cecilia, and Sarah M. Lakhani. "Transformative Effects of Immigration Law: Immigrants' Personal and Social Metamorphoses Through Regularization." *American Journal of Sociology* 121, no. 6 (2016): 1818–55. https://doi.org/10.1086/685103.

Mercado, Alfonso, Frances Morales, Andy Torres, and Amanda Palomin. "¿Dónde Está Mi Mamá? Clinical Implications of Family Separations." *Journal of Health Service Psychology* 48, no. 2 (2022): 49–58.

Mettler, Suzanne. *Divided Citizens: Gender and Federalism in New Deal Public Policy.* Ithaca, NY: Cornell University Press, 1998.

Metzger, Andy. "Baker Vows Veto of Senate Immigration Bill." State House News Service. *Sentinel & Enterprise* (Fitchburg, MA), May 25, 2018. http://www.sentinelandenterprise.com/news/ci_31901806/baker-vows-veto-senate-immigration-bill.

Metzger, Andy. "Mass. Residents Overburdened by Health Costs." *Commonwealth Magazine*, October 22, 2019. https://commonwealthmagazine.org/health-care/mass-residents-overburdened-by-health-costs/.

Metzl, Jonathan. *Dying of Whiteness: How the Politics of Racial Resentment Is Killing America's Heartland.* New York: Basic Books, 2019.

Migration Policy Institute. "State Demographics Data Profiles—Massachusetts." n.d., accessed November 15, 2023. https://www.migrationpolicy.org/data/state-profiles/state/demographics/MA.

Miles, Matthew, and A. Michael Huberman. *An Expanded Sourcebook: Qualitative Data Analysis.* 2nd ed. Thousand Oaks, CA: Sage Publications, 1994.

Miller, Alexander, Julia Meredith Hess, Deborah Bybee, and Jessica Goodkind. "Understanding the Mental Health Consequences of Family Separation for Refugees: Implications for Policy and Practice." *American Journal of Orthopsychiatry* 88, no. 1 (2018): 26.

Miller, Leila. "Trump Administration's 'Public Charge' Rule Has Chilling Effect on Benefits for Immigrants' Children." *Los Angeles Times*, September 3, 2019.

Miller, Sarah. "The Effect of the Massachusetts Reform on Health Care Utilization." *Journal of Health Care Organization, Provision, and Financing* 49, no. 4 (2012): 317–26.

Milligan, Susan. "Trump's First TV Ad: A Wall, a Ban, and a Beheading." *US News*, January 4, 2016. http://www.usnews.com/news/articles/2016/01/04/donald-trumps-inaugural-tv-ad-a-wall-a-muslim-ban-and-beheading-isis.

Miroff, Nick, and Devlin Barrett. "ICE Preparing Targeted Arrests in 'Sanctuary Cities,' Amplifying President's Campaign Theme." *Washington Post,* September 29, 2020. https://www.washingtonpost.com/immigration/trump-ice-raids

-sanctuary-cities/2020/09/29/99aa17f0-0274-11eb-8879-7663b816bfa5_story
.html.

Mohl, Bruce. "Virus Notes: Baker Hits Trump Immigration Stance." *CommonWealth
Beacon*, April 21, 2020. https://commonwealthbeacon.org/politics/virus-notes
-baker-hits-trump-immigration-stance/.

Mohl, Bruce. "Mass. Welcome Mat for Migrants Starting to Fray." *CommonWealth
Beacon*, September 12, 2023. https://commonwealthbeacon.org/politics/mass
-welcome-mat-for-migrants-starting-to-fray/.

Molina, Natalia. *Fit to be Citizens? Public Health and Race in Los Angeles, 1879–1939*.
Berkeley: University of California Press, 2006.

Molina, Natalia. *How Race Is Made in America: Immigration, Citizenship, and the
Historical Power of Racial Scripts*. Berkeley: University of California Press, 2014.

Monroe, Carla, and Ronald Hall. "Colorism and U.S. Immigration: Considerations
for Researchers." *American Behavioral Scientist* 62 (2018): 2037–54.

Montalvo, Frank. "Surviving Race: Skin Color and the Socialization and Acculturation of Latinas." *Journal of Ethnic and Cultural Diversity in Social Work* 13, no. 3
(2005): 25–43.

Montoya-Galvez, Camilo. "Administration Reinstates Protections from Deportation
for Sick Immigrants After Massive Uproar." *CBS News*, September 20, 2019.
https://www.cbsnews.com/news/medical-deferred-action-trump-administration
-reinstates-deportation-relief-for-sick-immigrants-after-uproar/.

Montoya-Galvez, Camilo. "Immigrants in ICE Custody Clash with Massachusetts
Jail Officials in Latest Disturbance over Coronavirus." *CBS News*, May 2, 2020.
https://www.cbsnews.com/news/immigrants-in-ice-custody-clash-with
-massachusetts-jail-officials-in-latest-disturbance-over-coronavirus/.

Montoya-Galvez, Camilo. "Biden Administration Stops Enforcing Trump-Era
'Public Charge' Green Card Restrictions Following Court Order." *CBS News*,
March 10, 2021. https://www.cbsnews.com/news/immigration-public-charge
-rule-enforcement-stopped-by-biden-administration/.

Mora, G. Cristina. *Making Hispanics: How Activists, Bureaucrats, and Media Constructed a New American*. Chicago: University of Chicago Press, 2014.

Morgante, Victoria. "Make America Hate Again: A Quantitative Analysis on the
Effects of Presidential Rhetoric During the Obama and Trump Administration."
PhD diss., Rutgers University, 2021.

Motomura, Hiroshi. *Immigration Outside the Law*. New York: Oxford University
Press, 2014.

Moura, Paula. "Brazilian Immigrants Requesting More Asylum Status in the US."
Folha de S.Paulo, July 3, 2019. https://www1.folha.uol.com.br/internacional/en
/world/2019/07/brazilian-immigrants-requesting-more-asylum-status-in-the
-us.shtml.

Muñoz, Ana Patricia, Marlene Kim, Mariko Chang, Regine Jackson, Darrick
Hamilton, and William Darity, Jr. *The Color of Wealth in Boston*. Federal Reserve
Bank of Boston, March 25, 2015. https://www.bostonfed.org/publications/one
-time-pubs/color-of-wealth.aspx.

Murguia, Edward, and Edward Telles. "Phenotype and Schooling Among Mexican Americans." *Sociology of Education* 69, no. 4 (1996): 276–89.

Musich, Shirley, Shaohung Wang, Kevin Hawkins, and Andrea Klemes. "The Impact of Personalized Preventive Care on Health Care Quality, Utilization, and Expenditures." *Population Health Management* 19, no. 6 (2016): 389–97. https://doi.org/10.1089/pop.2015.0171.

Naderifar, Mahin, Hamideh Goli, and Fereshteh Ghaljaie. "Snowball Sampling: A Purposeful Method of Sampling in Qualitative Research." *Strides in Development of Medical Education* 14, no. 3 (2017). https://doi.org/10.5812/sdme.67670.

National Academies of Sciences, Engineering, and Medicine. *The Integration of Immigrants into American Society*. The National Academic Press, 2015. https://nap.nationalacademies.org/catalog/21746/the-integration-of-immigrants-into-american-society.

National Immigration Forum. *Fact Sheet: Deferred Enforced Departure (DED)*. March 12, 2021. https://immigrationforum.org/article/fact-sheet-deferred-enforced-departure-ded/.

Naylor, Brian, and Tamara Keith. "Kamala Harris Tells Guatemalans Not to Migrate to the United States." *NPR*, June 7, 2021. https://www.npr.org/2021/06/07/1004074139/harris-tells-guatemalans-not-to-migrate-to-the-united-states.

Negrón-Gonzales, Genevieve. "The Making and Unmaking of Common Sense: Undocumented Latino Youth and Political Consciousness." PhD diss., University of California, Berkeley, 2011.

Neufeld, Anne, Margaret Harrison, Miriam Stewart, Karen Hughes, and Denise Spitzer. "Immigrant Women: Making Connections to Community Resources for Support in Family Caregiving." *Qualitative Health Research* 12, no. 6 (2002): 751–68.

Ngai, Mae. *Impossible Subjects: Illegal Aliens and the Making of Modern America*. Princeton, NJ: Princeton University Press, 2004.

Ngai, Mae. "Birthright Citizenship and the Alien Citizen." *Fordham Law Review* 75 (2007): 2521–3295. http://ir.lawnet.fordham.edu/flr/vol75/iss5/10.

Nguyen, Geoffrey, Thomas LaVeist, Mary Harris, Lisa Datta, Theodore Bayless, and Steven Brant. "Patient Trust-in-Physician and Race Are Predictors of Adherence to Medical Management in Inflammatory Bowel Disease." *Inflammatory Bowel Diseases* 15, no. 8 (2009): 1233–39.

Nguyen, Mai Thi, and Hannah Gill. "Interior Immigration Enforcement: The Impacts of Expanding Local Law Enforcement Authority." *Urban Studies* 53, no. 2 (2016): 302–23.

Nichols, Vanessa Cruz, Alana LeBrón, and Francisco Pedraza. "Policing Us Sick: The Health of Latinos in an Era of Heightened Deportations and Racialized Policing." *PS: Political Science & Politics* 51, no. 2 (2018): 293–97. https://doi.org/10.1017/S1049096517002384.

Northridge, M. E., A. Kumar, and R. Kaur. "Disparities in Access to Oral Health Care." *Annual Review of Public Health* 41 (2020): 513–35. https://doi.org/10.1146/annurev-publhealth-040119-094318.

Norton, Michael, and Matt Murphy. "Baker Still Opposed to Immigrant Driver's License Bill." *Herald News*, February 6, 2020. https://www.heraldnews.com /story/news/2020/02/06/baker-still-opposed-to-immigrant/1751334007/.

Novak, Nicole, Arline Geronimus, and Aresha Martinez-Cardoso. "Change in Birth Outcomes Among Infants Born to Latina Mothers After a Major Immigration Raid." *International Journal of Epidemiology* 46, no. 3 (2017): 839–49. https://doi .org/10.1093/ije/dyw346.

Nuila, Ricardo. *The People's Hospital: Hope and Peril in American Medicine*. New York: Scribner, 2022.

Obama, Barack. "United States Health Care Reform: Progress to Date and Next Steps." *Journal of the American Medical Association* 316, no. 5 (2016): 525–32.

Obinna, Denise N. "Confronting Disparities: Race, Ethnicity, and Immigrant Status as Intersectional Determinants in the COVID-19 Era." *Health Education & Behavior* 48, no. 4 (2021): 397–403.

Oboler, Suzanne. "The Politics of Labeling: Latino/a Cultural Identities of Self and Others." *Latin American Perspectives* 19, no. 4 (1992): 18–36. http://www.jstor .org/stable/2633842.

Oboler, Suzanne. *Ethnic Labels, Latino Lives: Identity and the Politics of (Re)Presentation in the United States*. Minneapolis: University of Minnesota Press, 1995.

Ochoa, Gilda. "Mexican Americans' Attitudes Toward and Interactions with Mexican Immigrants: A Qualitative Analysis of Conflict and Cooperation." *Social Science Quarterly* 81, no. 1 (2000): 84–105.

Oliver, Melvin, and Thomas Shapiro. *Black Wealth / White Wealth: A New Perspective on Racial Inequality*. New York: Routledge, 1995.

Olmos, Daniel "Racialized Im/migration and Autonomy of Migration Perspectives: New Directions and Opportunities." *Sociology Compass* 13 (2019): e12729. https://doi.org/10.1111/soc4.12729.

Omi, Michael, and Howard Winant. *Racial Formation in the United States: From the 1960s to the 1990s*. New York: Routledge, 1994.

Ong, Aihwa, Virginia Dominguez, Jonathan Friedman, Nina Glick Schiller, Verena Stolcke, David Wu, and Hu Ying. "Cultural Citizenship as Subject-Making: Immigrants Negotiate Racial and Cultural Boundaries in the United States." *Current Anthropology* 37, no. 5 (1996): 737–62.

Ornstein, Charles. "Epic Fail: Where Four States Health Exchanges Went Wrong." *ProPublica*, February 6, 2014. https://www.propublica.org/article/epic-fail -where-four-state-health-exchanges-went-wrong.

Orris, Allison, April Grady, and Cindy Mann. *Public Charge Rule Would Have Significant, Negative Impact on Immigrants' Health Care and the Safety-Net Delivery System*. Commonwealth Fund, 2018. https://www.commonwealthfund .org/blog/2018/public-charge-rule-negative-impact-immigrants-health-care.

Ortega, Alexander, Jessie Kemmick Pintor, Brent Langellier, Arturo Vargas Bustamante, Maria-Elena De Trinidad Young, Michael Prelip, Cinthya Alberto, and Steven Wallace. "Cardiovascular Disease Behavioral Risk Factors Among Latinos by Citizenship and Documentation Status." *BMC Public Health* 20, no. 629 (2020): 1–9. https://doi.org/https://doi.org/10.1186/s12889-020 -08783-6.

Ortega, Alexander, Ryan McKenna, Jessie Kemmick Pintor, Brent Langellier, Dylan Roby, Nadereh Pourat, Arturo Vargas Bustamante, and Steven Wallace. "Health Care Access and Physical and Behavioral Health Among Undocumented Latinos in California." *Medical Care* 56, no. 11 (2018): 919–26. https://doi.org/10.1097 /MLR.0000000000000985.

Ortega, Alexander, Hector Rodriguez, and Arturo Vargas Bustamante. "Policy Dilemmas in Latino Health Care and Implementation of the Affordable Care Act." *Annual Review of Public Health* 18, no. 36 (2015): 525–44.

Osborn, Robin, David Squires, Michelle Doty, Dana Sarnak, and Eric Schneider. "In New Survey of Eleven Countries, US Adults Still Struggle with Access to and Affordability of Health Care." *Health Affairs* 35, no. 12 (2016). https://doi.org /10.1377/hlthaff.2016.1088.

Page, Kathleen, Maya Venkataramani, Chris Beyrer, and Sarah Polk. "Undocumented U.S. Immigrants and COVID-19." *New England Journal of Medicine* 382, no. 21 (2020): e62. https://doi.org/10.1056/NEJMp2005953.

Paik, A. Naomi. "Abolitionist Futures and the US Sanctuary Movement." *Race & Class* 59, no. 2 (2017): 3–25.

Palloni, Alberto, and Elizabeth Arias. "Paradox Lost: Explaining the Hispanic Adult Mortality Advantage." *Demography* 41, no. 3 (2004): 385–415.

Palmer, Richard, Deborah Ismond, Erik Rodriguez, and Jay Kaufman. "Social Determinants of Health: Future Directions for Health Disparities Research." Supplement, *American Journal of Public Health* 109, no. 1 (2019): S70–S71. https://ajph.aphapublications.org/doi/pdf/10.2105/AJPH.2019.304964.

Panikkar, Bindu, Mark Woodin, Doug Brugge, Anne Marie Desmarais, Raymond Hyatt, Rose Goldman, Alex Pirie, et al. "Occupational Health and Safety Experiences Among Self-Identified Immigrant Workers Living or Working in Somerville, MA by Ethnicity, Years in the US, and English Proficiency." *International Journal of Environmental Research and Public Health* 9, no. 12 (2012): 4452–69. https://www.mdpi.com/1660-4601/9/12/4452.

Papanicolas, Irene, Liana Woskie, and Ashish Jha. "Health Care Spending in the United States and Other High-Income Countries." *JAMA* 319, no. 10 (2018): 1024–39. https://doi.org/doi:10.1001/jama.2018.1150.

Park, Lisa Sun-Hee. *Entitled to Nothing: The Struggle for Immigrant Health Care in the Age of Welfare Reform.* New York: New York University, 2011.

Park, Lisa Sun-Hee, Erin Hoekstra, and Anthony M. Jiménez. *The Third Net: The Hidden System of Migrant Health Care.* New York: New York University Press, 2024.

Parker, Ashley, and Steve Eder. "Inside the Six Weeks Donald Trump Was a Nonstop 'Birther.'" *New York Times*, July 2, 2016. https://www.nytimes.com /2016/07/03/us/politics/donald-trump-birther-obama.html.

Parmet, Wendy. "Immigration and Health Care Under the Trump Administration." *Health Affairs*, January 18, 2018. https://www.healthaffairs.org/do/10.1377 /forefront.20180105.259433/.

Parmet, Wendy, and Lorianne Sainsbury-Wong, "Restoring Legal Immigrants' State Health Insurance—the Finch Case." *Boston Health Law Reporter* 7, no. 3 (2012): 6–10. https://papers.ssrn.com/sol3/papers.cfm?abstract_id=2117815.

Patel, Kavita, and John McDonough. "From Massachusetts to 1600 Pennsylvania Avenue: Aboard the Health Reform Express." *Health Affairs* 29, no. 6 (2010): 1106–11. https://doi.org/10.1377/hlthaff.2010.0429.

Patler, Caitlin, and Gabriela Gonzalez. "Compounded Vulnerability: The Consequences of Immigration Detention for Institutional Attachment and System Avoidance in Mixed-Immigration-Status Families." *Social Problems* 68, no. 4 (2021): 886–902. https://doi.org/10.1093/socpro/spaa069.

Patton, M. Q. "Enhancing the Quality and Credibility of Qualitative Analysis." *Health Services Research* 34, no. 5 (1999): 1189–208.

Pear, Robert, Sharon LaFraniere, and Ian Austen. "From the Start, Signs of Trouble at Health Portal." *New York Times*, October 12, 2013. https://www.nytimes.com/2013/10/13/us/politics/from-the-start-signs-of-trouble-at-health-portal.html.

Pedraza, Silvia. "Beyond Black and White: Latinos and Social Science Research on Immigration, Race, and Ethnicity in America." *Social Science History* 24 (2000): 697–726.

Peffley, Mark, Jon Hurwitz, and Paul Sniderman. "Racial Stereotypes and Whites' Political Views of Blacks in the Context of Welfare and Crime." *American Journal of Political Science* 41, no. 1 (1997): 30–60.

Peña, Lorgia García. *The Borders of Dominicanidad: Race, Nation, and Archives of Contradiction*. Durham, NC: Duke University Press, 2016.

Peña, Lorgia García. *Translating Blackness: Latinx Colonialities in Global Perspective*. Durham, NC: Duke University Press, 2022.

Pérez, Debra Joy, Lisa Fortuna, and Margarita Alegría. "Prevalence and Correlates of Everyday Discrimination Among U.S. Latinos." *Journal of Community Psychology* 36, no. 4 (2008): 421–33.

Peterson, Andrea. "Why It's So Hard to Find a Therapist Who Takes Insurance." *Wall Street Journal*, October 5, 2021. https://www.wsj.com/articles/why-its-so-hard-to-find-a-therapist-who-takes-insurance-11633442400.

Pham, Huyen, and Pham Hoang Van. "Subfederal Immigration Regulation and the Trump Effect." *New York University Law Review* 94, no. 1 (2019): 125–70. https://www.nyulawreview.org/issues/volume-94-number-1/subfederal-immigration-regulation-and-the-trump-effect/.

Phelan, Jo, and Bruce Link. "Controlling Disease and Creating Disparities: A Fundamental Cause Perspective." *Journals of Gerontology: Series B* 60, Special Issue 2 (2005): S27–S33. https://doi.org/10.1093/geronb/60.Special_Issue_2.S27.

Pierce, Sarah and Andrew Selee. *Immigration Under Trump: A Review of Policy Shifts in the Year Since the Election*. Migration Policy Institute, December 2017. https://www.migrationpolicy.org/research/immigration-under-trump-review-policy-shifts.

Pierson, Paul. "Federalism, Race, and the American Welfare State." In *Federalism and the Welfare State in a Multicultural World*, edited by Elizabeth Goodyear-Grant,

Richard Johnston, Will Kymlicka and John Myles, 131–50. Montreal, CAN: McGill-Queen's University Press, 2018.

Pillai, Drishti, and Samantha Artiga. *2022 Changes to the Public Charge Inadmissibility Rule and the Implications for Health Care,* Kaiser Family Foundation, 2022. https://www.kff.org/racial-equity-and-health-policy/issue-brief/2022-changes-to -the-public-charge-inadmissibility-rule-and-the-implications-for-health-care/.

Pillai, Drishti, and Samantha Artiga. *Florida's Recent Immigration Law Could Have Stark Impacts for Families and the State's Economy.* Kaiser Family Foundation, 2023. https://www.kff.org/policy-watch/floridas-recent-immigration-law-could -have-stark-impacts-for-families-and-the-states-economy/.

Politi, Emanuele, Adrian Lüders, Sindhuja Sankaran, Joel Anderson, Jasper Van Assche, Eva Spiritus-Beerden, Antoine Roblain, et al. "The Impact of COVID-19 on the Majority Population, Ethno-Racial Minorities, and Immigrants: A Systematic Literature Review on Threat Appraisals from an Inter-group Perspective." *European Psychologist* 26, no. 4 (2021): 298–309.

Porter, Michael. "What Massachusetts Can Teach America." *Boston Globe*, January 28, 2020. https://www.bostonglobe.com/2020/01/28/opinion/what -massachusetts-can-teach-america/.

Portes, Alejandro, Patricia Fernández-Kelly, and Donald Light. "Life on the Edge: Immigrants Confront the American Health System." *Ethnic and Racial Studies* 35, no. 1 (2012): 3–22.

Portes, Alejandro, and Rubén Rumbaut. *Immigrant America: A Portrait.* Berkeley: University of California Press, 2006.

Portes, Alejandro, and Min Zhou. "The New Second Generation: Segmented Assimilation and Its Variants." *Annals of the American Academy of Political and Social Science* 530, no. 1 (1993): 74–96.

Preloran, H. M., C. H. Browner, and E. Lieber. "Strategies for Motivating Latino Couples' Participation in Qualitative Health Research and Their Effects on Sample Construction." *American Journal of Public Health* 91, no. 11 (2001): 1832–41.

Preston, Julia. "New York Times: Immigration Program Is Rejected by Third State, Massachusetts." United Farm Workers, June 6, 2011. https://ufw.org/New-York -Times-Immigration-Program-Is-Rejected-by-Third-State-Massachusetts/.

Preston, Julia. "Despite Opposition, Immigration Agency to Expand Fingerprint Program." *New York Times*, May 11, 2012. https://www.nytimes.com/2012/05 /12/us/ice-to-expand-secure-communities-program-in-mass-and-ny.html.

Prewitt, Kenneth. "Racial Classification in America: Where Do We Go from Here?" *Daedalus* 134, no. 1 (2005): 5–17.

Provine, Doris, and Roxanne Doty. "The Criminalization of Immigrants as a Racial Project." *Journal of Contemporary Criminal Justice* 27, no. 3 (2011): 261–77.

Quisumbing King, Katrina. "Recentering U.S. Empire: A Structural Perspective on the Color Line." *Sociology of Race and Ethnicity* 5, no. 1 (2018): 11–25. https:// journals.sagepub.com/doi/10.1177/2332649218761977.

Rabin, David L., Anuradha Jetty, Stephen Petterson, and Allison Froehlich. "Under the ACA Higher Deductibles and Medical Debt Cause Those Most Vulnerable to

Defer Needed Care." *Journal of Health Care for the Poor and Underserved* 31, no. 1 (2020): 424–40. https://muse.jhu.edu/article/747797.

Raff, Jeremy. "How Fear Spreads the Coronavirus." *The Atlantic*, May 29, 2020. https://www.theatlantic.com/politics/archive/2020/05/immigrants-sick-covid -19-are-scared-seek-help/612142/.

Ramos, Tere. *Language Rights of Limited English Proficient Individuals*. Massachu- setts Law Reform Institute, May 16, 2016.

Rampell, Catherine "Trump Didn't Build His Border Wall with Steel. He Built It out of Paper." *Washington Post*, October 29, 2020. https://www.washingtonpost.com /opinions/2020/10/29/trump-immigration-daca-family-separation/?arc404 =true&s=03.

Rascoe, Ayesha, and Angela Kocherga. "The Biden Administration Is Building a Controversial Part of the Border Wall in Texas." *NPR*, October 8, 2023. https:// www.npr.org/2023/10/08/1204545880/the-biden-administration-is-building-a -controversial-part-of-the-border-wall-in-.

Raudenbush, Danielle. *Health Care Off the Books: Poverty, Illness, and Strategies of Survival in Urban America*. Berkeley: University of California Press, 2020.

Ray, Victor. "A Theory of Racialized Organizations." *American Sociological Review* 84, no. 1 (2019): 26–53.

Ray, Victor. *On Critical Race Theory: Why It Matters and Why You Should Care*. New York: Penguin Random House, 2022.

Ray, Victor, Pamela Herd, and Donald Moynihan. "Racialized Burdens: Applying Racialized Organization Theory to the Administrative State." *Journal of Public Administration Research and Theory* 33, no. 1 (2023): 139–52. https://doi.org/10 .1093/jopart/muac001.

Reeves, Aaron, Martin McKee, and David Stuckler. "The Attack on Universal Health Coverage in Europe: Recession, Austerity, and Unmet Needs." *European Journal of Public Health* 25, no. 3 (2015): 364–65.

Reilly, Adam. "In Everett's Mayoral Race, Identity and Governing Style Are Both on the Ballot." *WGBH News*, September 9, 2021. https://www.wgbh.org/news /politics/2021/09/09/in-everetts-mayoral-race-identity-and-governing-style -are-both-on-the-ballot.

Reingold, Beth, and Adrienne Smith. "Welfare Policymaking and Intersections of Race, Ethnicity, and Gender in U.S. State Legislatures." *American Journal of Political Science* 56, no. 1 (2012): 131–47.

Reinhart, R. J. "In the News: Americans' Satisfaction with Their Healthcare." *Gallup*, February 2, 2018. https://news.gallup.com/poll/226607/news -americans-satisfaction-healthcare.aspx.

Reverby, Susan. *Examining Tuskegee: The Infamous Syphilis Study and Its Legacy*. Chapel Hill: University of North Carolina Press, 2009.

Rhodan, Maya, and Elizabeth Dias. "Immigration Agents Arrested Men Outside a Church. But Officials Say It Was Just a Coincidence." *Time*, February 17, 2017. https://time.com/4674729/immigrations-church-sensitive-policy -concerns/.

Rhodes, Scott, Lilli Mann, Florence Simán, Eunyoung Song, Jorge Alonzo, Mario Downs, Emma Lawlor, et al. "The Impact of Local Immigration Enforcement Policies on the Health of Immigrant Hispanics/Latinos in the United States." *American Journal of Public Health* 105, no. 2 (2015): 329–37.

Rice, Thomas, Pauline Rosenau, Lynn Unruh, Andrew Barnes, Richard Saltman, and Ewout van Ginneken. "United States of America: Health System Review." *Health Systems in Transition* 15, no. 3 (2013): 1–431.

Rikard, R. V., Maxine S. Thompson, Julie McKinney, and Alison Beauchamp. "Examining Health Literacy Disparities in the United States: A Third Look at the National Assessment of Adult Literacy (NAAL)." *BMC Public Health* 16, no. 1 (2016): 975–11.

Rios, Simon. "Trump's Border Policies Mean Tougher Path for Brazilian Immigrants in Mass." *WBUR*, July 24, 2018. https://www.wbur.org/news/2018/07/24 /brazilian-immigrants-massachusetts.

Robertson, David. *Federalism and the Making of America.* New York: Routledge, 2017.

Robeznieks, Andis. *Doctor Shortages Are Here—and They'll Get Worse If We Don't Act Fast.* American Medical Association, 2022. https://www.ama-assn.org/practice -management/sustainability/doctor-shortages-are-here-and-they-ll-get-worse -if-we-don-t-act.

Rocheleau, Matt. "Greater Boston Home to 180,000 Undocumented Immigrants, Report Finds." *Boston Globe,* February 17, 2017. https://www.bostonglobe.com /metro/2017/02/17/greater-boston-home-undocumented-immigrants-report -finds/dFVIV8Qf3HjsxVeFYEgbAP/story.html.

Rodriguez, Clara. *Changing Race: Latinos, the Census and the History of Ethnicity.* New York: New York University Press, 2000.

Rodriguez, Michael, Kathryn Kietzman, Brenda Morales, and Nadereh Pourat. *Despite Documented Status, Many California Immigrants Have Negative Perceptions or Experiences of Public Charge Policy.* Health Policy Fact Sheet, UCLA Center for Health Policy Research, April 13, 2022. https://healthpolicy.ucla.edu /publications/Documents/PDF/2022/CA-Immigrants-Public-Charge-Policy -factsheet-apr2022.pdf.

Rodriguez, Robert, Jesus Torres, Jennifer Sun, Harrison Alter, Carolina Ornelas, Mayra Cruz, Leah Fraimow-Wong, et al. "Declared Impact of the US President's Statements and Campaign Statements on Latino Populations' Perceptions of Safety and Emergency Care Access." *PLOS ONE* 14, no. 10 (2019): e0222837. https://doi.org/10.1371/journal.pone.0222837.

Rodríguez-Muñiz, Michael. *Figures of the Future: Latino Civil Rights and the Politics of Demographic Change.* Princeton, NJ: Princeton University Press, 2021.

Romero, Simon, Caitlin Dickerson, Miriam Jordan, and Patricia Mazzei. "It Feels Like Being Hunted: Latinos Across U.S. In Fear After El Paso Massacre." *New York Times,* August 6, 2019a. https://www.nytimes.com/2019/08/06/us/el-paso -shooting-latino-anxiety.html.

Romero, Simon, Zolan Kanno-Youngs, Manny Fernandez, Daniel Borunda, Aaron Montes, and Caitlin Dickerson. "Hungry, Scared and Sick: Inside the Migration Detection Center in Clint, Tex." *New York Times*, July 7, 2019b. https://www.nytimes.com/interactive/2019/07/06/us/migrants-border-patrol-clint.html.

Rose, Carol, and Laura Rotolo. "Somerville's Smart Immigration Move—and Why the Rest of Mass. Should Follow." *WBUR*, May 21, 2014. https://www.wbur.org/cognoscenti/2014/05/21/secure-communities-carol-rose-and-laura-rotolo.

Rose, Joel. "Some Republicans Blame Migrants for COVID-19 Surges. Doctors Say They're Scapegoating." *NPR*, August 10, 2021. https://www.npr.org/2021/08/10/1026178171/republicans-migrants-covid-19-surges.

Roth, Wendy. *Race Migrations: Latinos and the Cultural Transformation of Race*. Palo Alto, CA: Stanford University Press, 2012.

Roy, Ananya. "The City in the Age of Trumpism: From Sanctuary to Abolition." *Environment and Planning D: Society and Space* 37, no. 5 (2019): 761–78. https://doi.org/10.1177/0263775819830969.

Rudowitz, Robin, Elizabeth Williams, Elizabeth Hinton, and Rachel Garfield. *Medicaid Financing: The Basics*. Kaiser Family Foundation, April 13, 2023, https://www.kff.org/medicaid/issue-brief/medicaid-financing-the-basics/#:~:text=Medicaid%20accounted%20for%207%20percent,federal%20government%20and%20the%20states.

Russell, Jenna. "As Migrants Are Placed Around Massachusetts, Towns Are Welcoming but Worried." *New York Times*, September 10, 2023. https://www.nytimes.com/2023/09/10/us/migrant-crisis-massachusetts-woburn.html.

Ryan, Jillian, Luke Lopian, Brian Le, Sarah Edney, Gisela Van Kessel, Ronald Plotnikoff, Corneel Vandelanotte, Tim Olds, and Carol Maher. "It's Not Raining Men: A Mixed-Methods Study Investigating Methods of Improving Male Recruitment to Health Behavior Research." *BMC Public Health* 19, no. 814 (2019): 1–9. https://doi.org/10.1186/s12889-019-7087-4.

Sacchetti, Maria, and Marissa Lang. "On Immigration, Patrick Is Measured." *Boston.com*, July 22, 2010. http://archive.boston.com/news/local/massachusetts/articles/2010/07/22/on_immigration_patrick_is_measured/.

Sadler, Georgia Robins, Hau-Chen Lee, Rod Seung-Hwan Lim, and Judith Fullerton. "Recruitment of Hard-to-Reach Population Subgroups via Adaptions of the Snowball Sampling Strategy." *Nursing and Health Sciences* 12, no. 3 (2010): 369–74. https://doi.org/https://doi.org/10.1111/j.1442-2018.2010.00541.x.

Sáenz, Rogelio, and Karen Manges Douglas. "A Call for the Racialization of Immigration Studies: On the Transition of Ethnic Immigrants to Racialized Immigrants." *Sociology of Race and Ethnicity* 1, no. 1 (2015): 166–80.

Saha, Somnath, Jose J. Arbelaez, and Lisa A. Cooper. "Patient-Physician Relationships and Racial Disparities in the Quality of Health Care." *American Journal of Public Health* 93, no. 10 (2003): 1713–19. https://doi.org/10.2105/ajph.93.10.1713.

Sainato, Michael. "'Your Mouth Becomes a Minefield': The Americans Who Can't Afford the Dentist." *The Guardian*, May 4, 2021. https://www.theguardian.com/us-news/2021/may/04/americans-dental-dentist-teeth-health-insurance.

Salkeld, Glenn. "What Are the Benefits of Preventive Health Care?" *Health Care Analysis* 6 (1998): 106–12. https://doi.org/10.1007/BF02678116.

Salsberg, Edward, Chelsea Richwine, Sara Westergaard, Maria Portela Martinez, Toyese Oyeyemi, Anushree Vichare, and Candice Chen. "Estimation and Comparison of Current and Future Racial/Ethnic Representation in the US Health Care Workforce." *JAMA Network Open* 4, no. 3 (2021): e213789. https://doi.org/10.1001/jamanetworkopen.2021.3789.

Sanchez, Gabriel, Natalie Masuoka, and Brooke Abrams. "Revisiting the Brown-Utility Heuristic: A Comparison of Latino Linked Fate in 2006 and 2016." *Politics, Groups, and Identities* 7, no. 3 (2019): 673–83. https://doi.org/10.1080/21565503.2019.1638803.

Sanchez, Gabriel, and Patricia Rodriguez Espinosa. "Does the Race of the Discrimination Agent in Latinos' Discrimination Experiences Influence Latino Group Identity?" *Sociology of Race and Ethnicity* 2, no. 4 (2016): 531–47. https://doi.org/10.1177/2332649215624237.

Sanchez, Gabriel, Edward Vargas, Melina Juarez, Barbara Aguinaga-Gomez, and Francisco Pedraza. "Nativity and Citizenship Status Affect Latinos' Health Insurance Coverage Under the ACA." *Journal of Ethnic and Migration Studies* 43, no. 12 (2017): 2037–54.

Sanchez, Gabriella, and Mary Romero. "Critical Race Theory in the US Sociology of Immigration." *Sociology Compass* 4 (2010): 779–88.

Sands, Geneva. "Arrests of Brazilian Migrants Entering US Illegally Spiked in 2019 Amid Border Surge." *CNN.com*, December 11, 2019. https://www.cnn.com/2019/12/11/politics/arrests-brazilian-migrants-spiked-2019-border-surge/index.html.

Sangalang, Cindy, David Becerra, Felicia Mitchell, Stephanie Lechuga-Peña, Kristina Lopez, and Isok Kim. "Trauma, Post-Migration Stress, and Mental Health: A Comparative Analysis of Refugees and Immigrants in the United States." *Journal of Immigrant and Minority Health* 21, no. 5 (2019): 909–19.

Sangaramoorthy, Thurka. *Landscapes of Care: Immigration and Health in Rural America*. Chapel Hill, NC: University of North Carolina Press, 2023.

Santana, Emilce. "Situating Perceived Discrimination: How Do Skin Color and Acculturation Shape Perceptions of Discrimination Among Latinos?" *Sociological Quarterly* 59, no. 4 (2018): 655–77.

Sarría-Santamera, Antonio, Ana Isabel Hijas-Gómez, Rocío Carmona, and Luís Andrés Gimeno-Feliú. "A Systematic Review of the Use of Health Services by Immigrants and Native Populations." *Public Health Reviews* 37, no. 1 (2016): 1–29.

Schinkel, Sanne, Barbara Schouten, Fatmagül Kerpiclik, Bas Van Den Putte, and Julia Van Weert. "Perceptions of Barriers to Patient Participation: Are They Due to Language, Culture, or Discrimination?" *Health Communication* 34, no. 12 (2018): 1469–81. https://doi.org/10.1080/10410236.2018.1500431.

Schmidt, Laura. "Unequal Coverage: The Experience of Health Care Reform in the United States." *Medical Anthropological Quarterly* 33, no. 3 (2019).

Schneider, Eric, Arnav Shah, Michelle Doty, Roosa Tikkanen, Katharine Fields, and Reginald D. Williams II. *Mirror, Mirror 2021—Reflecting Poorly: Health Care in the*

U.S. Compared to Other High-Income Countries. Commonwealth Fund, August 2021. https://www.commonwealthfund.org/sites/default/files/2021-08/Schneider_Mirror_Mirror_2021.pdf.

Schoen, Cathy, Robin Osborn, David Squires, Michelle Doty, Roz Pierson, and Sandra Applebaum. "How Health Insurance Design Affects Access to Care and Costs, by Income, in Eleven Countries." *Health Affairs* 29, no. 12 (2010): 2323–34. https://www.healthaffairs.org/doi/abs/10.1377/hlthaff.2010.0862.

Schoenberg, Shira. "Gov. Charlie Baker on ICE Raids: Feds Should Focus on Criminals." *Mass Live,* September 29, 2017. https://www.masslive.com/politics/2017/09/gov_charlie_baker_on_ice_raids.html.

Schut, Rebecca Anna, and Courtney Boen. "State Immigration Policy Contexts and Racialized Legal Status Disparities in Health Care Utilization Among US Agricultural Workers." *Demography* 59, no. 6 (2022): 2079–107.

Seifert, Robert, and Kelly Anthoula Love. *What to Know About ACOs: An Introduction to MassHealth Accountable Care Organizations.* Blue Cross Blue Shield of Massachusetts Foundation, 2018. https://www.bluecrossmafoundation.org/publication/what-know-about-acos-introduction-masshealth-accountable-care-organizations.

Sekhavat, Sarang. "Public Charge." Presentation at Health Care for All Democracy School, Boston, MA, May 16, 2019.

Selod, Saher. *Forever Suspect: Racialized Surveillance of Muslim Americans in the War on Terror.* New Brunswick, NJ: Rutgers University Press, 2018.

Sewell, Alyasah Ali. "The Racism–Race Reification Process: A Mesolevel Political Economic Framework for Understanding Racial Health Disparities." *Sociology of Race and Ethnicity* 2, no. 4 (2016): 402–32.

Sewell, Alyasah Ali, Justin M. Feldman, Rashawn Ray, Keon L. Gilbert, Kevin A. Jefferson, and Hedwig Lee. "Illness Spillovers of Lethal Police Violence: The Significance of Gendered Marginalization." *Ethnic and Racial Studies* 44 (2020): 1089–114. https://doi.org/10.1080/01419870.2020.1781913.

Shamsi, Hilal, Abdullah Almutairi, Sulaiman Al Mashrafi, and Talib Al Kalbani. "Implications of Language Barriers for Healthcare: A Systematic Review." *Oman Medical Journal* 35, no. 2 (2020): e122. https://doi.org/10.5001/omj.2020.40.

Shavers, Vickie, Fagan Pebbles, Dionne Jones, William Klein, Josephine Boyington, Carmen Moten, and Edward Rorie. "The State of Research on Racial/Ethnic Discrimination in the Receipt of Health Care." *American Journal of Public Health* 102, no. 5 (2012): 953–66.

Shaw, April, and Leila Barraza. *The Public Charge Rule and the Threat to Public Health.* Network for Public Health Law, 2020. https://www.networkforphl.org/resources/the-public-charge-rule-and-the-threat-to-public-health/?blm_aid=145255774.

Shear, Michael, and Miriam Jordan. "Undoing Trump's Anti-Immigrant Policies Will Mean Looking at the Fine Print." *New York Times,* February 10, 2021. https://www.nytimes.com/2021/02/10/us/politics/trump-biden-us-immigration-system.html.

Shoichet, Catherine. "As the US Rolls Out the Welcome Mat for Ukrainian Refugees, Some See a Double Standard at the Border." *CNN.com*, March 29, 2022. https://www.cnn.com/2022/03/29/us/ukrainians-us-mexico-border-cec/index.html.

Silver, Alexis. *Shifting Boundaries: Immigrant Youth Negotiating National, State, and Small-Town Politics*. Palo Alto, CA: Stanford University Press, 2018.

Simmons-Duffin, Selena. "Trump Is Trying Hard to Thwart Obamacare. How's That Going?" *NPR*, October 14, 2019. https://www.npr.org/sections/health-shots/2019/10/14/768731628/trump-is-trying-hard-to-thwart-obamacare-hows-that-going.

Singh, Maanvi. "'I Have a Broken Heart': Trump Policy Has Immigrants Backing Away from Healthcare Amid Crisis." *The Guardian*, March 29, 2020. https://www.theguardian.com/world/2020/mar/29/i-have-a-broken-heart-trump-policy-has-immigrants-backing-away-from-healthcare-amid-crisis.

Skloot, Rebecca. *The Immortal Life of Henrietta Lacks*. New York: Crown, 2010.

Slauson-Blevins, Kathleen, and Katherine Johnson. "Doing Gender, Doing Surveys? Women's Gatekeeping and Men's Non-Participation in Multi-Actor Reproductive Surveys." *Sociological Inquiry* 86, no. 3 (2016): 427–49.

Small, Mario Luis. "Neighborhood Institutions as Resource Brokers: Childcare Centers, Interorganizational Ties, and Resource Access Among the Poor." *Social Problems* 53, no. 2 (2006): 274–92. https://doi.org/10.1525/sp.2006.53.2.274.

Smedley, Brian, Adrienne Stith, and Alan Nelson, eds. *Unequal Treatment: Confronting Racial and Ethnic Disparities in Health Care*. National Academies of Sciences, Engineering, and Medicine, 2003. https://doi.org/10.17226/12875.

Smith, David Barton. *The Power to Heal: Civil Rights, Medicare, and the Struggle to Transform America's Healthcare System*. Nashville, TN: Vanderbilt University Press, 2016.

Smith, Rogers. *Civic Ideals: Conflicting Visions of Citizenship in US History*. New Haven, CT: Yale University Press, 1997.

Snowden, Lonnie, and Genevieve Graff. "The 'Undeserving Poor,' Racial Bias, and Medicaid Coverage of African Americans." *Journal of Black Psychology* 45, no. 3 (2019): 130–42.

Snyder, C. R., B. K. Frogner, and S. M. Skillman. "Facilitating Racial and Ethnic Diversity in the Health Workforce." *Journal of Allied Health* 47, no. 1 (2018): 58–65.

Solberg, Robert, Brandy Edwards, Jeffrey Chidester, Debra Perina, William Brady, and Michael Williams. "The Prehospital and Hospital Costs of Emergency Care for Frequent ED Patients." *American Journal of Emergency Medicine* 34, no. 3 (2016): 459–63. https://www.sciencedirect.com/science/article/pii/S0735675715010529.

Sommers, Benjamin. "The Perils of a Patchwork System." *Boston Globe*, December 16, 2019. https://www.bostonglobe.com/2019/12/16/opinion/perils-patchwork-system/.

Sommers, Benjamin, Robert Blendon, E. John Orav, and Arnold Epstein. "Changes in Utilization and Health Among Low-Income Adults After Medicaid Expansion or Expanded Private Insurance." *JAMA Internal Medicine* 176, no. 10 (2016): 1501–509.

Sommers, Benjamin, Bethany Maylone, Robert Blendon, E. John Orav, and Arnold Epstein. "Three-Year Impacts of the Affordable Care Act: Improved Medical Care and Health Among Low-Income Adults." *Health Affairs* 36, no. 6 (2017): 1119–28.

Sørensen, Kristine, Stephan Van den Broucke, James Fullam, Gerardine Doyle, Jürgen Pelikan, Zofia Slonska, and Helmut Brand. "Health Literacy and Public Health: A Systematic Review and Integration of Definitions and Models." *BMC Public Health* 12, no. 1 (2012): 80.

Soss, Joe, Sanford Schram, Thomas Vartanian, and Erin O'Brien. "The Hard Line and the Color Line: Race, Welfare, and the Roots of Get-Tough Reform." In *Race and the Politics of Welfare Reform*, edited by Sanford F. Schram, Joe Soss, and Richard C. Fording, 225–53. Ann Arbor: University of Michigan Press, 2003.

Sparer, Michael, George France, and Chelsea Clinton. "Inching Toward Incrementalism: Federalism, Devolution, and Health Policy in the United States and the United Kingdom." *Journal of Health Policy, Politics, and Law* 36, no. 1 (2011): 33–57. https://doi.org/10.1215/03616878-1191099.

Spithoven, Antoon. "The Influence of Vested Interests on Healthcare Legislation in the USA, 2009–2010." *Journal of Economic Issues* 50, no. 2 (2016): 630–38. https://doi.org/10.1080/00213624.2016.1179073.

Spocchia, Gino. "Final Tally of Lies: Analysts Say Trump Told 30,000 Mistruths— That's 21 a Day—During Presidency." *The Independent*, January 21, 2021. https://www.independent.co.uk/news/world/americas/us-election-2020/trump -lies-false-presidency-b1790285.html.

Stargardter, Gabriel. "A Brazilian Town Empties as Migration to U.S. Accelerates." *Reuters*, November 30, 2021. https://www.reuters.com/world/americas /brazilian-town-empties-migration-us-accelerates-2021-11-30/.

Starr, Paul. *The Social Transformation of American Medicine*. New York: Basic Books, 1982.

Steinberg, Emma, Doris Valenzuela-Araujo, Joseph Zickafoose, Edith Kieffer, and Lisa Ross DeCamp. "The 'Battle' of Managing Language Barriers in Health Care." *Clinical Pediatric* 55, no. 14 (2016): 1318–27.

Stepanikova, Irena, and Gabriela Oates. "Perceived Discrimination and Privilege in Health Care: The Role of Socioeconomic Status and Race." *American Journal of Preventative Medicine* 52, no. 1 (2017): S86–S94.

Strauss, Anselm, and Juliet Corbin. *Basics of Qualitative Research: Techniques and Procedures for Developing Grounded Theory*. 3rd ed. New York: Sage Publications, 1998.

Struyk, Ryan. "67 Times Donald Trump Tweeted About the 'Birther' Movement." *ABC News*, September 17, 2016. https://abcnews.go.com/Politics/67-times -donald-trump-tweeted-birther-movement/story?id=42145590.

Stumpf, Juliet. "The Crimmigration Crisis: Immigrants, Crime, and Sovereign Power." *American University Law Review* 56, no. 2 (2006): 367–419.

Sullivan, Laura, Tatjana Meschede, Lars Dietrich, and Thomas Shapiro. *The Racial Wealth Gap: Why Policy Matters.* Institute for Assets and Social Policy, Brandeis University, 2015.

Sun, Ken Chih-Yan. *Time and Migration: How Long-Term Taiwanese Migrants Negotiate Later Life.* Ithaca, NY: Cornell University Press, 2021.

Suro, Roberto, and Hannah Findling. *State and Local Aid for Immigrants During the COVID-19 Pandemic: Innovating Inclusion.* Center for Migration Studies, July 8, 2020. https://cmsny.org/publications/state-local-aid-immigrants-covid-19 -pandemic-innovating-inclusion/.

Swartz, Katherine. *Reinsuring Health: Why More Middle-Class People Are Uninsured and What Government Can Do.* New York: Russell Sage Foundation, 2006.

Tamborrino, Kelsey. "Trump Administration Officials Defend Mississippi Immigration Raids." *Politico,* August 11, 2019. https://www.politico.com/story/2019/08 /11/trump-immigration-raids-mississippi-1457761.

Tartaglia, Mike. "Private Prisons, Private Records." *Boston University Law Review* 94, no. 5 (2014): 1689–744. https://www.proquest.com/docview/1626355719.

Teles, Steven. "Kludgeocracy in America." *National Affairs* (Fall 2013). https://www .nationalaffairs.com/publications/detail/kludgeocracy-in-america.

Telles, Edward, and Project on Ethnicity and Race in Latin America (PERLA). *Pigmentocracies: Social Science Findings from the Project on Ethnicity and Race in Latin America.* Chapel Hill: University of North Carolina Press, 2014.

Terrazas, Aaron. *Salvadoran Immigrants in the United States in 2008.* Migration Policy Institute, 2010. https://www.migrationpolicy.org/article/salvadoran -immigrants-united-states-2008.

Terriquez, Veronica, and Tiffany Joseph. "Ethnoracial Inequality and Insurance Coverage Among Latino Young Adults." *Social Science & Medicine* 168 (2016): 150–58.

Terui, Sachiko. "Conceptualizing the Pathways and Processes Between Language Barriers and Health Disparities: Review, Synthesis, and Extension." *Journal of Immigrant and Minority Health* 19, no. 1 (2017): 215–24.

Thompson, Frank. "Medicaid Rising: The Perils and Potential of Federalism." In *Medicare and Medicaid at 50,* edited by Alan Cohen, David Colby, Keith Wailoo, and Julian Zelizer, chapter 9. New York: Oxford University Press, 2015.

Tikkanen, Roosa, and Melinda Abrams. *U.S. Health Care from a Global Perspective, 2019: Higher Spending, Worse Outcomes?* Commonwealth Fund, January 30, 2020. https://www.commonwealthfund.org/publications/issue-briefs/2020/jan /us-health-care-global-perspective-2019.

Tolbert, Jennifer, Kendal Orgera, Natalie Singer, and Anthony Damico. *Key Facts About the Uninsured Population.* Kaiser Family Foundation, 2019.

Tomes, Nancy. "The Social Transformation of American Medicine: An Historical Perspective." *Sociology of Health and Illness* 7, no. 2 (1985): 248–59. https://doi .org/https://doi.org/10.1111/1467-9566.ep10949093.

Torres-Ardila, Fabián, Iris Gómez, Philip Granberry, and Vicky Pulos. "The Effect of Proposed Changes in Federal Public Charge Policy on Latino U.S. Citizen Children in Massachusetts." *Gastón Institute Publications* 230 (2018). https://scholarworks.umb.edu/cgi/viewcontent.cgi?article=1231&context=gaston_pubs.

Toussaint-Comeau, Maude. "The Occupational Assimilation of Hispanic Immigrants in the U.S.: Evidence from Panel Data." *International Migration Review* 40, no. 3 (2006): 508–36.

Tracy, Natalycia. "Supporting Immigrant Communities in the COVID Pandemic Panel (Virtual)," June 1, 2021.

Trust for America's Health. *The Impact of Chronic Underfunding on America's Public Health System: Trends, Risks, and Recommendations, 2021.* May 2021. https://www.tfah.org/wp-content/uploads/2021/05/2021_PHFunding_Fnl.pdf.

Tu, Tianna, David Muhlestein, S. Lawrence Kocot, and Ross White. *The Impact of Accountable Care: Origins and Future of Accountable Care Organizations.* Brookings Institution, May 2015. https://www.brookings.edu/wp-content/uploads/2016/06/Impact-of-Accountable-CareOrigins-052015.pdf.

Tuan, Mia. *Forever Foreigners or Honorary Whites? The Asian Ethnic Experience Today.* New Brunswick, NJ: Rutgers University Press, 1999.

Tully, Tracey, and Michael Gold. "Long Lines as Undocumented Immigrants in N.Y. Rush to Get Licenses." *New York Times,* December 16, 2019. https://www.nytimes.com/2019/12/16/nyregion/undocumented-immigrant-drivers-license-ny-nj.html.

Tuohy, Brian. "Health Without Papers: Immigrants, Citizenship, and Health in the 21st Century." *Social Forces* 98, no. 3 (2020): 1052–73. https://doi.org/10.1093/sf/soz048.

Ugas, Mohamed, Mackinnon, Rebecca, Amadasun, Shawn, Escamilla, Zaira, Gill, Bhajan, Guiliani, Meredith, Fazelzad, Rouhi, Martin, Hilary, Samoil, Diana, and Papadakos, Janet. "Associations of Health Literacy and Health Outcomes Among Populations with Limited Language Proficiency: A Scoping Review." *Journal of Health Care for the Poor and Underserved* 34, no. 2 (2023): 731–57. https://doi.org/doi:10.1353/hpu.2023.0039.

Uggen, Christopher, and Jeff Manza. "Democratic Contraction? The Political Consequences of Felon Disenfranchisement in the United States." *American Sociological Review* 67, no. 6 (2002): 777–803. https://www.researchgate.net/publication/238215000_Democratic_Contraction_The_Political_Consequences_of_Felon_Disenfranchisement_in_the_United_States.

US Census Bureau. "Quick Facts: Massachusetts." July 1, 2019. https://www.census.gov/quickfacts/fact/table/MA,US/COM100221.

US Census Bureau. "Quick Facts: Boston, Massachusetts." 2021. https://www.census.gov/quickfacts/fact/map/US,bostoncitymassachusetts/AGE295218.

US Citizenship and Immigration Services (USCIS). "Refugees and Asylum." 2015. https://www.uscis.gov/humanitarian/refugees-asylum.

USCIS. "Early American Immigration Policies." 2020. https://www.uscis.gov/about-us/our-history/overview-of-ins-history/early-american-immigration-policies.

USCIS. "Chapter 2: Grounds for Revocation of Naturalization." 2022. https://www
.uscis.gov/policy-manual/volume-12-part-l-chapter-2.

USCIS. "Temporary Protected Status." 2024, accessed July 1, 2024. https://www
.uscis.gov/humanitarian/temporary-protected-status.

USCIS. "Chapter 3—Continuous Residence." 2023b, accessed October 30, 2023.
https://www.uscis.gov/policy-manual/volume-12-part-d-chapter-3.

US Department of Health and Human Services. *National Action Plan to Improve
Health Literacy*. Office of Disease Prevention and Health Promotion, 2010.

US Department of Health and Human Services. "New HHS Data Show More
Americans Than Ever Have Health Coverage through the Affordable Care Act."
June 5, 2021. https://www.cms.gov/newsroom/press-releases/new-hhs-data
-show-more-americans-ever-have-health-coverage-through-affordable-care-act.

US Department of State. *Report of the Visa Office 2016*. Bureau of Consular Affairs,
2016.

US Department of State. "Directory of Visa Categories." n.d., accessed October 30,
2023. https://travel.state.gov/content/travel/en/us-visas/visa-information
-resources/all-visa-categories.html.

Uzogara, Ekeoma. "Who Desires In-Group Neighbors? Associations of Skin Tone
Biases and Discrimination with Latinas' Segregation Preferences." *Group
Processes & Intergroup Relations* 22, no. 8 (2019): 1196–214. https://doi.org/10
.1177/1368430218788154.

Valdez, Zulema. *The New Entrepreneurs: How Race, Class, and Gender Shape American
Enterprise*. Palo Alto, CA: Stanford University Press, 2011.

Valencia, Milton. "Facing Deadline, City Council Makes Moves on Immigration,
Wetlands, Taxes." *Boston Globe,* December 11, 2019. https://www.bostonglobe
.com/metro/2019/12/11/facing-deadline-city-council-makes-moves
-immigration-wetlands-taxes/tbUulJHQswhPFCKYDxvb6K/story.html.

Valencia, Milton. "Immigrant Advocates Concerned with Public Charge Rule."
Boston Globe, February 24, 2020. https://www.bostonglobe.com/2020/02/24
/metro/immigrant-advocates-concerned-with-public-charge-rule/.

Valle, Ariana. "Race and the Empire-State: Puerto Ricans' Unequal U.S. Citizenship." *Sociology of Race and Ethnicity* 5, no. 1 (2018): 26–40. https://doi.org/10
.1177/2332649218776031.

Vandenbroucke, Jan, Erik von Elm, Douglas Altman, Peter Gøtzsche, Cynthia
Mulrow, Stuart Pocock, Charles Poole, James Schlesselman, and Matthias
Egger. "Strengthening the Reporting of Observational Studies in Epidemiology
(Strobe): Explanation and Elaboration." *PLOS Medicine* 4, no. 10 (2007): e297.
https://doi.org/10.1371/journal.pmed.0040297.

Van Natta, Meredith. "First Do No Harm: Medical Legal Violence and Immigrant
Health in Coral County, USA." *Social Science & Medicine* 235 (2019). https://doi
.org/10.1016/j.socscimed.2019.112411.

Van Natta, Meredith. *Medical Legal Violence: Health Care and Immigration Enforcement Against Latinx Noncitizens*. New York: New York University Press, 2023.

Van Natta, Meredith, Nancy Burke, Irene Yen, Mark Fleming, Christoph Hanss-mann, Maryani Palupy Rasidjan, and Janet Shim. "Stratified Citizenship, Stratified Health: Examining Latinx Legal Status in the U.S. Healthcare Safety Net." *Social Science & Medicine* 220 (2019): 49–55.

Vargas, Edward, Gabriel Sanchez, and Melina Juárez. "The Impact of Punitive Immigrant Laws on the Health of Latina/O Populations." *Politics & Policy* 45, no. 3 (2017): 312–37. https://onlinelibrary.wiley.com/doi/abs/10.1111/polp.12203.

Vargas, Robert. *Uninsured in Chicago: How the Social Safety Net Leaves Latinos Behind*. New York: New York University Press, 2022.

Varsanyi, Monica. *Taking Local Control: Immigration Policy Activism in U.S. Cities and States*. Palo Alto, CA: Stanford University, 2010.

Varsanyi, Monica, P. G. Lewis, D. M. Provine, and S. Decker. "A Multilayered Jurisdictional Patchwork: Immigration Federalism in the United States." *Law & Policy* 34, no. 2 (2012): 138–58.

Vesely, Colleen, Diamond Bravo, and Mariana Guzzardo. *Immigrant Families Across the Life Course: Policy Impacts on Physical and Mental Health*. National Council on Family Relations, July 9, 2019. https://www.ncfr.org/resources/research-and-policy-briefs/immigrant-families-across-life-course-policy-impacts-physical-and-mental-health.

Viladrich, Anahí. "Beyond Welfare Reform: Reframing Undocumented Immigrants' Entitlement to Health Care in the United States, a Critical Review." *Social Science & Medicine* 74, no. 6 (2012): 822–29. http://dx.doi.org/10.1016/j.socscimed.2011.05.050.

Viladrich, Anahí, and Barbara Tagliaferro. "Picking Fruit from Our Backyard's Trees: The Meaning of Nostalgia in Shaping Latinas' Eating Practices in the United States." *Appetite* 97 (2016): 101–10. https://doi.org/10.1016/j.appet.2015.11.017.

Villalobos, Bianca, Juventino Hernandez Rodriguez, and Cynthia Funes. "Prejudice Regarding Latinx-Americans." In *Prejudice, Stigma, Privilege, and Oppression*, edited by L. Benuto, M. Duckworth, A. Masuda, and W. O'Donohue, 77–90. New York: Springer International Publishing, 2020.

Villarosa, Linda. *Under the Skin: The Hidden Toll of Racism on American Lives and on the Health of Our Nation*. New York: Doubleday Press, 2022.

Villazor, Rose Cuison. "'Sanctuary Cities' and Local Citizenship." *Fordham Urban Law Journal* 37, no. 2 (2010): 573–98.

Villazor, Rose Cuison, and Kevin Johnson. "The Trump Administration and the War on Immigration Diversity." *Wake Forest Law Review* 54, no. 2 (2019): 575–616.

Virdee, Satnam, and Brendan McGeever. "Racism, Crisis, Brexit." *Ethnic and Racial Studies* 41, no. 10 (2018): 1802–19. https://doi.org/10.1080/01419870.2017.1361544.

Viruell-Fuentes, E. A., P. Y. Miranda, and S. Abdulrahim. "More than Culture: Structural Racism, Intersectionality Theory, and Immigrant Health." *Social Science & Medicine* 75, no. 12 (2012): 2099–106.

Vujicic, Marko, and Chelsea Fosse. "Time for Dental Care to Be Considered Essential in US Health Care Policy." *AMA Journal of Ethics* 24, no. 1 (2022): E57–63. https://doi.org/doi: 10.1001/amajethics.2022.57.

Waldinger, Roger. "A Cross-Border Perspective on Migration: Beyond the Assimilation/Transnationalism Debate." *Journal of Ethnic and Migration Studies* 43 (2017): 3–17. https://www.tandfonline.com/doi/full/10.1080/1369183X.2016.1238863.

Walsh, Martin. "Amendments to 'Boston Trust Act' Announced." City of Boston, June 14, 2019.

Ward, Nicole, and Jeanne Batalova. *Frequently Requested Statistics on Immigrants and Immigration in the United States.* Migration Policy Institute, March 14, 2023. https://www.migrationpolicy.org/article/frequently-requested-statistics-immigrants-and-immigration-united-states#unauthorized.

Warner, David. "Access to Health Services for Immigrants in the USA: From the Great Society to the 2010 Health Reform Act and After." *Ethnic and Racial Studies* 35 (2012): 40–55.

Watkins-Hayes, Celeste. *The New Welfare Bureaucrats: Entanglements of Race, Class, and Policy Reform.* Chicago: University of Chicago Press, 2009.

Watts, Johnathan. "Operation Car Wash: Is This the Biggest Corruption Scandal in History?" *The Guardian*, June 1, 2017. https://www.theguardian.com/world/2017/jun/01/brazil-operation-car-wash-is-this-the-biggest-corruption-scandal-in-history.

WBUR Newsroom. "The Mass. Medicaid Program Is Changing How It Delivers Health Care." *WBUR*, March 1, 2018. https://www.wbur.org/commonhealth/2018/03/01/masshealth-restructuring-acos.

Welsh, Teresa. "Boston Bombings Trip Up Immigration Debate." *U.S. News & World Report*, April 23, 2013. https://www.usnews.com/opinion/articles/2013/04/23/will-the-boston-bombings-derail-immigration-reform.

Whatley, Monica, and Jeanne Batalova. *Limited English Proficient Population of the United States in 2011.* Migration Policy Institute, 2013. https://www.migrationpolicy.org/article/limited-english-proficient-population-united-states-2011.

White, Augustus. *Seeing Patients: Unconscious Bias in Health Care.* Cambridge, MA: Harvard University Press, 2011.

White, Kari, Valerie Yeager, Nir Menachemi, and Isabel Scarinci. "Impact of Alabama's Immigration Law on Access to Health Care Among Latina Immigrants and Children: Implications for National Reform." *American Journal of Public Health* 104, no. 3 (2014): 397–405.

Willen, Sarah. "Migration, Illegality, and Health: Mapping Embodied Vulnerability and Debating Health Related-Deservingness." *Social Science & Medicine* 74, no. 6 (2012): 805–11.

Williams, David, and Chiquita Collins. "Racial Residential Segregation: A Fundamental Cause of Racial Disparities in Health." *Public Health Reports* 116, no. 5 (2001): 404–16. https://www.ncbi.nlm.nih.gov/pmc/articles/PMC1497358/.

Williams, David, and Lisa Cooper. "Reducing Racial Inequities in Health: Using What We Already Know to Take Action." *International Journal of Environmental Research and Public Health* 16, no. 4 (2019): 606. https://doi.org/10.3390/ijerph16040606.

Williams, David, and Selina Mohammed. "Discrimination and Racial Disparities in Health: Evidence and Needed Research." *Journal of Behavioral Medicine* 32, no. 1 (2009): 20–47.

Williams, David, Selina A. Mohammed, Jacinta Leavell, and Chiquita Collins. "Race, Socioeconomic Status, and Health: Complexities, Ongoing Challenges, and Research Opportunities." *Annals of the New York Academy of Sciences* 1186, no. 1 (2010): 69–101. https://doi.org/10.1111/j.1749-6632.2009.05339.x.

Wilson, Fernando, Leah Zallman, Jose Pagan, Yang Wang, Moosa Tatar, and Jim Stimpson. "Comparison of Use of Health Care Services and Spending for Unauthorized Immigrants vs. Authorized Immigrants or US Citizens Using a Machine Learning Model." *JAMA Network Open* 3, no. 12 (2020): 1–11.

Wilson, Jennifer Fisher. "Massachusetts Health Care Reform Is a Pioneer Effort, but Complications Remain." *Annals of Internal Medicine* 148, no. 6 (2008): 489–92.

Wilson, Jill. *Investing in English Skills: The Limited English Proficient Workforce in U.S. Metropolitan Areas*. Brookings Institution, September 24, 2014, https://www.brookings.edu/articles/investing-in-english-skills-the-limited-english-proficient-workforce-in-u-s-metropolitan-areas/.

Winters, Mike. "Over Half of Americans Have Medical Debt, Even Those with Health Insurance—Here's Why." *CNBC.com*, March 11, 2022. https://www.cnbc.com/2022/03/11/why-55percent-of-americans-have-medical-debt-even-with-health-insurance.html.

Wolcott, Harry. *Transforming Qualitative Data: Description, Analysis, and Interpretation*. Thousands Oak, CA: Sage Publishing, 1994.

Wolfe, Mary, Noreen McDonald, and G. Mark Holmes. "Transportation Barriers to Health Care in the United States: Findings from the National Health Interview Survey, 1997–2017." *American Journal of Public Health* 110, no. 6 (2020): 815–22.

Wong, Tom, and Angela García. "'UnDACAmented' Youth and the Determinants of Applying for Deferred Action: A Nationwide Empirical Analysis of DACA Applications." Presentation at Illegality, Youth, and Belonging Conference, Harvard Graduate School of Education, Cambridge, MA, October 25–26, 2013.

Wong, Tom, Angela García, Marisa Abrajano, David Fitzgerald, Karthick Ramakrishnan, and Sally Le. *Undocumented No More: A Nationwide Analysis of Deferred Action for Childhood Arrivals, or DACA*. Center for American Progress, September 20, 2013. https://www.americanprogress.org/article/undocumented-no-more/.

Wong, Tom, Deborah Kang, Carolina Valdivia, Josefina Espino, Michelle Gonzalez, and Elias Peralta. "How Interior Immigration Enforcement Affects Trust in Law Enforcement." *Perspectives on Politics* 19, no. 2 (2021): 357–70.

Woolf, S. H., and L. Y. Aron. "The U.S. Health Disadvantage Relative to Other High-Income Countries: Findings from a National Research Council / Institute of Medicine Report." *JAMA* 309, no. 8 (2013): 771–72.

World Bank Group. "World Bank in Dominican Republic: Overview." 2020. https://www.worldbank.org/en/country/dominicanrepublic/overview.

Wouters, Olivier J. "Lobbying Expenditures and Campaign Contributions by the Pharmaceutical and Health Product Industry in the United States, 1999–2018." *JAMA Internal Medicine* 180, no. 5 (2020): 688–97. https://doi.org/10.1001/jamainternmed.2020.0146.

Wray-Lake, Laura, Rachel Wells, Lauren Alvis, Sandra Delgado, Amy Syvertsen, and Aaron Metzger. "Being a Latinx Adolescent under a Trump Presidency: Analysis of Latinx Youth's Reactions to Immigration Politics." *Children and Youth Services Review* 87 (April 2018): 192–204.

Wright, B. "Who Governs Federally Qualified Health Centers?" *Journal of Health Politics, Policy, and Law* 38, no. 1 (2013): 27–55. https://doi.org/10.1215/03616878-1898794.

Wu, Connor Y. H., Benjamin F. Zaitchik, Samarth Swarup, and Julia M. Gohlke. "Influence of the Spatial Resolution of the Exposure Estimate in Determining the Association Between Heat Waves and Adverse Health Outcomes." *Annals of the American Association of Geographers* 109, no. 3 (2019): 875–86.

Yazdiha, Hajar. "Exclusion Through Acculturation? Comparing First- and Second-Generation European Muslims' Perceptions of Discrimination Across Four National Contexts." *Ethnic and Racial Studies* 42, no. 5 (2018): 782–800. https://www.tandfonline.com/doi/full/10.1080/01419870.2018.1444186.

Yazdiha, Hajar. "Toward a Du Boisian Framework of Immigrant Incorporation: Racialized Contexts, Relational Identities, and Muslim American Collective Action." *Social Problems* 68, no. 2 (2021): 300–320.

Yee, Vivian. "A Marriage Used to Prevent Deportation. Not Anymore" *New York Times*, April 19, 2018. https://www.nytimes.com/2018/04/19/us/immigration-marriage-green-card.html.

Zallman, L., Lila Flavin, Danny McCormick, and J. Wesley Boyd. "Medical Expenditures on and by Immigrant Populations in the United States: A Systematic Review." *International Journal of Health* 48, no. 4 (2018): 601–21. https://doi.org/10.1177/0020731418791963.

Zallman, L., Fernando Wilson, James Stimpson, Adriana Bearse, Lisa Arsenault, Blessing Dube, David Himmelstein, and Steffie Woolhandler. "Unauthorized Immigrants Prolong the Life of Medicare's Trust Fund." *Journal of General Internal Medicine* 31 (2016): 122–27. https://doi.org/10.1007/s11606-015-3418-z.

Zallman, L., S. Woolhandler, D. Himmelstein, D. Bor, and D. McCormick. "Immigrants Contributed an Estimated $115.2 Billion More to the Medicare Trust Fund than They Took Out in 2002–2009." *Health Affairs* 32, no. 6 (2013): 1153–60.

Zhang, Xiaoming, Daniel Lin, Hugh Pforsich, and Vernon Lin. "Physician Workforce in the United States of America: Forecasting Nationwide Shortages."
Human Resources for Health 18, no. 1 (2020): 8–9.

Zhao, Yue, Norman Segalowitz, Anastasiya Voloshyn, Estelle Chamoux, and
Andrew Ryder. "Language Barriers to Healthcare for Linguistic Minorities: The
Case of Second Language-Specific Health Communication Anxiety." *Health
Communication* 36, no. 3 (2019): 334–46. https://doi.org/10.1080/10410236
.2019.1692488.

Zimmerman, Wendy, and Karen Tumlin. *Patchwork Policies: State Assistance for
Immigrants Under Welfare Reform*. Urban Institute, 1999. http://webarchive
.urban.org/publications/309007.html.

Zolberg, Aristide. *A Nation by Design: Immigration Policy in the Fashioning of America*.
Cambridge, MA: Harvard University Press, 2006.

Zubaran, Carlos. "The Quest for Recognition: Brazilian Immigrants in the United
States." *Transcultural Psychiatry* 45, no. 4 (2008): 590–610.

INDEX

Abbott, Greg, 8
Abrego, Leisy, 44, 49, 111
ACA. *See* Affordable Care Act (ACA)
Accountable Care Organizations (ACOs), 166, 269n18
administrative burdens, 50–51, 84–92, 106, 118, 158, 190–91, 192, 201, 207, 237; reductions in, 210; RLS and, 52, 195–98, 207
advocacy organizations. *See* immigrant and health advocates
Affordable Care Act (ACA), 190, 208, 250n20; administrative burdens, 50–51; coverage gap provisions, 69; eligibility, 5, 70; federal health reform under, 236–46; immigrants' exclusion, 5; immigrants' knowledge of, 84, 124, 153; legislative restrictions, 28; model for, 8, 69, 216; Republican opposition to, 166–67, 187; state residency-based access, 117; Trump administration's opposition, 5, 31, 116, 134–35, 157, 166–67, 185, 187; 2013 rollout, 50–51, 65, 69, 265n14; uninsured population under, 28, 70, 165, 166, 205; website crash, 122, 265n14. *See also* MA health coverage system, Latinx immigrants' access (2015–2016); individual mandate, tax penalties
African immigrants, 4, 202
Aliens with Special Status, 236
American Civil Liberties Union, 247
American Medical Association (AMA), 23, 24, 25

arrests, by immigration enforcement, 58, 99, 105, 106, 113, 153–54, 172, 181, 191; in "sensitive locations," 170, 179, 246; of students, 169–70
Asad, Asad, 37, 111, 139–40, 143
Asian, Middle Eastern, or Northern African (MENA) heritage, 202
Asian immigrants, 4, 38–39, 41
asylees, 55, 56, 57, 72–73, 116, 120, 129, 163; health coverage eligibility and options, 27, 67, 68, 70, 87, 118; psychological evaluations, 185–86

Baker, Charlie, 116, 149, 150, 154–55, 160, 235, 252n72, 264n2
Biden administration, immigration policy, 5, 107, 193, 252n76, 263n110
Black Americans: discrimination and racism toward, 20–21, 37, 58, 96, 98, 108, 176, 178, 199, 214; distrust of healthcare system, 25; exclusion from citizenship, 41, 140, 178, 203; exclusion from welfare state, 41; healthcare inequities, 20–21, 25, 98; health coverage enrollment obstacles, 125; as immigrant advocates, 171; immigrants of color misrecognized as, 36; incarceration, 42; infant and maternal mortality rate, 214; as physicians, 23, 25; police violence toward, 178–79, 203
Black Bostonians, household median net worth, 133

Black ethnoracial classification, 38–39, 133, 174–75, 180. *See also under specific immigrant groups*

Blue Cross Blue Shield, 23, 97; of Massachusetts, 98, 258n5

Bolsonaro, Jair, 13

border (US), 8, 34, 71, 141, 240, 245; crossings by unaccompanied minors, 116, 128–30, 141, 153; family separations at, 183, 246–47; mistreatment of immigrants at, 5, 243, 246–47, 263n110; walls, 107, 134

Border Security, Economic Opportunity, and Immigration Modernization Act, 72–73, 241

Boston, MA, 141, 204; immigrants' contributions to, 6–7; immigrants' countries of origin, 250n25; racism and segregation in, 6; sanctuary policy, 111, 169–70, 200–201, 212, 245–46; Trust Act, 169–70, 245–46. *See also* Latinx immigrants, in Greater Boston

Boston Health Coalition (BHC) providers: demographics, 177–78, 217, 221, 222, 252n71; discriminatory medical encounters with, 103–4; RLS-based discrimination toward, 177–78

Boston Health Coalition (BHC) providers, opinions on Latinx immigrants' healthcare issues, 14, 17, 19, 216–19, 220–22; ACA implementation, 220; anti-immigrant rhetoric, 60–61; CelticCare, 236; healthcare affordability, 128; health literacy, 77–78; ICE raids, 107–8, 141; immigrant healthcare access, 88, 109, 114, 115, 125–26, 166, 189, 194; immigrants' working conditions, 82; interview protocol and, 227; language obstacles to health care, 52, 89; Latinx ethnoracial classification, 177–78; medical interpreters, 100–103, 263n103; mental health conditions, 83; naturalized citizens' health care discrimination, 33, 35; primary care physicians, 94; public policy structural racism, 45–47; RLS-based discrimination, 47–48, 174, 176; structural racism, 45–47, 108; Trump administration policies, 167, 185–86, 187–88

Boston Marathon bombing, 72–73, 103

Boston Police Department, 169–70, 179, 245

Brazilian immigrants, in Greater Boston, 7, 12–14, 54, 116–17, 118, 138, 156, 189, 215–16, 223; administrative burdens, 195; Amarelo/Yellow/Asian ethnoracial classification, 75, 260n40, 261n63, 266n32; Black ethnoracial classification, 21, 79, 81, 96, 101, 107, 133, 134–35, 137, 148, 174, 261n63; co-ethnic discrimination toward, 138; demographic characteristics, 10, 11, 13–14, 15–16, 75, 116, 124; discriminatory medical encounters, 103–4; English language proficiency, 124, 261n64, 268n4; ethnoracial classification as immigrants, 105–6, 132; ethnoracial self-classification, 130–32, 224–25, 266nn36–37; health coverage prevalence, 65, 76, 93, 96, 126, 159, 260n56, 265n21, 268n3; health literacy, 77–78, 200; Hispanic ethnoracial classification, 131, 134–35, 226; Latinx/Latino ethnoracial classification, 10, 14, 79, 81, 83, 93, 96, 101, 131, 135–36, 173, 200, 226, 261n63; LEP status, 99–100, 135, 175; LPR status, 13–14, 79, 95–96, 110, 116, 231–32; mental health conditions, 82–83, 142–43; naturalized citizens, 54, 60, 136; Pardo ethnoracial classification, 74–75, 79, 95–96, 224; perceived as different from Latinos, 77–78, 138, 200; postmigration health/healthcare experiences, 81–82, 142–43, 147–48, 158–59, 267n58, 268n2; premigration ethnoracial racial classification, 74–75; premigration health/healthcare experiences, 64, 74–75, 76–78, 79, 94, 95–96, 147–48, 198, 199, 223, 260n39, 265n21; racial profiling, 105; return immigration, 215, 250n57; RLS-based discrimination toward, 62, 105–6, 135–36, 173–74, 176, 177–78, 200, 267n49; skin color/physical appearance, 13, 14, 83, 105–6, 112–13, 138, 148, 199–200, 223–24; socioeconomic status and education, 75, 78, 81–82, 112–13, 130, 159, 198, 199, 223, 260n39, 265n21, 268n4; suicide rates, 154; undocumented, 13–14, 81, 93, 105,

Democratic Party, 8, 65, 134, 149, 154, 160, 194–95

dental care, 86, 96, 101, 119, 127, 183–84, 253n99, 261nn71–73, 262n89

deportation, 12, 19, 42–43, 59, 106, 144, 154, 201, 220, 237, 240n21, 244; for criminal behavior, 55, 72, 73, 212; documentation status and, 55–57, 198, 231–32, 257n77; family preparedness plans for, 163–64; fingerprint database-based, 72, 244; health services use as risk factor for, 32, 99, 109, 110, 113, 147, 157, 191, 193, 204; racially privileged status and, 55; racial profiling and, 38, 57–58, 105, 153–54; RLS discrimination and, 57–59, 172, 191; system embeddedness avoidance and, 111; TPS status and, 57, 130

deportation policies, 5, 36, 38, 50, 107–8, 237, 244; affecting DACA recipients, 245, 252n76; Biden administration, 107, 263n110; Bush administration, 244, 245; Obama administration, 73, 106–7, 141, 245, 272n19; Trump administration, 106–7, 180–81, 193, 237

DeSantis, Ron, 8

detention, 19, 58, 106, 107–8, 141, 180, 220, 237; centers, 49–50, 58, 180, 185; documentation status and, 50, 57, 58, 106, 140, 231; health services use as risk factor for, 107, 109, 113, 147, 191, 204–5; law enforcement encounters-based, 42–43, 58, 105, 107–8, 113, 172, 181; of LPRs, 231; racial profiling and, 105, 153–54; of US-born citizens, 140

Development, Relief, and Education for Alien Minors (DREAM) Act, 241, 245

Disproportionate Share Hospital program, 29

documentation status, as barrier to health coverage access, 26–30, 117–18, 194, 202, 223–24; under ACA, 28, 70, 115, 118, 120–21; continuum, 231–32, 265n13; immigrants' perception of, 48–50; intersection with federal immigration policy, 40–41, 61; macro-level policy positions, 40–41, 61, 208–9; under Massachusetts health reform, 66–69, 118–21, 209; Medicare and Medicaid eligibility and, 26–27, 29,

165, 209; private health insurance and, 27–28; public benefits access and, 30, 40–41, 43, 44; relation to racially privileged status, 55–61, 198; removal of, 208–9; RLS-based discrimination and, 35, 36, 51, 110–11, 139–40; under Trump administration, 180–81. *See also* lawful permanent residents (LPRs); naturalized citizens; refugees; temporary protected status (TPS) recipients; undocumented immigrants

documented noncitizens, 8, 49–50, 58, 69, 160, 164, 180–81

domestic violence, 72, 171

Dominican immigrants, in Greater Boston, 7, 118; administrative burdens, 195; Black ethnoracial classification, 7, 10, 21, 75, 79, 105, 131, 132, 133, 134–35, 147–48, 154, 198–99, 200, 260n40; co-ethnic discrimination toward, 138–39; demographic characteristics, 11, 15–16, 75–76, 116, 124; discriminatory medical encounters, 104; English language proficiency, 124, 261n64, 268n4; ethnoracial classification as immigrants, 132; ethnoracial self-classification, 130–32, 224–25, 266n36; health care access inequities, 1–3, 33, 53; health coverage costs, 97–98; health coverage prevalence, 65, 76, 93, 96, 126, 159, 260n56, 265n21, 268n3; health profiles, 65; Hispanic ethnoracial classification, 131, 134–35, 147, 173, 198; Latinx/Latino/Latina ethnoracial classification, 10, 48–49, 105, 131, 134–35, 147, 154, 173, 198, 200; LEP status, 135, 175; LPR status, 10, 53, 104–5, 112, 144–45, 198; Moreno ethnoracial classification, 74–75, 79, 224; naturalized citizens, 10, 49–50, 53, 60, 97–98, 112, 116, 124–25, 127, 147, 154; non-White ethnoracial classification, 34; Pardo ethnoracial classification, 74–75; postmigration health/healthcare experiences, 79–81, 112, 142, 147–48, 158–59, 267n58; premigration health/healthcare experiences, 64, 74–76, 77, 78, 94, 147–48, 198, 260n39, 265n21; racialization as immigrants, 105–6; racial profiling, 105; RLS-based discrimination toward, 33, 34, 39–40, 53, 59, 60, 104–6, 135–36, 173, 198–99, 267nn49–50; skin color/physical appearance, 7, 10, 75, 77, 79, 104, 105–6, 112, 143–44, 223–24; socioeconomic status and education, 75–76, 78, 81–82, 112, 159, 165n21, 198, 260n39, 268n4; undocumented, 48–49, 77, 104; White ethnoracial classification, 131, 260n40

double consciousness theory, 37, 178

drivers' licenses, 137, 146, 172, 177–78; for undocumented immigrants, 17, 73, 82–83, 89, 116, 187, 194–95, 252n72

Du Bois, W. E. B., 37, 178

Emergency Medical Treatment and Labor Act, 29, 254n110

emergency room (ER) care, 76, 95, 104, 271n21

employment, of immigrants, 1, 14, 173; during COVID-19 pandemic, 28, 206; effect of RLS-based discrimination on, 136; effect on health status, 80, 82, 142, 146–47, 154; employment authorizations, 223; racialized disparities, 108, 132, 208; undocumented immigrants' access, 48–49; undocumented income from, 90; workplace experiences, 60–61, 169, 183–84, 199, 206

English language proficiency, 124, 265n19, 268n4; learning programs, 210–11, 244. See also limited English proficiency (LEP) entries

ethnoracial classifications, 249nn2–3; public policy related to, 41; self-classification, 130–32, 224–26, 258n4, 266n36; US Census Bureau-based, 40, 131, 226. See also specific ethnoracial classifications

European immigrants, 38–39, 250n25

Feagin, Joseph, 45

Federal Bureau of Investigation (FBI), 71–72, 244

federalism, policy implications of, 40–50, 190–91, 192–95. See also macro-level (government policies) RLS

federal poverty level (FPL), 26, 86, 87, 119, 237, 253n92, 261n72, 264n11

fingerprint databases, 71–72, 244

Flores, Jose Martin Paz, 169

Flores-Gonzalez, Nilda, 140

Florida, 8, 13, 256n50; racial profiling policy, 42

Free Care. See Health Safety Net (HSN)

García, Angela, 172–73

Gateway Cities Program, 244

gender, relation to citizenship, 39

gentrification, 10, 38, 80, 133–34, 198, 232

Golash-Boza, Tanya, 37

green card holders. See lawful permanent residents (LPRs)

green cards, 49, 145, 162; Diversity Immigrant Visa ("green card lottery"), 266n24; eligibility, 40, 162, 266n24; as health coverage eligibility documentation, 88

Haitian immigrants, 7–8, 250n25

Harris, Kamala, 263n110

hate crimes, 172, 175–76, 187

Healey, Maura, 8, 195, 270n43

health, social determinants, 3–4, 190, 203, 208, 211–12

healthcare access: in home countries, postmigration, 201, 270n49, 271n21; as right, 114, 163. See also racialized legal status (RLS), as constraint on healthcare access

Health Care for All helpline, 210

Healthcare.gov website, 122

healthcare providers: cooperation with immigration enforcement, 107, 147, 179–80; cultural sensitivity, 2, 148, 149, 211–12; ethnoracial diversity, 106, 211–12; Hispanic, 2; immigrants' access to, 81, 98, 126, 142, 226; quality of interactions with, 1–2, 32, 53–54, 98, 99–100, 101, 103, 106, 112, 147–49, 270n49; responses to Trump administration policies, 159–64. See also Boston Health Coalition (BHC) providers

healthcare system (US): multiple stakeholders, 23–24, 25, 29–30; overview, 22–25; recommended policies for reform of, 211–12

Health Connector, 85–87, 89, 151, 166, 179–80

health coverage, 258n2; under comprehensive health reforms, 32; macro-level policy recommendations for, 208–11; origin and development, 22–25; US-international comparison, 4

health exchanges, 28, 70, 88, 115, 117, 128, 167, 209, 235

health insurance, 258n2. *See also* health coverage; private health insurance coverage

Health Insurance Portability and Accountability Act (HIPAA), 109–10, 263n116

health literacy, 77–78, 84, 93, 112, 113, 207, 210

health outcomes: US-international comparison, 4. *See also* health status, of immigrants

health policy: influence of corporations on, 29–30; intersection with immigration policy, 40–41, 70–72, 144–47, 164, 168–72, 190–91; policy landscape changes (2012–2019), 189–90, 233–47; recommendations for, 208–14

Health Safety Net (HSN), 66, 67, 68, 70, 85, 116, 125, 258n2; application process, 85–92; denial /loss of coverage under, 88, 165–66; discontinued state funding, 19, 150–52, 154–55, 165–66, 187, 213; eligibility, 86, 87, 88, 89, 118, 119, 127, 150, 213; Free Care predecessor, 84–85, 92, 93–94, 109, 259n16; healthcare costs coverage, 126–27, 150; income-based eligibility, 90–91; policy recommendations for, 213

health status, of immigrants, 53, 55, 225; comparison with US-born population, 209; effect of inadequate healthcare on, 204–5; effect of RLS-related stress on, 82, 142–43, 146–47, 154, 183–84, 204; postmigration, 78–83, 112, 121–22, 142–43, 146–48, 158–59, 226–27, 267n58, 268n2; premigration, 64, 74–78, 94, 95–96, 142, 147–48, 198, 199, 223, 260n39, 265n21; racialized disparities, 108

helplines, for health coverage access, 89, 166, 197, 219

Herd, Pamela, 50–51, 197–98

HIPAA. *See* Health Insurance Portability and Accountability Act (HIPAA)

Hispanic ethnoracial classification, 79, 137, 175, 226, 249n2. *See also under specific immigrant groups*

Hispanic immigrants, 137, 138, 165

Hispanic population, of US, 5

Hodgson, Thomas, 180

Honduran immigrants, 130

hospitals, 22–23, 25, 29, 252n61, 254n110

housing: discrimination/segregation in, 41, 48–49, 51, 137, 204, 208, 232; insecurity, 3–4, 38, 132–33, 137, 142, 190, 232

ICE. *See* Immigration and Customs Enforcement

identification (ID) documentation, 14, 174; for health coverage eligibility, 49, 109, 110–11, 120, 122–23, 129; municipal ID cards, 172; as protection against RLS-based discrimination, 177–78

Illegal Immigration Reform and Immigrant Responsibility Act (IIRIRA), 69, 71, 244

Illinois, Medicaid expansion and access, 42, 194, 209

immigrant and health advocates, 236–37, 238; demographics and positionality, 17, 177–78, 217, 221, 228; interventions with immigration officials, 144; interview protocol with, 18–19, 228; lawsuit against Trump administration, 247; perceptions of immigrant groups, 200

immigrant and health advocates, opinions on Latinx immigrants' healthcare issues, 21, 68, 73, 159, 197, 218; anti-immigrant sociopolitical climate, 136–37, 139–40; discrimination in health care, 53–54, 96–97; health care/coverage access, 62, 68, 73, 88–89, 92, 94, 97, 120, 122–24, 145–46, 190; health coverage cost, 90–91; health status, 146–47; housing insecurity, 133–34; HSN changes, 150–51, 152, 165–66; immigration enforcement practices, 146, 171; language barriers, 121; mental health conditions, 142–43; RLS-based discrimination, 175, 177–80; structural racism, 45–47; Trump administration policies, 35, 135, 156, 157, 159–64, 183, 184–85, 187–88; unaccompanied minors, 128–29; working conditions, 82, 136

Immigration and Customs Enforcement (ICE), 49, 161, 201; cooperation with local law enforcement, 63–64, 71, 73, 107–8, 111, 150, 169–70, 212; Secure Communities (S-Comm) program, 71–72, 73, 107–8, 170, 241, 244, 245, 259n29. *See also* raids

Immigration and Naturalized Services (INS), 49–50

immigration documents, fraudulent, 71

immigration enforcement: as obstacle to healthcare access, 144–45, 146, 200–201; post-9/11, 241, 244; racialized, 6, 46, 106–11, 113, 157. *See also* Immigration and Customs Enforcement; immigration policy; law enforcement *entries*

immigration policy, 4, 5, 40, 46; alignment with criminal law, 37–38; Biden administration, 5, 107, 193, 252n76, 263n110; Bush (George W.) administration, 244, 245, 259n29; Clinton administration, 145–46, 209, 240, 244, 245; effect of ethnoracial demographics on, 46; effect on US social order, 40; federal authority over, 164, 255n18; intersection with health policy, 40–41, 70–72, 144–47, 164, 168–72, 190–91; intersection with other policy domains, 40–41, 43, 194, 255n33; of Massachusetts, 149–51, 237, 240–44, 245; Obama administration, 5, 18, 72, 73, 106–7, 116, 141, 145–46, 153, 170, 241, 245, 272n19; post-9/11, 50, 107–8; Reagan administration, 209, 240; recommended reform, 209; restrictive, 64; state and federal disconnections, 42–43, 90, 172; of state governments, 42–43; Trump administration, 5, 31, 35, 46, 54, 90, 116, 157, 160–88, 246–47

incarceration, 38, 42, 58, 108, 144, 180

Indigenous ancestry, 7, 12, 54, 55, 74–75, 165, 182, 212, 225, 249n3

Indigenous languages, 12, 102

individualism, 207

individual mandate, tax penalties, 19, 91, 112, 122, 125, 127–28, 145, 167, 235

interpreters: medical, 14, 64, 89, 94, 100–103, 106, 121, 211, 216–17, 222, 263n103; for public benefits access, 46–47, 88–89

intersectionality, of RLS, 8–9, 36, 37, 38, 58, 63, 122, 195, 202–3, 250n23

Islamophobia, 244

Janey, Kim, 250n27

Johnson, Lyndon B., 29

Kennedy, Ted, 244

Lacks, Henrietta, 253n87

language(s): as barrier to healthcare access, 63, 106; discrimination based on, 35–36, 46–47, 105; as race and ethnicity marker, 35, 105–6, 107, 134, 158, 175–76. *See also* limited English proficiency (LEP) populations; Portuguese language, of Brazilian immigrants; Spanish language, of Latinx immigrants

language access, as civil right, 46–47, 52, 99, 121, 210

Latina ethnoracial classification, 1–3, 137, 147, 165, 174, 249n2

Latinx ethnoracial classification, 174. *See also under specific immigrant groups*

Latinx immigrants, 4, 5; anti-immigrant rhetoric toward, 98–99; co-ethnic discrimination among, 138–39, 176–77

Latinx immigrants, in Greater Boston, 6, 7–9; co-ethnic discrimination among, 138–39; geographic shifts, 232; heterogeneity, 7, 199–201; uninsured status, 126

Latinx immigrants, in Greater Boston, health coverage access study, 6, 8–9; data transcription and analysis protocol, 20, 218, 228–30; interview protocol, 6, 9–10, 17, 18–19, 222–28; interview protocol (advocates), 18–19, 228; interview protocol (BHC providers),

Medicaid patients, 125; role in healthcare system development, 22–25; shortage, 24–25; White, 21

police. *See* law enforcement *entries*

Portuguese language, of Brazilian immigrants, 7, 13, 14, 17, 79, 89, 138, 141, 142, 158, 221, 222–23, 224–25, 229, 230, 251n39, 266n33; as barrier to healthcare and coverage, 64, 197, 199; healthcare providers' lack of proficiency in, 52, 93–94, 100, 101

preexisting conditions, 117, 205–6

pregnant women, health coverage, 26, 68, 76, 161, 238, 253n94, 254n110, 264nn10–11

premiums, 4, 95–96, 122, 239, 258n2; ACA-related increase, 127–28; as obstacle to health coverage, 4, 97–98, 205; of private health insurance, 27, 28, 126

preventive care, 19, 26, 32, 68, 116, 126, 204–5, 208–9, 253n99, 259n17

Priority Enforcement Program, 73

private health insurance coverage, 16, 17, 24, 26, 66, 88, 260n56, 262n85; cost as obstacle to, 27–28, 91, 97–98; healthcare quality under, 96; post-ACA implementation, 117; premigration, 76–77, 78; subsidies for, 87

privilege, racialized, 13, 54–61, 55–61, 199–200, 256n39

profiling, ethnoracial, 38, 42, 57–60, 71, 82, 105, 108, 137, 153–54, 194–95

PRUCOL. *See* Permanent Residence Under Color of Law

PRWORA. *See* Personal Responsibility and Work Opportunity Act

public benefits access and use: administrative burdens, 50–54, 61; bureaucratic disentitlement in, 91–92; citizenship criterion, 34; disenrollment, 162, 193; documentation status-based, 40–41, 48–49; eligibility criteria, 34, 50, 55, 244; ethnoracial classification-based, 6, 41; immigrants' declining of, 144; for LPRs, 55; overlapping policy domains, 42, 43; PRUCOL-based eligibility, 27; state government policies, 41, 42, 244; under Trump administration, 160–61

public charge rule, 31, 46, 55, 71, 90, 109–10, 197, 228, 268n8; under Biden administration, 193; under Trump administration, 5, 31, 46, 90, 161–63, 167–68, 185, 187, 193, 197, 243, 250n22, 268nn7–8

public health system: funding, 23, 29, 205–6, 211, 244; immigrants' access to, 79

public policy, relation to healthcare and public benefits access, 6; influence of federalism on, 40–50; race-neutral policies, 35, 37, 45, 46, 51, 195, 202; resource allocation domains, 42–44. *See also* health policy; immigration policy

Puerto Ricans, 7, 12, 104, 139, 171, 176

race: as construct, 38; relationship to poverty, 46

race-neutral policies, 35, 37, 45, 46, 51, 195, 202

race scholarship, 37–38

racialization, definition, 3

racialized legal status (RLS), as constraint on healthcare access, 6, 112, 117, 122, 131–38, 148–49, 190–91, 192, 195; anti-immigrant rhetoric and, 134–38; definition of RLS, 2–3, 4, 5, 34; future research recommendations for, 202–3; intersectionality, 8–9, 36, 37, 38, 58, 63, 122, 164, 191, 195, 202–3, 250n23; national implications, 201–7; origins, 30–31, 37–40; resource allocation impact, 42–44; structural racism and, 30–31, 35; theoretical framework, 34–40. *See also* macro-level (government policies) RLS; meso-level (bureaucracies and institutions) RLS; micro-level (individual interactions) RLS; RLS-based discrimination *under specific immigrant groups and specific topics*

racism, 2–3, 34, 35–37, 45, 48, 59, 78–79, 173–74; systemic, 44–45, 195, 202. *See also* structural racism

raids, by immigration enforcement, 58–59 63, 72, 107–8, 141, 242, 243, 244, 246, 267n56; as healthcare access obstacle, 107–8, 154, 200–201; warnings about, 146, 154, 163, 197, 201

Ray, Victor, 45, 51, 197–98

recession (2008), 123, 244

policies, 50–51; Medicaid administration role, 26; public benefits policies, 41, 42, 45, 71

structural racism, 3, 4–5, 35–37, 39–40, 61, 195; BHC providers on, 45–47; in healthcare system, 25, 202; in housing, 133, 198; racialized burdens concept, 51; relation to systemic racism, 44–45

Student Immigrant Movement (SIM), 164

subsidized health coverage, 26, 67, 98; under ACA, 28, 115, 117, 126–27, 165, 264n8; administrative burdens, 84; application process, 85–87; documentation status and, 34; healthcare costs under, 97–98, 126; income-level-based ineligibility, 62, 112; Medicare Part D, 268n8; noncitizen's exclusion/restricted access, 34, 41, 91, 165, 264n6; private health insurance, 28, 66, 68, 87

suicide, 82, 142–43, 154

Sun, Ken, 203

tax contributions, of immigrants, 6, 27, 62, 87, 138, 167, 208–9

tax credits, advance premium, 122

Tax Cuts and Jobs Act, 19, 167

tax penalties, under individual mandate, 19, 91, 112, 122, 125, 127–28, 145, 167, 235

temporary protected status (TPS) recipients, 9, 16, 56, 57, 185, 224; children of, 128–29; discrimination toward, 138; health coverage options, 67, 68; liminally legal status, 12, 57, 129–30; Medicaid and Medicare ineligibility, 70; public benefits access, 129; Trump administration policies toward, 243

Trujillo, Rafael, 10, 75–76

Trump, Donald, 5; campaign and election (2016), 19, 116, 117, 152, 153, 156–57, 159, 162, 182, 220; racist and anti-immigrant rhetoric, 47–48, 60–61, 106–7, 134–38, 140, 141, 143, 153–54

Trump administration: health providers' and advocates' responses to, 159–64; immigration policy, 5, 31, 35, 46, 54, 90, 116, 157, 160–88, 246–47; RLS-based discrimination under, 19, 172–81.

See also MA health coverage system, Latinx immigrants' access (2019)

Tuskegee Syphilis Study, 253n87

undocumented immigrants, 3, 16, 250n25; denial of rights, 36; detention/deportation risk, 56, 57, 58, 163–64; family preparedness plans, 163–64; health coverage eligibility, 27, 42, 70, 86, 87, 88, 89–90, 118, 166, 191; in-state tuition rate eligibility, 73, 270n9; path to citizenship, 73, 209; physical features, 54–56; private insurance coverage, 118; public benefits access, 43, 44; racial profiling risk, 58; stereotypes, 37, 107, 108–9; subsidized hospital care, 29

undocumented status: immigrants' perceptions of, 48–49; as obstacle to health care, 85; public misperceptions, 107; of TPS recipients, 57. *See also under specific immigrant groups*

uninsured populations, 28, 235; ACA-related reduction, 16, 28, 70, 165, 166; Latinx, 8, 65, 126; in MA, 8, 11, 16, 17, 62–63, 65, 66, 69, 91, 152, 165, 234, 269n11; medical exploitation, 25; under Trump administration, 168

US-born citizens: deportation/detention risk, 55, 56, 57–58, 140; health coverage options, 67

US Citizenship and Immigration Services (USCIS), 171

US Congress, 29–30, 45

US Constitution, 45, 164

US Department of Homeland Security (DHS), 71–72, 110, 141, 162, 180, 240, 244, 253n93, 268n7, 270n43

US Supreme Court, 29–30, 45, 117, 166; *Shelby v. Holder*, 45; *Students for Fair Admissions v. Harvard*, 45

Valle, Ariana, 140

Van Natta, Meredith, 79, 111, 143, 145

Varsanyi, Monica, 43

Venezuelan immigrants, 7–8, 263n110

visas/visa holders, 27, 57, 70, 223, 224; religious, 15; student, 16, 67, 70, 124, 257n76; tourist, 14, 15, 81, 257n76; work, 16, 67, 70, 257n76

voting rights, 45, 55, 172

Walsh, Marty, 160, 250n27, 264n2
welfare: benefits, 42; reform, 55, 69, 71; state, 41
White Americans, 34, 38, 41; concerns about ethnoracial demographics, 46, 134; healthcare quality, 96–97; public benefits access, 43, 44; White privilege, 44, 55–56, 96–97, 98, 258n87; White supremacy, 3, 4–5, 34, 36, 38, 44, 45, 46, 108, 157

White ethnoracial classification, 174–75, 258n87. *See also under specific immigrant groups*
work permits, 18, 130, 136, 223, 224, 245, 252n76
Wu, Michelle, 6–7

young adults, 37, 117, 193–94, 209, 213